Acute Care Surgery Handbook

Salomone Di Saverio • Fausto Catena
Luca Ansaloni • Federico Coccolini
George Velmahos
Editors

Acute Care Surgery Handbook

Volume 1 General Aspects, Non-gastrointestinal and Critical Care Emergencies

Foreword by David Feliciano

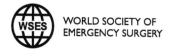
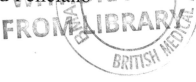 WORLD SOCIETY OF
EMERGENCY SURGERY

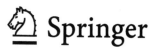 Springer

Editors

Salomone Di Saverio
Emergency and Trauma Surgery
Service
C.A. Pizzardi Maggiore Hospital
AUSL Bologna
Bologna, Italy

Fausto Catena
Emergency and Trauma Surgery
Maggiore Hospital of Parma
Parma, Italy

Luca Ansaloni
General, Emergency and Trauma
Surgery
Papa Giovanni XXIII Hospital
Bergamo, Italy

Federico Coccolini
General, Emergency and Trauma
Surgery
Papa Giovanni XXIII Hospital
Bergamo, Italy

George Velmahos
Trauma, Emergency Medicine
Harvard Medical School
Massachusetts General Hospital
Boston, Massachusetts
USA

ISBN 978-3-319-15340-7   ISBN 978-3-319-15341-4   (eBook)
DOI 10.1007/978-3-319-15341-4

Library of Congress Control Number: 2016960296

Printed on acid-free paper

This Springer imprint is published by Springer Nature
The registered company is Springer International Publishing AG
The registered company address is: Gewerbestrasse 11, 6330 Cham, Switzerland

With deep gratitude I'd like to dedicate this book the memory of my father, Tito, who recognized my inclinations early on, and who encouraged and supported me in my pursuit of a medical and surgical career. His constant presence in my youth is for me still a model for how to lead my own life. I also wish to thank my mother Gabriella, who has always been the beacon of light guiding me morally and culturally. She remains my mentor in logic and the humanities, sharing the wisdom of her beloved Greek and Latin masters. Last but not least, I am grateful to and dedicate this book to my devoted wife Omeshnie, who is constantly supporting me with patience and love

Salomone Di Saverio

To my parents who served as my life's springboard and to my wife and children who serve as my life's compass

George Velmahos

To my family that tolerates me and my job every day....

Fausto Catena

To my wife Anna

Federico Coccolini

Foreword

As specialization in general surgery has continued to increase around the world, it has become obvious that patients with injuries and those with acute surgical conditions benefit from care by surgical specialists with training and continuing interest in these fields. The specialty of acute care surgery (ACS), now approximately 10 years old, has evolved rapidly. There are now fellowships for postresidency training in the field, designated ACS Services in most academic and large community hospitals, and surgical organizations such as the World Society of Emergency Surgery to encourage best practices and continuing research and development in the field. Having a standard textbook in the field of acute care surgery is a necessary next step.

Dr. Salomone Di Saverio from Bologna, Italy, and colleagues from the World Society of Emergency Surgery have now authored the *Acute Care Surgery* manual. Volume 1 of this comprehensive manual provides the perspective on ACS around the world, the history of the specialty, opportunities for research in the field, organization of an in-hospital ACS service, and describes the use of checklists to enhance patient safety. The remainder of the text focuses on management of patients with a variety of ACS conditions from the head and neck to the anus to the peripheral vascular system. In addition, there are comprehensive chapters on resuscitation, use of ultrasound, use of antibiotics, management of septic shock, nutrition, other areas of surgical critical care, and the role of interventional radiology in ACS. Finally, there are chapters highlighting the care of special patient groups such as children, pregnant women, geriatric patients, burn patients, transplant patients, and any patients requiring damage control operations or developing the abdominal compartment syndrome.

This manual is a broad overview of the field of acute care surgery written by many individuals who have contributed to the rapid development of the field. Dr. Di Saverio and his colleagues have taken their extensive experience in acute care surgery and have consolidated and organized it into this comprehensive and readable manual. This will soon be a standard text used by surgeons who practice acute care surgery around the world, and it was a privilege to review it.

David V. Feliciano, MD, FACS
Battersby Professor and Director of General Surgery
IUH (Indiana University Health) Methodist Hospital
Emeritus Chief, Division of General Surgery
Department of Surgery
Emeritus Chief of Surgery
Indiana University Hospital
Indiana University Medical Center
Indianapolis, IN, USA

Preface

The World Society of Emergency Surgery (WSES) was established in 2007 and its aim was clearly declared: "The overall goals include the promotion of the specialty of emergency surgery as part of the emerging discipline of acute care surgery via academic exchange in an effort to further training and education as well as translational research in the specialty".

Since 2011, the core group of Acute Care and Trauma Surgeons, founder members of World Society of Emergency Surgery, had the feeling of a strong need for improving education in the field of Acute Care and Trauma surgery, especially for the younger surgeons or any doctors and professional, approaching for the first time this discipline and the complex management of trauma and acute care (non-trauma) patients.

We have therefore had the idea of writing initially a book of trauma surgery, aiming to offer a practical manual of procedures, techniques, and operative strategies, which was published 2 years ago.

Following this preliminary and successful project, we have decided to proceed further with the project of a comprehensive acute care surgery manual, covering the whole aspects of the treatment of acute surgical patients, with a worldwide perspective. In different nations and continents, the emergency surgical care may vary widely. Being a group of World Emergency

Surgeon, we would like to provide suggestions and skills that are valid and therefore can be used everywhere, as well as to give a picture of several different options and perspectives in acute care surgery.

After more than a year of hard work, it is now with great pleasure that we are announcing the completion of our further ambitious project of an acute care surgery manual, where most of the renowned acute care surgeons and physicians from all over the world have made an appreciated and highly valuable contribution, with the intent not to merely describe in academic fashion the most recent surgical techniques, but rather to suggest the best surgical and/or endoscopic and/or interventional radiology strategies, with the final of keeping the things simple but effective when in treating a patient in acute care setting. The contributing professionals are herewith sharing their expertise for achieving a wise clinical judgment and good common sense. We hope this manual may represent a real "vademecum," especially for young physicians and trainees, with the specific aim of giving a fresh view and practical suggestions for best managing acute patients and improving the skills of their treating surgeons and physicians.

This Volume 1 of the manual is dealing with non-GI injuries in acute care surgery, offering an overview of the most common problems in thoracic, obstetric, gynecologic, anorectal, vascular, and skin surgery. Chapters on complications in postoperative bariatric surgery, antibiotic management, nutrition, and interventional radiology in acute care surgery are also included. This practical and complete guide stems from the partnership and collaboration between the members of World Society of Emergency Surgery (WSES) and other internationally recognized experts in the field; its aim is to provide general surgeons as well as emergency physicians, gastroenterologists and professionals from many other specialties, residents and trainees with a complete and up-to-date overview of the most relevant operative techniques and with useful "tips and tricks" for their daily clinical practice.

Once again, I would like to thankfully acknowledge the excellent level of scientific quality and educational value of the content that each chapter's author have contributed. The material received is, once again, extremely extensive in terms of quantity and quality that the contents have been apportioned between two volumes.

We are moreover very glad that this project, conducted in cooperation with our World Society of Emergency Surgery and its Journal, has truly joined together not only acute care surgeons, but also surgeons and physicians from other surgical specialties, such as thoracic and vascular surgery, ObGy, urology, pediatrics, ENT, as well as gastroenterology, gastrointestinal endoscopy, and interventional radiology, from all over the world sharing our experiences in the management of the acutely ill patients. The multidisciplinary board of authors, editors, and foreword writers of this book is truly International with contributors from the Americas, Europe, Africa, Australasia, and Asia. This is the most heartening and promising signal for a worldwide collaboration.

This is the second of the planned WSES Books series, starting the WSES Educational Program for the next future years. This project aims to link together WSES courses, WSES Guidelines, and WSES books to give complete educational tools to the next generation of emergency and trauma surgeons.

WSES is demonstrating to act as the first scientific world society capable to develop a systematic scientific and education program with the aim of science progress according to evidence-based medicine and experience sharing program among professionals.

I would also like to acknowledge the invaluable foreword contributions from two masters, Dr. Kenneth Mattox MD FACS and Dr. David Feliciano MD FACS, emanating from their extensive experiences.

Last but not least, I am deeply grateful to the board of Directors of AUSL Bologna for their continuing commitment in improving Public Health and the care of Acute Surgical patients.

Special mention to the Director General of AUSL Bologna, Dr. Chiara Gibertoni, the Health Director Dr. Angelo Fioritti, the Administrative Director Dr. AM. Petrini, the Directors of the Department of Emergency Dr. Giovanni Gordini and Department of Surgery Prof Elio Jovine, and the chief of the Trauma Surgery Unit Dr. Gregorio Tugnoli. With the contribution and cooperation of all these professionals, an outstanding model of Acute Care Surgery and Trauma Center for a modern and multidisciplinary care of the Acute Surgical Patients has been developed in the Province of Bologna, including a functional model of "Hub and Spoke" and a convenient system of Tertiary Referral Care. I am sincerely proud to be part of this exciting multidisciplinary team of AUSL Bologna dedicated to the improvement of Acute Care Surgery model, within a northern Italian province of Emilia Romagna region!

We look forward to a successful and worldwide ongoing cooperation within our international family of enthusiastic acute care and emergency surgeons, aiming to provide a better care for the acutely ill surgical patients.

Bologna, Italy   Salomone Di Saverio, MD, FACS, FRCS

Contents

Chapter 1
Acute Care Surgery Around the World: Future Perspectives

Rao R. Ivatury and Fausto Catena

Increasing specialization and fragmentation of 'general surgery' has reduced the role of surgeons to care for patients with acute surgical emergencies. The need for such services, however, has escalated due to the population living to older age with increasingly complex diseases and co-morbidities. Compounding the problem is the mounting number of severely injured patients in the emergency departments which are already filled to capacity by non-emergency patients. Other factors have also contributed to the emergence of the new specialty of 'acute care surgery'. These include the dissatisfaction of surgeons with trauma as a career in the current era of non-operative management of many traumatic injuries; the loss of traditional general surgery cases to 'organ-specific practices' (e.g. colon and rectal surgery, upper

R.R. Ivatury, MD, FACS, FCCM (✉)
Department of Surgery, Virginia Commonwealth University,
Richmond, VA, USA
e-mail: raoivatury@gmail.com

F. Catena, MD
Emergency Surgery Department, Parma University Hospital, Parma, Italy

© Springer International Publishing Switzerland 2017
S. Di Saverio et al. (eds.), *Acute Care Surgery Handbook*,
DOI 10.1007/978-3-319-15341-4_1

1.1.3   United Kingdom

Emergency Surgery in the United Kingdom has always been a contentious issue with notable differences to elective surgery. The NHS Confederation has an initiative called 'Leading edge publications' to stimulate debate. First in this series is by Andy Black on the future of acute care [26]. In this monograph, he makes a strong argument that emergency care needs to be modified with new approaches to emergency assessment with integration of medical and surgical teams. Specific to emergency surgery, the Nuffield Trust was commissioned by The Royal College of Surgeons of England to explore the challenges facing emergency general surgery (EGS) and identify opportunities to overcome them [27]. In an elaborate process with peer reviews, expert panels and new analyses, the report exposed the pitfalls in emergency surgery and summarized the many challenges facing emergency general surgery in the United Kingdom. They suggested potential opportunities to address these, including the systematic use of protocols and pathways, increased use of network-based approaches, development of new non-medical roles and new training models. This is a fascinating report that describes in detail the suboptimal status of the emergency surgical care in the United Kingdom. A recent article confirmed the greater need for EGS positions in the United Kingdom, despite a lack of training and certification [28]. The authors surveyed consultant members and UK trainees and noted, over a 6 year study period, that there were 1240 consultant job adverts in a general surgical specialty. The number of EGS adverts increased significantly in 2012–2014 compared to 2009–2011 ($p=0.008$). Only 21 % of trainees believed EGS will be delivered by EGS consultants in the future while only 8.2 % of trainees stated EGS as their career plan. Less than half of all UK consultant surgeons see

Chapter 1
Acute Care Surgery Around the World: Future Perspectives

Rao R. Ivatury and Fausto Catena

Increasing specialization and fragmentation of 'general surgery' has reduced the role of surgeons to care for patients with acute surgical emergencies. The need for such services, however, has escalated due to the population living to older age with increasingly complex diseases and co-morbidities. Compounding the problem is the mounting number of severely injured patients in the emergency departments which are already filled to capacity by non-emergency patients. Other factors have also contributed to the emergence of the new specialty of 'acute care surgery'. These include the dissatisfaction of surgeons with trauma as a career in the current era of non-operative management of many traumatic injuries; the loss of traditional general surgery cases to 'organ-specific practices' (e.g. colon and rectal surgery, upper

R.R. Ivatury, MD, FACS, FCCM (✉)
Department of Surgery, Virginia Commonwealth University,
Richmond, VA, USA
e-mail: raoivatury@gmail.com

F. Catena, MD
Emergency Surgery Department, Parma University Hospital, Parma, Italy

© Springer International Publishing Switzerland 2017   1
S. Di Saverio et al. (eds.), *Acute Care Surgery Handbook*,
DOI 10.1007/978-3-319-15341-4_1

GI surgery, endocrines) and highly specialized techniques (minimally invasive surgery, organ transplantation, and robotic surgery). Even non-surgical specialties, for example interventional radiology and gastrointestinal endoscopy have eroded the modern surgical practice [1]. The time was ripe for the creation of a new specialty, acute care surgery, created and developed by the American Association of Surgery for Trauma (AAST).

Current Status of ACS in the United States   LD Britt, former President of AAST, architect of the name 'acute care surgery' and the 'creator of AAST Congress of Trauma and acute care surgery' [2] expounded on the current status of the specialty in his Fitts oration to the AAST last year. He also elaborated on his vision of the future challenges and impediments to the success of this specialty and potential strategies for the AAST to pursue. This specialty is not to be confused with 'surgical hospitalists' [3] who only provide in-hospital coverage of emergency general surgical services, but have no specialized expertise. As also underscored by Britt [2], ACS '"will gain the ultimate recognition for its impact and value that it brings to the optimal care of the severely injured and critically ill surgical patients, by promulgating the brand and "chronicle and publish well-documented improved outcome results, and advance the science by rigorous studies….."'.

In fact, several recent studies have documented that the concept of ACS has lead to improved, perhaps optimal care of the surgical patient. Many academic centres in the USA have replaced 'general surgery' divisions with a Division of ACS [3–15], recognizing that there is no question that the establishment of both the Acute Care Surgery model and the Acute Care Surgery fellowship is the paramount advancement needed to begin addressing the health care disparities in acute surgical care [2]. Several tertiary hospitals appear to subscribe to this concept that the ACS teams are now the 'general surgeons' of the department with their three pillars of expertise: trauma, emergency general surgery and in certain settings, surgical critical care [2, 4–15]. The last mentioned pillar of expertise appears to be more prevalent in the United States rather than other countries, where medical intensivists and anaesthesiologists serve the critically injured or ill patient.

Of great interest, even though there was initial opposition for the ACS model voiced by many, more recent experience has the support of the model from 'specialty surgeons' as well as hospital administrators [4–15]. There is tremendous variation in the implementation of ACS models still in the USA. For instance, Santry and colleagues [16] documented that in the ACS hospitals 25 % do emergency general surgery (EGS) alone, 21 % perform EGS and trauma, 17 % EGS and elective surgery, while 30 % perform all three. ACS model was adopted by nearly one-third of US university-affiliated hospitals and the model was more prevalent among urban, university-based level-I trauma centres [16]. Investigating the impact of ACS service on trauma volumes and outcomes, one study found that despite a 60 % increase in total patient volume and a 233 % increase in operative volume, the addition of EGS to a trauma service did not compromise trauma patient outcomes [8]. Similar to other series, Machailidu and associates [10] found that during ACS period time to gall bladder surgery was shorter (20.8 h vs. 25.7 h, $p=0.007$), more patients had surgery within 24 h (75 % vs. 59 %, $p=0.004$) and there were more operations between 12:00 MN and 7:00 AM (25 % vs. 6.4 %, $p<0.001$). These translated into shorter hospital stay at an average cost savings of $ 1000 per patient. In the context of finances, several studies documented a positive contribution margin from ACS model [11–14].

The impact of ACS service on the elective surgical case load was investigated by Miller and Meredith [13]. They found that the number of operations by ACS group increased significantly compared with the mean of the 2 years preceding the service creation (1,639 vs 790/year; $p=0.007$) There was no change in total operations done by the elective surgery group (2,763 vs

2,496/year; $p=0.13$). Caseload did increase by 23 % in the elective surgery group. They concluded that ACS creation took emergency business from the elective group, but this was replaced with elective cases. This resulted in higher collections for both groups and a resultant significant increase in collections in aggregate.

Addressing the question whether the ACS paradigm is applicable to smaller community hospitals, Kalina and Johnson [17] reported that the model can be successfully implemented and maintained at a non-trauma centre with potentially $2 million savings in a single year. The key to success is creation of a system that standardizes high-quality care, collaboration between acute care surgeons, non-surgical intensivists, elective general surgeons and medical staff administration. Similar sustainability and success of this model was confirmed in a non-trauma setting by O'Mara and colleagues [14].

Of note, there is also evidence that the ACS model has become increasingly popular for resident trainees. The attractive features for in-training residents include team work, shift work, exposure to more operative cases than trauma surgery will ever provide and the resolution by the ACS model of the many 'lifestyle' issues that trauma as a career would pose. In essence, ACS represents the natural maturation of the field of general surgery, and the ACS specialist comes the closest to the traditional concept of the true 'general' surgeon [1, 17, 18]. Cherry-Bukowiec and co-authors [17] documented that the non-trauma emergency surgery service provided ample opportunity for complex decision making, operative procedures, advanced surgical critical care management, acute care faculty surgical skills: all excellent for general and ACS residency training. In fact, the Acute Care Surgery Ad Hoc Committee of EAST [18] conducted a survey of all its members who opined that the biggest incentive to a career in ACS was that it was a challenging and exciting activity; the biggest disincentive was working at night. Seventy-two percent expressed satisfaction with their career profile, and 92 % were either very or somewhat happy with their career. The authors concluded that, compared with their previous survey, overall career satisfaction seemed stable. They suggested focus on surgeon satisfaction may lead to enhancements in patient care.

ACS seems to resonate well with medical students as well in their choice of a surgical career. A recent study [19] surveyed medical students with interest in surgery as a career asking them to rank factors and experiences influencing career selection on a scale of no influence to 10 (critical). Among 337 responses, the three most popular career choices were orthopaedics (16 %), Trauma/ACS (12 %) and paediatric surgery (8 %). Overall, 115 students (34 %) selected emergent surgery (Trauma/ACS) as one of their top three career choices. Factors that were ranked significantly higher by the students interested in T/ACS were related to professional satisfaction. Lifestyle factors received lower emphasis when choosing a surgical career. This appears to be a significant change from surveys in late 1990s that documented the lack of interest in trauma as a career.

The ultimate role for the acute care surgeon is in 'surgical rescue', as observed by Peitzman and his group [20]. They noted that the expertise of acute care surgeons was required to find, treat and salvage patients from post-operative, serious complications. In their experience, this was required, on an average, for one such patient per day. More than 80 % of them required surgical treatment. More than half of them needed multiple procedures to be rescued from their complication. Half of these patients are from other services (the majority surgical) within the authors' hospital. The other half were equally from regional hospitals and the authors' own service. They concluded that early consultation, detection and intervention by the acute care surgery team provide the best chance for optimal recovery of these patients. This can be pronounced as the 'ultimate' contribution of ACS for the care of the severely injured or ill.

1.1 Acute Care Surgery Around the World

1.1.1 Canada

There is a renewed interest in the paradigm of acute care surgery in Canada [21–23]. Excellent outcomes (reduced time to consult and reduced hospital LOS) were documented post ACS implementation. These good results appear to be based on three notable changes brought about by the ACS paradigm: improved access to prompt high-quality surgical intervention for patients with time-dependent illnesses such as severe sepsis and septic shock, quality control by defining and standardizing best practices in surgical complications and the initiation of ACS registry that will define optimal care. Many Canadian surgeons believe that acute care surgery may provide a framework for general surgeons to work together. It can bring advances in techniques and strategy from all general surgical sub-specialties back to our roots [22]. At the same time, it is realized that, pragmatically, this requires the commitment of all sub-specialties of surgery. Also crucial is the institutional commitment to provide ancillary supportive services and economic incentive for the model to succeed. The benefits to the surgeon-in-training are already becoming increasingly evident, especially for the trauma surgeon who had become a non-operating surgeon prior to the onset of ACS [21–23]. The same concepts of ACS are increasingly becoming pertinent to the smaller community hospitals [21–23].

1.1.2 European Model

Trauma and emergency surgery practice is quite variable in different parts of Europe [24]. While general surgery is a recognized specialty, visceral/abdominal surgery is a specialty in some countries and traumatology and trauma have different connotation in different countries. For example, the traumatologist/trauma surgeon treats skeletal trauma in Austria and Slovenia, whereas an orthopaedist does this in Finland, France, Italy, Norway, Portugal, Romania, Spain and Turkey; a general surgeon in Greece and Switzerland does trauma surgery, while visceral trauma is treated by a general surgeon in Austria, Croatia, Finland, Greece, Italy, Luxembourg, the Netherlands, Norway, Portugal, Romania, Switzerland, Spain and Turkey; by a visceral and/or trauma surgeon in Czech Republic, Germany, France and Slovenia. Abdominal emergencies are mostly handled by general surgeons in the majority of European countries. Specialty emergencies (thoracic and vascular are mostly treated by specialty or trauma or general surgeons) are treated by general surgeons. Some large hospitals in Germany have a central unit for all acute care, whether medical or surgical, while most of other countries have no separate departments or divisions. The specialists routinely involved in surgical acute care are traumatologists/orthopaedists in 13 countries, general surgeons in 11, anaesthesiologists/ intensivists in 10 countries and visceral/abdominal surgeons in 4 countries. There is little or no interest in acute care surgery (as a sub-specialty) in Austria and Slovenia, while there are signs of a trend toward the same in Finland, Germany. There appears to be no unified system of acute care surgery in Europe at the present time [24].

Currently, there is a tremendous interest in addressing the problem of emergency surgery. The European Union of Medical Specialists (UEMS) have formed a Working Group on Emergency Surgery and summarized their initial findings: 'organisation of emergency surgical care is complex; training surgeons to provide emergency care is challenging; a flexible training model to accommodate international differences and improve standards may be the solution; a transferrable competence will be easier to implement than a new specialty' [25]. Similar efforts are under way in the United Kingdom.

1.1.3 United Kingdom

Emergency Surgery in the United Kingdom has always been a contentious issue with notable differences to elective surgery. The NHS Confederation has an initiative called 'Leading edge publications' to stimulate debate. First in this series is by Andy Black on the future of acute care [26]. In this monograph, he makes a strong argument that emergency care needs to be modified with new approaches to emergency assessment with integration of medical and surgical teams. Specific to emergency surgery, the Nuffield Trust was commissioned by The Royal College of Surgeons of England to explore the challenges facing emergency general surgery (EGS) and identify opportunities to overcome them [27]. In an elaborate process with peer reviews, expert panels and new analyses, the report exposed the pitfalls in emergency surgery and summarized the many challenges facing emergency general surgery in the United Kingdom. They suggested potential opportunities to address these, including the systematic use of protocols and pathways, increased use of network-based approaches, development of new non-medical roles and new training models. This is a fascinating report that describes in detail the suboptimal status of the emergency surgical care in the United Kingdom. A recent article confirmed the greater need for EGS positions in the United Kingdom, despite a lack of training and certification [28]. The authors surveyed consultant members and UK trainees and noted, over a 6 year study period, that there were 1240 consultant job adverts in a general surgical specialty. The number of EGS adverts increased significantly in 2012–2014 compared to 2009–2011 ($p=0.008$). Only 21 % of trainees believed EGS will be delivered by EGS consultants in the future while only 8.2 % of trainees stated EGS as their career plan. Less than half of all UK consultant surgeons see

EGS as a sub-specialty. The authors concluded there is an increasing societal need for EGS consultants over the last 6 years and that Emergency Surgery has emerged as a new sub-specialty. Much work needs to be done for optimization of emergency surgical care.

1.1.4 Italy

As the pioneers of the World Society of Emergency Surgery (WSES), Italy has been at the forefront of refining the emergency general surgery component of acute care surgery [29, 30]. The editors of the World Journal of Emergency Surgery (WJES), official organ of WSES, often bemoaned the suboptimal care of the emergency surgery patients all over Europe. They exposed the lack of wide use of minimum standards set for emergency surgery and re-emphasized the need for the development of widely accepted guidelines for urgent surgical intervention as well as optimal post-operative care.

The WSES has indeed accomplished these goals very effectively for the past decade, publishing in the WJES these guidelines for a variety of emergent clinical problems. In a recent editorial, Salomone and colleagues, thought leaders in the WSES, opined in an editorial that there is increasing evidence in the literature showing that acute care surgical patients are best approached and managed only by attending surgeons with appropriate expertise in the field of Emergency and Trauma Surgery.

This approach is necessary to prevent complications, recognize them promptly and treat them appropriately [31].

The present manual, designed and executed by the leaders of the WSES is a vivid example of the contributions of the Society to ACS.

1.1.5   Israel

In Israel, the benefits of acute care surgery model are very appealing for surgeons, hospitals and clinical researchers [32]. Practicing general surgeons do take emergency department calls, sometimes forcing sub-specialty surgeons as a back-up for patients beyond their expertise and area of interest. This is a prime example of a flexible model of ACS, adopted to the area and the institution under question, with differing layers of emphasis on the two predominant parts of ACS: trauma and emergency surgery (the critical care component, as in Europe and South America, belongs to non-surgeons, e.g. anaesthetists or medical intensivists). Clearly, structured training fellowships should be provided and encouraged to produce a sufficient workforce of young, interested acute care surgeons. As the model matures, the impact of an ACS service on the clinical productivity of surgeons will be realized. The continuing contributions of Israeli surgical leaders to the WSES and their enthusiasm for the ACS paradigm bodes well for its success in Israel.

1.1.6   Australia and New Zealand

There is enthusiasm for the acute surgical unit (ASU) model of care in Australasia [33–35]. Increasingly positive experiences in terms of faster response to emergency department review, shorter time to emergency surgery and a reduction in hospital length of stay are being reported with the ASU model, at least in the larger centres. In a meta-analysis of ASU versus traditional 'on-call' model of care, Nagaraja and associates [35] reported on 18 studies; appendectomy ($n=9$), acute cholecystitis ($n=7$). In the appendectomy cohort, proportion of perforation, negative appendectomy rate, conversion rate to open surgery were similar in pre-ASU and ASU period. Complications, however, were significantly lower in the ASU group; 14.5 % pre-ASU and 10.9 % post-ASU ($p=0.009$). Proportion of night-time operations reduced significantly in the ASU period (OR 1.9, 95 % CI 1.32–2.74, $p=0.001$). These results are similar to other reviews of ACS in other countries. It is certain that ACS has a bright future in Australasia.

1.1.7 South America

Latin America and the Caribbean have a tremendous burden of violence, and, along with road traffic incidents, trauma is a serious health care problem. Poor preventive efforts in trauma as well as general health make emergency surgical care and trauma enormous problems. At the present time, there is a lack of statewide system development. While there is widespread enthusiasm for ACS paradigm among surgeons, South America has many difficult hurdles for instituting it.

1.1.8 Low and Middle Income Countries (LMIC)

Emergency surgical care and injury continue to be major health care problems in LMIC. Many efforts are under way to address them. These include creating an acute care service delivery model to function in parallel with preventive and primary services, and improving coordination between various health care specialists who deliver this care. Data systems are being improved to define the problem and integrate acute care burden with the rest of the health system [36]. The African Federation for Emergency Medicine and the Academic Emergency Medicine Consensus Conference (devoted to 'Global health and emergency care: a research agenda for M') held in 2013 focussed on some of these aspects [37].

The second edition of 'Disease control priorities in developing countries' has chapters on surgery, emergency medical systems and injury [38]. Emergency obstetric care and essential trauma guidelines are both being used to evaluate surgical needs in LMICs. WHO established a Global Initiative on Emergency and Essential Surgical Care (GIESSC). For these reasons – large burden, attractive cost-effectiveness and past neglect – the Copenhagen Consensus in May 2008 considered essential surgery as a potential priority investment for the world's poor.

In a recent article, Zakrison [39] argues that it is irresponsible to ignore the larger social, political and economic context of global surgical disease when this is merely another manifestation of poverty in its worst form. How to gain access to ACS? Some believe that it should be delivered one patient at a time. Others maintain that this effort is useless, and prefer to re-direct scarce funds to high-technology endeavours. Happily, the common perception that surgical care is merely a luxury in poor countries is being reconsidered and its essential role in global public health is being acknowledged [39].

1.1.9 Summary of the Nature of ACS and Future Considerations

In an outstanding communication, 'A qualitative analysis of acute care surgery in the United States: It's more than just "a competent surgeon with a sharp knife and a willing attitude"', Santry and colleagues [40] detailed the results of their interviewees of 18 ACS leaders from geographically distributed areas in the USA. All respondents described ACS as a specialty treating "time-sensitive surgical disease including trauma, emergency general surgery (EGS), and surgical critical care (SCC); 11 of 18 combined trauma and EGS into a single clinical team; 9 of 18 included elective general surgery……Eight of 18 ACS teams had scheduled EGS operating room time....13 of 18 shared EGS due to volume, human resources, or competition for revenue. Only 12 of 18 had formal sign out rounds; only 2 of 18 had prospective EGS data registries.......

ACS was described as the "last great surgical service' reinvigorated to provide 'timely', cost-effective EGS by experts in 'resuscitation and critical care' and to attract 'young, talented, eager surgeons' to trauma/SCC (surgical critical care); however, there was concern that ACS might become the 'wastebasket for everything that happens at inconvenient times " [40]. The authors gave direct quotations of fascinating opinions of these leaders, expanding on the benefits and challenges of the ACS model (Table 1.1). This paper is an excellent summary of ACS, a required reading for all who want to know about this new model.

In summary, current consensus appears to confirm that the ACS model is one of inclusion rather exclusion. It has to be designed with flexibility, based on local, regional needs and the type of patients and the level of the institution (university, community centres). It may have different identities in different countries. In some, as for example in the university-based centres in the USA, ACS will have all three components (trauma, emergency surgery and surgical critical care). In other countries, ACS may only refer to emergency general surgery, while in still others it may focus on emergency general surgery and trauma. Whatever the wrinkle, it definitely has an impressive role for patient well-being, physician and professional satisfaction and administrative support.

With elective general surgery teams, sub-specialists in surgery, surgically minded intensivists and knowledgeable administrators cheering on, ACS has the potential to dramatically improve the care of emergency surgery and trauma patients and bring broad-based general surgery back to the future., it is worthwhile, however, to keep in mind this admonition from LD Britt [2]: 'Yes, the "table has been set" but the maturation process must continue and do so on the right trajectory.'

Table 1.1 Benefits and challenges of ACS Santry et al. [40]

Benefits:
Frees up elective surgeon
Job satisfaction
Lifestyle
Increased revenue
Resident education
Interest in ACS
Expedites care
Critical Care expertise
Evidence based standards
Research
Stand-by help
Emergency Department satisfaction
Hospital reputation
Access to emergency GS care
Expedited referrals
Challenges:
Not enough manpower
Poor continuity
Lack of OR availability
Intrusion of non-acute care surgeons

References

1. Søreide K. Trauma and the acute care surgery model – should it embrace or replace general surgery? Scand J Trauma Resusc Emerg Med. 2009;17:4.
2. Britt LD. Acute care surgery: is it time for a victory lap? J Trauma Acute Care Surg. 2016;80(1):8–15.
3. Maa J, Carter JT, Gosnell JE, et al. The surgical hospitalist: a new model for emergency surgical care. J Am Coll Surg. 2007;205(5):704–11.
4. Quereshi A, Smith A, Wright F, et al. The impact of an acute care emergency surgical service on timely surgical decision making and emergency department overcrowding. J Am Coll Surg. 2011;213(2):284–93.
5. Ingraham AM, Cohen ME, Raval MV, et al. Comparison of hospital performance in emergency versus elective general surgery operations at 198 hospitals. J Am Coll Surg. 2011;212(1):20–8.

6. Ciesla DJ, Cha JY, Smith JS, et al. Implementation of an acute care surgery service at an academic trauma center. Am J Surg. 2011;202(6):779–85.
7. Tisherman SA, Ivy ME, Frangos SG, et al. Acute care surgery survey: opinions of surgeons about a new training paradigm. Arch Surg. 2011;146(1):101–6.
8. Branco BC, Inaba K, Lam L, et al. Implementing acute care surgery at a level I trauma center: 1-year prospective evaluation of the impact of this shift on trauma volumes and outcomes. Am J Surg. 2013;206(1):130–5.
9. Privette AR, Evans AE, Moyer JC, et al. Beyond emergency surgery: redefining acute care surgery. J Surg Res. 2015;196(1):166–71.
10. Michailidou M, Kulvatunyou N, Friese RS, et al. Time and cost analysis of gallbladder surgery under the acute care surgery model. J Trauma Acute Care Surg. 2014;76(3):710–4.
11. Procter L, Kearney P, Korosec RL, et al. An acute care surgery service generates a positive contribution margin in an appropriately staffed hospital. J Am Coll Surg. 2013;216(2):298–301.
12. Alexander MS, Nelson C, Coughenour J. Acute care surgery practice model: targeted growth for fiscal success. Surgery. 2013;154(4):867–72.
13. Miller PR, Wildman EA, Chang MC, et al. Acute care surgery: impact on practice and economics of elective surgeons. J Am Coll Surg. 2012;214:531.
14. O'Mara MS, Scherer L, Wisner D, et al. Sustainability and success of the acute care surgery model in the nontrauma setting. J Am Coll Surg. 2014;219:90–100.
15. Kalina M. Implementation of an Acute Care Surgery Service in a Community Hospital: impact on hospital efficiency and patient outcomes. Am Surg. 2016;82(1):79–84.
16. Santry HP, Madore JC, Collins CE, et al. Variations in the implementation of acute care surgery: results from a national survey of university-affiliated hospitals. J Trauma Acute Care Surg. 2015;78(1):60–7.
17. Cherry-Bukowiec JR, Miller BS, Doherty GM, et al. Nontrauma emergency surgery: optimal case mix for general surgery and acute care surgery training. J Trauma. 2011;71(5):1422–6.
18. Lissauer ME, Schulze R, May A, et al. Update on the status and future of acute care surgery: 10 years later. J Trauma Acute Care Surg. 2014;76(6):1462–6.
19. Moore PK, Grant AR, Tello TL, et al. Future of acute care surgery: a perspective from the next generation. J Trauma Acute Care Surg. 2012;72(1):94–9.

20. Peitzman AB, Sperry JL, Kutcher ME, et al. Redefining acute care surgery: surgical rescue. J Trauma Acute Care Surg. 2015;79:327.

21. Ball CG, Hameed SM, Brenneman FD. Acute care surgery: a new strategy for the general surgery patients left behind. Can J Surg. 2010;53:84–5.

22. Hameed SM, Brenneman FD, Ball CG. General surgery 2.0: the emergence of acute care surgery in Canada. Can J Surg. 2010;53:79–83.

23. Wanis KN, Hunter AM, Harington MB, et al. Impact of an acute care surgery service on timeliness of care and surgeon satisfaction at a Canadian academic hospital: a retrospective study. World J Emerg Surg. 2014;9:4.

24. Uraneus S, Lamont E. Acute care surgery: the European model. World J Surg. 2008;32:1605–12.

25. Tilsed J. Emergency surgery in Europe: the UEMS perspective. https://www.uems.eu/__.../18-09-2015. Accessed 23 Apr 2016.

26. Black A. The future of acute care. www.durrow.org.uk/resources/publications/The-future-of-acute-care.pdf. Accessed 23 Apr 2016.

27. Emergency general surgery: challenges and opportunities www.nuffieldtrust.org.uk/Publications/Ourpublications. Accessed 23 Apr 2016.

28. Pearce L, Smith SR, Parkin E, et al. Emergency general surgery: evolution of a subspecialty by stealth. World J Emerg Surg. 2016;11:2.

29. Catena F, Moore EE. Emergency surgery, acute care surgery and the boulevard of broken dreams. World J Emerg Surg. 2009;4:4.

30. Catena F, Moore F, Ansaloni L, et al. Emergency surgeon: "last of the mohicans" 2014–2016 editorial policy WSES- WJES: position papers, guidelines, courses, books and original research; from WJES impact factor to WSES congress impact factor. World J Emerg Surg. 2014;9(1):14.

31. Di Saverio S, Tugnoli G, Catena F, et al. Surgeon accountability for patient safety in the Acute Care Surgery paradigm: a critical appraisal and need of having a focused knowledge of the patient and a specific subspecialty experience. Patient Saf Surg. 2015;9:38.

32. Kashuk JL, Klein Y, Bacchus H, et al. Acute care surgery: what's in a name? A new specialty comes of age. Isr Med Assoc J. 2013;15:213–7.

33. Hsee L, Devaud M, Middelberg L, et al. Acute surgical unit at Auckland City Hospital: a descriptive analysis. ANZ J Surg. 2014;84(1–2):25–30.

34. Page DE, Dooreemeah D, Thiruchelvam D. Acute surgical unit: the Australasian experience. ANZ J Surg. 2014;84(1–2):25–30.

35. Nagaraja V, Eslick GD, Cox MR. The acute surgical unit model verses the traditional "on call" model: a systematic review and meta-analysis. World J Surg. 2014;38(6):1381–7.
36. Debas H, Gosselin R, McCord C, Thind A. Surgery. In: Jamison D, editor. Disease control priorities in developing countries. 1st ed. New York: Oxford University Press; 2006; 2006ue with high-risk surgery. Med Care. 2011;49:107 6Y1081.
37. Aufderheide TP, Nolan JP, Jacobs IG, et al. Global health and emergency care: a resuscitation research agenda – Part 1. Acad Emerg Med. 2013;20(12):1289–96.
38. Ozgediz D, Jamison D, Cherianc M, et al. The burden of surgical conditions and access to surgical care in low- and middle-income countries. Bull World Health Organ. 2008;86(8):646.
39. Zakrison TL. Global acute care surgery–a public health intervention or a tool for social change? Trop Med Surg. 2013;1:4–133.
40. Santry HP, Pringle PL, Collins CE, et al. A qualitative analysis of acute care surgery in the United States: it's more than just "a competent surgeon with a sharp knife and a willing attitude". Surgery. 2014;155(5):809–25.

Chapter 2
A History of Acute Care Surgery (Emergency Surgery)

Matthew E. Kutcher and Andrew B. Peitzman

2.1 Introduction

The broader field of surgery has made significant strides over the past two decades in both the understanding of surgical disease as well as in the technical conduct of operations. However, a significant portion of surgical patients present with "time-sensitive surgical disease" requiring immediate evaluation and management, often at times of the day or in clinical settings in which a specialist is not immediately available [1]. As the number of surgeons trained and willing to provide comprehensive care for this population has declined while the clinical need continues to increase, the specialty of Acute Care Surgery (ACS; referred to as Emergency Surgery in Europe) was proposed by the American Association for the Surgery of Trauma

M.E. Kutcher, MD • A.B. Peitzman, MD (✉)
University of Pittsburgh, F-1281, UPMC-Presbyterian, 200 Lothrop Street, Pittsburgh, PA 15213, USA
e-mail: peitzmanab@upmc.edu

© Springer International Publishing Switzerland 2017
S. Di Saverio et al. (eds.), *Acute Care Surgery Handbook*,
DOI 10.1007/978-3-319-15341-4_2

(AAST). At its inception, ACS was initially comprised of trauma, emergency general surgery, and critical care. As the specialty has begun to mature, it has expanded its focus to include elective general surgery and surgical rescue (Fig. 2.1).

2.2 The Need for Acute Care Surgery

In the year 2000, an estimated 103.1 million Americans – more than one-third of the population of the United States – visited an emergency department for care. As this number continued to rise, 60 % of emergency centers reported running at capacity, and 40 % reported overcrowding on a daily basis. In 2006, the Institute of Medicine released a report describing "hospital-based emergency care at the breaking point," citing overcrowding of emergency departments, inadequate specialty provider availability, and inadequate compensation for care provided [2].

From a global perspective, the need for Emergency Surgery is enormous [3–5]. Five million deaths a year occur from injury, and 500,000 women die from complications of pregnancy annually. Excluding trauma and obstetrics, 900,000 more deaths occur from illnesses within the skill set of the emergency surgeon: peptic ulcer disease, abdominal aortic aneurysm, bowel obstruction, mesenteric ischemia, appendicitis, soft tissue infection, and abscesses [3–5]. Seventy percent of these deaths occur in low and middle income countries, which have the least capacity to provide care to these patients.

In the United States, a confluence of three key factors led to a need for the creation and branding of a new surgical discipline to care for these patients: (1) the changing face of trauma care, (2) decline in the general surgery workforce, and (3) the advent of the closed critical care model.

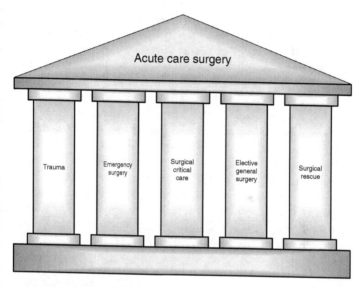

Fig. 2.1 The five pillars of Acute Care Surgery (Adapted from the upcoming edition of Mattox, Moore, Feliciano. TRAUMA. Lewis T, Rosengart MR, Peitzman AB, Acute Care Surgery, McGraw-Hill, New York, 2015)

2.2.1   The Changing Face of Trauma Care

The current practice of trauma surgery largely developed in response to an earlier Institute of Medicine report describing injury as "the neglected disease of modern society," circulated in 1966 [6]. In the decades since, a renaissance in the delivery of trauma care occurred in which the rate of injury-related mortality dropped precipitously, largely related to widespread regionalization and standardization of trauma systems. [7, 8] Despite these successes, by the early 2000s the field of trauma surgery became caught in "an identity crisis" [9]. With improvements in critical care and trends towards nonoperative management, many practicing trauma surgeons found their operative volumes decreasing, with the median caseload per surgeon reported as low as 50 per year in 2006 [10]. The ascendance of adjunct trauma specialties such as orthopedics and neurosurgery prompted some practitioners to comment that the days of the trauma surgeon as a master surgical technician were over [11], instead having devolved into serving as "house staff for the subspecialist" [12]. The specialty has also become plagued by long, unpredictable work hours and high levels of stress. In a 2006 survey of trauma surgeons concerning their future, 88 % reported feeling undervalued by society and the healthcare system [10]. However, despite these difficulties, nearly 90 % reported satisfaction with their career choice in trauma, 72 % reported being satisfied by their current trauma care practice, and 88 % called for change to revitalize the field.

2.2.2 Decline in the General Surgery Workforce

Overall, the number of general surgeons in the United States declined more than 25 % from 1981 to 2005, with losses noted in both rural and urban areas [13]. Compared to the recommended 6 general surgeons per 100,000 population [14], recent projections suggest that if current trends continue the United States will have a shortfall of between 23,000 and 32,000 surgeons by the year 2025 [15]. Compounding this problem, current general surgeons are aging, with more than 32 % of general surgeons older than 55 years and only 20 % younger than 35 years (2007 data) [16]. Clinically, this has led to a crisis in ensuring the availability of appropriate surgical care to the acutely ill and injured. A survey of emergency department directors conducted in 2010 revealed that 74 % of emergency departments reported difficulty with specialist coverage in a variety of disciples, 37 % of departments reported incomplete or no general surgery coverage, and 55 % documented inconsistent trauma coverage [17]. In the same study, 23 % of facilities had lost or downgraded their trauma center level designation due to inadequate surgical coverage [17].

In addition to overall workforce losses in general surgery, specialization has greatly reduced the number of surgeons available to provide emergency surgical care. Currently, more than 75 % of graduating general surgery residents pursue specialty training, and this number appears to be increasing [18]. Several reasons exist for surgeons to narrow their practices. Specialization allows selecting a limited number of procedures and body of literature to master, in the face of an otherwise rapidly expanding technical and knowledge base. Financial incentives exist as well, as in many settings subspecialists bill at higher fees than general surgeons performing similar procedures. As well, specialty practice is felt by many to be more conducive to limited work hours, family priorities, and general flexibility. As fewer graduates of surgical residency remain in the "core" practice of general surgery, they quickly lose their comfort in emergency general and trauma surgery [19].

2.2.3   The Closed Critical Care Model

In the United States, the Acute Care Surgeon is actively involved in ICU care. Similar to the workforce crisis in general surgery, data point to a worsening shortage of critical care providers despite an increasing need [20]. The demand for intensive care unit services is likely to continue to grow as the average acuity of hospitalized patients increases in parallel with the aging population [21], with a recent congressional report projecting shortages of up to 35 % in the intensivist workforce by the year 2020 [22]. In particular, there is a nationwide shortage of surgeons certified in critical care. While an intensivist-led model of critical care is associated with significant reductions in mortality risk (relative risk: 0.78), this effect appears to most profound in units led by *surgical* intensivists (relative risk: 0.67) [23]. Unfortunately, only 61 % of Level I and 22 % of Level II trauma centers provide this intensivist-led model of critical care delivery [24]. Given the expanding technical expertise and sizable, fast-moving body of literature associated with the field of critical care, data would suggest that it is no longer best practice for general surgeons to care primarily for surgical patients in an intensive care unit without formal training in critical care.

2.3 The Development of Acute Care Surgery

Given these clear challenges to provide adequate surgical and critical care for acutely ill and injured patients, the American Association for the Surgery of Trauma (AAST) convened an *ad hoc* Committee to Develop the Reorganized Specialty of Trauma, Surgical Critical Care, and Emergency Surgery to address these unmet needs in 2003. The committee, comprised of members of several prominent national and regional surgical and critical care organizations, was renamed the Acute Care Surgery Committee in 2005. As described in the group's 2005 publication in the Journal of Trauma [25], the AAST proposed to merge, re-brand, and codify the practice of trauma surgery, emergency general surgery, and surgical critical care into a single distinct specialty of Acute Care Surgery (ACS). An AAST retreat in 2007 was subsequently devoted to developing a curriculum, competency tools, a case registry, certification criteria, and mechanism for program site visits to support a complete educational program of ACS. Recognition of the need for Emergency Surgery has been thoughtfully documented in the United Kingdom, Australia, and multiple other countries globally [3–5, 26, 27].

2.4   The Current State of Acute Care Surgery

2.4.1   Training of Acute Care Surgeons

The AAST has designed and implemented an ACS curriculum at the fellowship level, consisting of a 2-year training program completed following completion of an American College of Graduate Medical Education-approved general surgery residency. The first year of the curriculum involves an American Board of Surgery-certified fellowship in surgical critical care, requiring 9 months of intensive care unit rotations; the remaining 3 months are devoted to the remainder of the ACS curriculum. Over the remaining 15 months, suggested rotations include 2–3 months on an acute care surgery service, 1–2 months of thoracic surgery, 1–2 months of transplant or hepatobiliary surgery, 1–2 months of vascular surgery, and 1–3 months of electives. Recommended electives include neurosurgery, orthopedics, burn surgery, and pediatric surgery. The focus of this aspect of training is to supplement the surgical experience of trainees in management of major thoracic, hepatic, and vascular injuries, and to ensure that any knowledge, experiential, or technical voids that existed during residency training are filled. In total, this constitutes 9 months of formal critical care training and 15 months of operative rotations. Additional essential components of an ACS fellowship include the practice of elective general surgery as well as a minimum of 52 trauma and emergency surgery night-time calls. At the present time, 19 ACS fellowships across the United States are accredited by the AAST.

The specific curriculum for ACS training continues to evolve. Despite the initial concept of ACS including technical training in emergency neurosurgical and orthopedic care, although only 6% of surveyed ACS leaders formally include these practices [1]; this aspect of ACS, although not formally realized, would present clear theoretical advantages to surgeons in rural or austere environments [28]. Some authors have also suggested a role for integration of a more knowledge-based curriculum into ACS training, addressing topics such as management of surgical infections, sepsis, multiple organ dysfunction, and acute kidney injury, although this has not yet become standard [29, 30].

Analysis of case logs from the first year of organized reporting on ACS fellowship trainees revealed that fellows performed an average of 195 cases per year, roughly 40 % of which were elective and 60 % emergent [31]. Requirements for the case mix achieved in ACS fellowship have been revised since their initial release in 2007 [32], now defining specific anatomic areas with minimum case requirements to ensure proficiency across anatomic regions. An additional category has been added to facilitate logging of diagnostic and therapeutic ultrasound procedures as well. Recent analysis suggests that ACS fellowship case mix continues to lack head and neck procedures, thoracic vascular exposures, and pediatric cases [33].

2.4.2   Implementation and Evolution of Acute Care Surgery

Despite the timely adoption and rapid growth of ACS as a field, its penetrance and implementation vary widely. Of 258 University Health Systems Consortium hospitals surveyed in 2015, 31 % had implemented a clinical ACS service, compared to 52 % maintaining a traditional general surgeon on-call model [34]. Of ACS services in this study, 67 % had dedicated emergency general surgery operative block time (versus 28 % of traditional models), and 93 % of ACS groups (versus 45 % of traditional models) provided intensive care unit coverage. In a separate survey study of ACS leaders, roughly 60 % of ACS teams subsume both trauma and emergency general surgery under the same clinical service, and about half include elective general surgery as well [1].

While the initial conception of ACS included only the triad of trauma, emergency general surgery, and surgical critical care, several practitioners feel that two additional key pillars of ACS practice exist. The fourth pillar of ACS consists of the practice of elective general surgery. Conceptually, much of the skill set for understanding and management of acute surgical emergencies is rooted in anatomic and physiological principles first learned in the elective surgery setting. To take the example of colon cancer, the elective colorectal surgeon has a thorough knowledge of the disease process and relevant anatomy, and is the ideal surgical specialist to counsel a patient with colon cancer and carry out the elective surgical options for its treatment; however, the same patient presenting with tumor-related perforation, intra-abdominal sepsis, and critical illness presents a different challenge, requiring the same knowledge base but an integrated acute management skill set such as that offered by an acute care surgeon. The fundamental surgical principles in both settings are rooted in an understanding of the elective surgical practice, while the optimal management is specific to the patient's presentation.

A second additional pillar of ACS similarly stems from a patient physiology-centered approach to management in the patient with a procedural complication. According to CDC figures, of more than 36 million inpatient hospital discharges, more than 900,000 are related to a complication of medical or surgical care: This is a more common discharge diagnosis than bowel obstruction, appendicitis, and cholelithiasis combined [35]. Based on data from the University of Pittsburgh, 20 % of the admissions and consult handled by a mature ACS service are for management of a medical or surgical complication: More than 80 % of patients require an operation, and more than half require multiple operations. Importantly, 50 % of these complications are referred to our service after a procedure performed by another interventional or surgical service at the same institution, 25 % are related to an ACS service complication, and 25 % are referred from another institution [36]. Several recent large studies demonstrate that incidence of surgical complications across surgical specialties at high-performing versus low-performing hospitals is not significantly different, but that differences in morbidity and mortality stem primarily from the capacity of high-performing hospitals to expeditiously and appropriately manage the complication [37–42]. The skills of the acute care surgeon are uniquely tailored to the management of time-sensitive physiology in the patient with a complication and play a critical role in maintaining institution-wide patient outcomes, especially in centers with multiple interventional and surgical specialty services.

2.4.3   Impact on Patient Outcome

In terms of addressing timeliness of care in patients with time-sensitive surgical disease, results have been encouraging. One institution's reported experience of the effect of implementing an ACS service on emergency department overcrowding found reductions in surgical decision time of 15 %, and reduction in emergency department "time-to-stretcher" of 20 % [43]. A second similar study showed significant improvements in time-to-operation (192 min versus 221 min) as well as proportionally fewer after-hours operative cases (60 % versus 72 %) after creation of an ACS service [44].

In terms of clinical outcomes at the patient level, the impact of ACS has been studied in the management of appendicitis as well as acute gallbladder disease. In an early cases series, patients with appendicitis treated by an ACS team compared to a traditional general surgery on-call practice model had significantly decreased time from consultation to operation (3.5 h versus 7.6 h) and from presentation to operation (10.1 h versus 14.0 h), significantly decreased rates of appendiceal rupture (12.3 % versus 23.3 %) and overall complications (7.7 % versus 17.4 %), and an overall significant decrease in hospital length of stay (2.3 days versus 3.5 days) [45]. Similar improvement in the care of patients with acute appendicitis has been seen in several other subsequent studies comparing ACS to a traditional general surgery call structure, with specific reductions in time-to-evaluation, time-to-operation, proportion of cases completed after-hours, length of stay, and overall health care costs [46–48]. Using cholecystectomy for acute biliary pathology as a benchmark, benefits in outcomes and processes of care have shown similar improvement with the advent of an ACS model. In one study, mean time-to-evaluation was reduced by 5.8 h, time-to-operation by 25 h, and hospital length of stay by 1.9 days, while fewer complications occurred at an overall cost savings of up to $3000 per patient [46]. In addition to improved time-to-operation, complication rate, and length of stay, a recent study further described a significantly increased proportion of cholecystectomy within 24 h of presentation (75 % versus 59 %) and fewer cases requiring conversion from a laparoscopic to open approach (4.2 % versus 11.6 %) [49]. As with appendicitis, several other studies have shown similar significant reductions in time-to-operation, complication rates, and proportion of cases completed after-hours in patient with acute biliary presentations treated by ACS surgeons [50–52]. Overall, a meta-analysis of 18 studies on management of appendicitis, acute cholecystitis, and small bowel obstruction under an ACS model compared to a traditional general surgery structure confirmed a reduction in complication rate for appendectomy and cholecystectomy, with a reduced laparoscopic-to-open conversion rate and shorter length of stay for patients with cholecystitis across all studies evaluated [53].

2.4.4 Impact on Practicing Surgeons

In the nearly one decade since its inception, the ACS model has achieved notable success in meaningfully changing the field, while challenges still exist. With the initial implementation of ACS models, concerns were raised that the merging of trauma and emergency surgery practices might negatively impact trauma outcomes, or reduce productivity in surgeons who practice as part of more traditional general surgery models. Fortunately, neither concern has borne out in the published literature. Multiple studies have shown that increases in workload associated with development of an ACS service do not affect time-to-operation, morbidity or mortality rates for injured patients cared for by the same service [54–56]. Furthermore, in one study, work relative value unit (RVU) production increased for both ACS *and* non-ACS surgeons after implementation of an ACS service, likely due to optimization of elective time usage facilitating a more focused practice for non-ACS general surgeons. Both ACS and non-ACS general surgeons showed improved job satisfaction after the advent of ACS in this study [57]. Another group found that ACS implementation did have modest (8%) RVU production losses for non-ACS surgeons, but these appeared to be counterbalanced by increased billing collections by both groups and an increase in elective caseload for non-ACS surgeons, overall resulting in an annual departmental revenue boost in excess of $2 million [58]. In terms of addressing job satisfaction, a survey of practicing acute care surgeons performed in 2013 reported that 71% were satisfied with their practice profile, and 92% report being happy with their work in general, although 66% reported some degree of burn-out [59].

2.4.5 Impact on Resident Training

Concern exists that, with declining operative volumes, general surgery residency does not adequately prepare trainees for independent practice, with substantial variation between residency programs as well as between trainees at any given program [60]. This reduced caseload and high degree of variability, in combination with trends towards nonoperative management of blunt trauma and a decreasing overall incidence of penetrating trauma, particularly effects resident education in trauma [61]. A study of the general surgery resident experience before and after implementation of an ACS service reported that consolidation of call responsibilities into a single ACS service reduced multiple surgical team overlap, thereby increasing efficiency while preserving operative and clinical volume, while also facilitating increasing didactic conference and clinic attendance as well as independent reading time [62]. Additional studies of general surgery operative case logs evaluating the impact of creation of an ACS service [63] and presence of an ACS fellow [64] did not appear to detract from resident case volume or complexity. In fact, resident survey data suggests that general surgery residents have a positive response to the presence of an ACS fellow [64]. From the resident career choice perspective, a recent survey of categorical general surgery residents revealed that more than 90 % had an appropriate understanding of the components of ACS, and nearly half had considered a career in ACS after graduating. Residents believed that ACS offers equivalent or better case complexity (88 %), scope of practice (84 %), case volume (75 %), and reimbursement (69 %) compared with general surgery [65].

2.5 Conclusion

The specialty of Acute Care Surgery has evolved to address the needs of critical patients with time-dependent surgical disease. Addressing paradigm shifts in the practice of trauma surgery as well as critical shortages in the general surgical and critical care workforce, ACS knits together the disciplines of trauma, emergency general surgery, and surgical critical care with the practice of elective general surgery and the skill set for surgical rescue of the patient with a complication to create a distinct and evolving specialty.

References

1. Santry HP, Pringle PL, Collins CE, et al. A qualitative analysis of acute care surgery in the United States: it's more than just "a competent surgeon with a sharp knife and a willing attitude". Surgery. 2014;155(5):809–25.
2. Institute of Medicine Committee on the Future of Emergency Care in the U. S. Health Care System. Hospital-based emergency care: at the breaking point. Washington, DC: National Academy Press; 2006.
3. Leppaniemi A. Emergency surgery at crossroads: is it enough just to plug the hole? Scand J Surg. 2007;96(3):182–3.
4. Peitzman AB, Leppaniemi A, Kutcher ME, et al. Surgical rescue: an essential component of acute care surgery. Scand J Surg. 2015;104(3):135–6.
5. Stewart B, Khanduri P, McCord C, et al. Global disease burden of conditions requiring emergency surgery. Br J Surg. 2014;101(1):e9–22.
6. Institute of Medicine. Accidental death and disability: the neglected disease of modern society. Washington, DC: National Academy Press; 1966.
7. Celso B, Tepas J, Langland-Orban B, et al. A systematic review and meta-analysis comparing outcome of severely injured patients treated in trauma centers following the establishment of trauma systems. J Trauma. 2006;60(2):371–8; discussion 378.
8. MacKenzie EJ, Rivara FP, Jurkovich GJ, et al. A national evaluation of the effect of trauma-center care on mortality. N Engl J Med. 2006;354(4):366–78.
9. Esposito TJ, Rotondo M, Barie PS, et al. Making the case for a paradigm shift in trauma surgery. J Am Coll Surg. 2006;202(4):655–67.
10. Esposito TJ, Leon L, Jurkovich GJ. The shape of things to come: results from a national survey of trauma surgeons on issues concerning their future. J Trauma. 2006;60(1):8–16.

11. Moore EE. Trauma surgery: is it time for a facelift? Ann Surg. 2004;240(3):563–4.
12. Ciesla DJ, Moore EE, Cothren CC, et al. Has the trauma surgeon become house staff for the surgical subspecialist? Am J Surg. 2006;192(6):732–7.
13. Lynge DC, Larson EH, Thompson MJ, et al. A longitudinal analysis of the general surgery workforce in the United States, 1981–2005. Arch Surg. 2008;143(4):345–50; discussion 351.
14. American College of Surgeons Health Policy Research Institute. The surgical workforce in the United States: profile and recent trends. Chapel Hill: American College of Surgeons Health Policy Research Institute; 2010.
15. IHS, Inc. The complexities of physician supply and demand: projections from 2013 to 2025. Washington, DC: Association of American Medical Colleges; 2015.
16. Fischer JE. The impending disappearance of the general surgeon. JAMA. 2007;298(18):2191–3.
17. Rao MB, Lerro C, Gross CP. The shortage of on-call surgical specialist coverage: a national survey of emergency department directors. Acad Emerg Med. 2010;17(12):1374–82.
18. Borman KR, Vick LR, Biester TW, et al. Changing demographics of residents choosing fellowships: longterm data from the American Board of Surgery. J Am Coll Surg. 2008;206(5):782–8; discussion 788–9.
19. Stitzenberg KB, Sheldon GF. Progressive specialization within general surgery: adding to the complexity of workforce planning. J Am Coll Surg. 2005;201(6):925–32.
20. Napolitano LM, Fulda GJ, Davis KA, et al. Challenging issues in surgical critical care, trauma, and acute care surgery: a report from the Critical Care Committee of the American Association for the surgery of trauma. J Trauma. 2010;69(6):1619–33.
21. Angus DC, Kelley MA, Schmitz RJ, et al. Caring for the critically ill patient. Current and projected workforce requirements for care of the critically ill and patients with pulmonary disease: can we meet the requirements of an aging population? JAMA. 2000;284(21):2762–70.
22. Health Resources and Services Administration. The critical care workforce: a study of the supply and demand for critical care physicians (Report to Congress). 2006.
23. Nathens AB, Rivara FP, MacKenzie EJ, et al. The impact of an intensivist-model ICU on trauma-related mortality. Ann Surg. 2006;244(4):545–54.

24. Nathens AB, Maier RV, Jurkovich GJ, et al. The delivery of critical care services in US trauma centers: is the standard being met? J Trauma. 2006;60(4):773–83; discussion 783–4.

25. Committee to Develop the Reorganized Specialty of Trauma, Surgical Critical Care, and Emergency Surgery. Acute care surgery: trauma, critical care, and emergency surgery. J Trauma. 2005;58(3):614–6.

26. Deane SA, MacLellan DG, Meredith GL, et al. Making sense of emergency surgery in New South Wales: a position statement. ANZ J Surg. 2010;80(3):139–44.

27. Pearse RM, Harrison DA, James P, et al. Identification and characterisation of the high-risk surgical population in the United Kingdom. Crit Care. 2006;10(3):R81.

28. Ciesla DJ. The acute care surgeon and emergency specialty procedures. J Am Coll Surg. 2007;205(1):187–9.

29. Kelly E, Rogers Jr SO. Graduate medical education in trauma/critical care and acute care surgery: defining goals for a new workforce. Surg Clin North Am. 2012;92(4):1055–64. x.

30. May AK, Cuschieri J, Johnson JL, et al. Determining a core curriculum in surgical infections for fellowship training in acute care surgery using the Delphi technique. Surg Infect (Larchmt). 2013;14(6):547–53.

31. Dente CJ, Duane TM, Jurkovich GJ, et al. How much and what type: analysis of the first year of the acute care surgery operative case log. J Trauma Acute Care Surg. 2014;76(2):329–38; discussion 338–9.

32. Davis KA, Dente CJ, Burlew CC, et al. Refining the operative curriculum of the acute care surgery fellowship. J Trauma Acute Care Surg. 2015;78(1):192–6.

33. Duane TM, Dente CJ, Fildes JJ, et al. Defining the acute care surgery curriculum. J Trauma Acute Care Surg. 2015;78(2):259–63; discussion 263–4.

34. Santry HP, Madore JC, Collins CE, et al. Variations in the implementation of acute care surgery: results from a national survey of university-affiliated hospitals. J Trauma Acute Care Surg. 2015;78(1):60–7; discussion 67–8.

35. Buie VC, Owings MF, DeFrances CJ, Golosinskiy A. National hospital discharge survey: 2006 annual summary. Vital Health Stat 2010;168:1–79.

36. Peitzman AB, Sperry JL, Kutcher ME, et al. Redefining acute care surgery: surgical rescue. J Trauma Acute Care Surg. 2015; 79(2):327.

37. Almoudaris AM, Burns EM, Mamidanna R, et al. Value of failure to rescue as a marker of the standard of care following reoperation for

complications after colorectal resection. Br J Surg. 2011;98(12): 1775–83.

38. Ferraris VA, Bolanos M, Martin JT, et al. Identification of patients with postoperative complications who are at risk for failure to rescue. JAMA Surg. 2014;149(11):1103–8.

39. Ghaferi AA, Birkmeyer JD, Dimick JB. Hospital volume and failure to rescue with high-risk surgery. Med Care. 2011;49(12):1076–81.

40. Taenzer AH, Pyke JB, McGrath SP. A review of current and emerging approaches to address failure-to-rescue. Anesthesiology. 2011;115(2):421–31.

41. Tamirisa NP, Parmar AD, Vargas GM, et al. Relative contributions of complications and failure to rescue on mortality in older patients undergoing pancreatectomy. Ann Surg. 2016;263(2):385–91. Doi: 10.1097/SLA.0000000000001093.

42. Wong SL, Revels SL, Yin H, et al. Variation in hospital mortality rates with inpatient cancer surgery. Ann Surg. 2015;261(4):632–6.

43. Qureshi A, Smith A, Wright F, et al. The impact of an acute care emergency surgical service on timely surgical decision-making and emergency department overcrowding. J Am Coll Surg. 2011;213(2):284–93.

44. Wanis KN, Hunter AM, Harington MB, et al. Impact of an acute care surgery service on timeliness of care and surgeon satisfaction at a Canadian academic hospital: a retrospective study. World J Emerg Surg. 2014;9(1):4.

45. Earley AS, Pryor JP, Kim PK, et al. An acute care surgery model improves outcomes in patients with appendicitis. Ann Surg. 2006;244(4):498–504.

46. Cubas RF, Gomez NR, Rodriguez S, et al. Outcomes in the management of appendicitis and cholecystitis in the setting of a new acute care surgery service model: impact on timing and cost. J Am Coll Surg. 2012;215(5):715–21.

47. Fu CY, Huang HC, Chen RJ, et al. Implementation of the acute care surgery model provides benefits in the surgical treatment of the acute appendicitis. Am J Surg. 2014;208(5):794–9.

48. Wright GP, Ecker AM, Hobbs DJ, et al. Old dogs and new tricks: length of stay for appendicitis improves with an acute care surgery program and transition from private surgical practice to multispecialty group practice. Am Surg. 2014;80(12):1250–5.

49. Michailidou M, Kulvatunyou N, Friese RS, et al. Time and cost analysis of gallbladder surgery under the acute care surgery model. J Trauma Acute Care Surg. 2014;76(3):710–4.

50. Britt RC, Bouchard C, Weireter LJ, et al. Impact of acute care surgery on biliary disease. J Am Coll Surg. 2010;210(5):595–9, 599–601.

51. Lau B, Difronzo LA. An acute care surgery model improves timeliness of care and reduces hospital stay for patients with acute cholecystitis. Am Surg. 2011;77(10):1318–21.

52. Lim DW, Ozegovic D, Khadaroo RG, et al. Impact of an acute care surgery model with a dedicated daytime operating room on outcomes and timeliness of care in patients with biliary tract disease. World J Surg. 2013;37(10):2266–72.

53. Nagaraja V, Eslick GD, Cox MR. The acute surgical unit model verses the traditional "on call" model: a systematic review and meta-analysis. World J Surg. 2014;38(6):1381–7.

54. Branco BC, Inaba K, Lam L, et al. Implementing acute care surgery at a level I trauma center: 1-year prospective evaluation of the impact of this shift on trauma volumes and outcomes. Am J Surg. 2013;206(1):130–5.

55. Matsushima K, Cook A, Tollack L, et al. An acute care surgery model provides safe and timely care for both trauma and emergency general surgery patients. J Surg Res. 2011;166(2):e143–7.

56. Pryor JP, Reilly PM, Schwab CW, et al. Integrating emergency general surgery with a trauma service: impact on the care of injured patients. J Trauma. 2004;57(3):467–71; discussion 471–3.

57. Barnes SL, Cooper CJ, Coughenour JP, et al. Impact of acute care surgery to departmental productivity. J Trauma. 2011;71(4):1027–32; discussion 1033–4.

58. Miller PR, Wildman EA, Chang MC, et al. Acute care surgery: impact on practice and economics of elective surgeons. J Am Coll Surg. 2012;214(4):531–5; discussion 536–8.

59. Lissauer ME, Schulze R, May A, et al. Update on the status and future of acute care surgery: 10 years later. J Trauma Acute Care Surg. 2014;76(6):1462–6.

60. Bell Jr RH, Biester TW, Tabuenca A, et al. Operative experience of residents in US general surgery programs: a gap between expectation and experience. Ann Surg. 2009;249(5):719–24.

61. Spain DA, Miller FB. Education and training of the future trauma surgeon in acute care surgery: trauma, critical care, and emergency surgery. Am J Surg. 2005;190(2):212–7.

62. Wood L, Buczkowski A, Panton OM, et al. Effects of implementation of an urgent surgical care service on subspecialty general surgery training. Can J Surg. 2010;53(2):119–25.

63. Hatch Q, McVay D, Johnson EK, et al. The impact of an acute care surgery team on general surgery residency. Am J Surg. 2014;208(5):856–9.
64. Dinan KA, Davis JW, Wolfe MM, et al. An acute care surgery fellowship benefits a general surgical residency. J Trauma Acute Care Surg. 2014;77(2):209–12.
65. Coleman JJ, Esposito TJ, Rozycki GS, et al. Acute care surgery: now that we have built it, will they come? J Trauma Acute Care Surg. 2013;74(2):463–8; discussion 468–9.

Chapter 3
Scientific Research in Emergency Surgery Setting

Federico Coccolini, Giulia Montori, Marco Ceresoli, Fausto Catena, and Luca Ansaloni

3.1 What Is Research?

To readers who are engaged in research this question may seem obvious. However, such a definition is needed in order to distinguish research from related activities such as audit or journalism. It is surprisingly difficult to find a definition that distinguishes satisfactorily between these things [1].

The following possible definitions can be taken into consideration [2]:

- A systematic investigation to establish facts
- An attempt to find out something in a systematic and scientific manner

F. Coccolini (✉) • G. Montori • M. Ceresoli • L. Ansaloni
General, Emergency and Trauma Surgery, Papa Giovanni
XXIII Hospital, Bergamo, Italy
e-mail: federico.coccolini@gmail.com

F. Catena
General and Emergency Surgery, Parma University Hospital, Parma, Italy

© Springer International Publishing Switzerland 2017
S. Di Saverio et al. (eds.), *Acute Care Surgery Handbook*,
DOI 10.1007/978-3-319-15341-4_3

39

- A systematic investigation designed to develop generalizable knowledge
- A focused systematic study undertaken to increase new knowledge and understanding
- A systematic study directed toward fuller scientific knowledge or understanding
- The collection of information about a particular subject
- An inquiry that involves seeking evidence to increase knowledge

Although these definitions capture elements that are common to many types of research, they fail to distinguish clearly between research and other activities [2].

The "European Textbook on Ethics in Research" [2] suggests that we should adopt an inclusive working definition of research, such as the following: "Research aims to generate (new) information, knowledge, understanding, or some other relevant cognitive good, and does so by means of a systematic investigation".

In emergency surgery field, the definition of research and the methods to be performed is a little more complicated. This is due to the peculiar subset of patients and the partially "research-hostile" clinical environment.

3.2 Why Is Research Important?

Several reasons show research is intrinsically necessary:

- Research gave us a better quality of life.
- A large number of lives have been saved thank to research-derived improvements.
- In some cases, knowledge may be considered at least good for its own sake.

Considering these three main reasons, we can conclude that from the ethical point of view the research must be performed and constantly improved in order to reach every time more advanced observational points. This will lead to a possible continuous improvement in quality of cure and consequently of life or disease status.

Considering the eventuality of a research goodness for its own sake the advancement of knowledge about an issue, even if apparently not immediately useful, for sure it contributes to increase the universal understanding of the mechanisms. This, associated to other subsequent discovers, could potentially in future find new understandings. This second justification provides a reason why research without any apparent anticipated applications or direct benefits may nonetheless be ethical.

It is always to be taken into account that the research process involves costs. These costs range from the participant time use to the eventual risks. Taking these into consideration is not acceptable to dissociate the research project from an ethical evaluation and an analysis if the research is in some way worthwhile. In fact, especially in emergency surgery setting, where economical and human resources are often too scarce to promote, plan, and realize a research project must take into account the necessity to utilize as less resources as possible. In fact, the major obstacle in realizing effective researches in emergency surgery is methodological. To have real and clinically/statistically significant results in this field, it needs at least the twofold of effort than in many other surgical fields.

For this and other reasons, emergency surgery setting often raises the question about whether research ethics committees (EC) should have a role in ensuring that research is not just ethically sound but also scientifically/methodologically sound. There is some debate about this question, since the operating principles for many ECs discourage them from looking at methodology as it is felt that they are not well constituted to make this judgement in relation to the wide range of projects that they assess [3]. On the other hand, given that both of the arguments in favour of allowing research depend on the research having some chance of successfully reaching its objectives, it would seem that research needs to be methodologically sound to be ethical – especially when it involves risks to the participants (15a). Lastly, stimulating high-quality research in emergency surgery would prevent from the possible future dangerous application of uncontrolled experimentations, as for example happened with the application of peritoneal washing in complicated diverticulitis.

3.2.1 Ethical Codes

Ethical codes and guidelines are necessary to establish the values of a particular institution or society. The most important examples of codes and laws which drive the research rules have been developed during the last century:

- The Nuremberg Code [4]
- The World Medical Association's Declaration of Helsinki [5]
- The Council for International Organizations of Medical Sciences' (CIOMS) International Ethical Guidelines for Biomedical Research Involving Human Subjects [6]
- The Charter of Fundamental Rights of the European Union [7]
- The European Convention on Human Rights [8]
- The European Union Good Clinical Practice Directive [9]
- The Convention for the Protection of Human Rights and Dignity of the Human Being with Regard to the Application of Biology and Medicine: Convention on Human Rights and Biomedicine (The Oviedo Convention) [10]
- The European Union Clinical Trials Directive [11]

Historically, the development of research ethics has been greatly influenced by examples of scandals and unethical research. In fact, the norms of modern research ethics were codified by the Nuremberg Code in 1947 in response to Nazi medical research and further developed by the World Medical Association's Declaration of Helsinki in 1964. Concerns about the effectiveness of the existing regulation arose when attention was drawn to various ethical concerns in ongoing research [12]. These concerns led to the 1975 revision of the Declaration of Helsinki, which introduced the requirement of a formal independent committee review of research protocols. Subsequent different conventions, charter, and directives have been progressively developed.

3.3 Study Phases

Different phases of clinical trials exist according to the developing step into which is situated the drug or the procedure to be investigated.

Phase 0: These trials (micro-dosing trials) are an interim step between preclinical and phase I studies, where a small number of human volunteers take small doses of experimental test article so there is little risk of toxicity. These trials have no therapeutic intent; the aim is to evaluate human pharmacology and identify any toxic effect.

Phase I: These trials represent the first stage of testing in human participants; they are generally associated with a higher risk of harm than any other trials, especially the so-called first-into-man trials and dose-escalating trials.

Phase II: During this phase, an experimental drug/procedure is tested for safety and efficacy in a larger population of individuals afflicted with the disease or condition for which the drug was developed. These trials generally involve around 200–600 participants.

Phase III: During this phase, after a drug/procedure is shown to be reasonably effective, it is compared with current standard treatments for the relevant condition in a large trial involving a substantial number of participants. Generally these trials are represented by major randomized controlled trials and usually involve 500–3,000 participants.

Phase IV: These trials begin after a drug/procedure has been definitively approved for distribution or marketing in case of drug or has been definitively recognized as safe and effective in case of a procedure. These trials represent substantially a population-based surveillance of the wide range application of the studied drug/procedure in order to have confirmation of the results with a wide sample of patients.

In emergency surgery field, the two last study phases are the most represented.

3.4 Main Types of Study Design

Many different designs exist for clinical studies. All of them can be applied with more or less difficulties in emergency surgery.

Observational trials have the aim to verify prospectively or retrospectively the application of a determined variable (drug/procedure) to a determined cohort of patients.

Active control trials that are designed to show that the efficacy of a drug/procedure is better or no worse than that of the active comparative treatment also exist. The last ones are the so-called non-inferiority trials.

Other trials called equivalence trials have the primary objective of showing that the response to two or more treatments does not significantly differ. This is usually demonstrated by showing that the true treatment difference is likely to lie between a lower and upper equivalence margin of clinically acceptable differences. The cohort of patients used as a control can be chosen within the patients treated in the same or in a previous period of time (historical control cohort).

The choice of the type of comparison has a strong influence on technical aspects of the study design, sample size, and statistical analysis.

Several designs of comparative clinical studies exist. The most common type uses two parallel groups: parallel group design. In most cases, trial participants are randomized to one of the two treatment groups, with randomization commonly giving each participant the same possibility or chance to be allocated to either treatment section. One group receives the test drug/procedure, and the other group receives another that could be also a placebo treatment or the current best available treatment on the market (standard treatment). It is also possible to give both groups the standard treatment with the addition – as an add-on treatment or as a combination therapy – of the studied drug/procedure for one of the two treatment groups. In emergency surgery, these are the most difficult studies to be performed. The impossibility, in the majority of situations, to give placebo and the difficulty to randomize emergency surgery patients lead to a great methodological and ethical effort in order to obtain a feasible protocol.

Another type of trial hardly applicable to the emergency surgery setting is the cross-over trial design. The enrolled patients receive both drug/procedure in sequence. In effect, each participant serves as his/her own control. It is important in a cross-over trial that the underlying condition – for instance, a disease – does not change over time, and that the effects of one treatment disappear before the next is applied. For this reason, this study design is hard to be applied in emergency surgery setting.

An increasing number of trials use the so-called adaptive clinical trial design who adjusts the design of the trial with the increasing of the number of participants and with the ongoing analysis about the efficacy of the drug/procedure. These kinds of designs are hardly applicable to emergency surgery.

Lastly, patients can be enrolled in one or in many centres. Multicentre trials are carried out for two reasons. First, they often allow the accrual of a sufficient number of patients to satisfy the trial objective in a reasonable amount of time. Second, they produce more general findings, with participants recruited from a wider population and a broader range of clinical settings. As a consequence, data obtained from multicenter trials are more easily applicable to the rest of population.

3.5 Endpoints

In general, and in emergency surgery in particular, the endpoints represent the main issue in designing a clinical trial. Methodological and endpoint set-up is one of the key to have success especially in emergency surgery trials. The three fundamental criteria for a trial endpoint are that it should be measurable and interpretable, sensitive to the objective of the trial and clinically relevant.

Endpoints are divided in order of importance into:

- *Primary endpoint*: The variable providing the most relevant and convincing evidence related to the prime objective of the trial.
- *Secondary endpoints*: Can data be obtained that support the primary objective or measurements of effects related to other secondary objectives. These should be pre-defined in the protocol, explaining their importance and role in interpreting trial results.

The main endpoints often evaluated in clinical trials are:

- *Mortality*: One of the main issues studied in emergency surgery is the immediate effect of a determined drug/procedure in reducing the mortality.
- *Efficacy*: More in general efficacy is an estimate of how effective studied drug/procedure is in eliminating/reducing the symptoms or long-term endpoints of the disease treated.
- *Safety* of the drug/procedure applied is as important as the treatment efficacy. All negative adverse reactions or events should be documented. The monitoring for adverse reactions or events is fundamental to determine patient safety during a clinical trial.
- *Quality of life* (*QoL*) is now a well-established matter of study. Issues included into the QoL evaluation are physical, mental and social well-being, and not just the absence of disease or illness. There are many different QoL measurements more or less specific for the disease or condition general (well-being QoL questionnaires) and there are disease-specific questionnaires that are more sensitive to treatment and disease influences. All questionnaires must be validated before to be inserted as an endpoint.

Moreover the endpoints can be divided into clinical and surrogate endpoints. In emergency surgery often, due to the impossibility to obtain definitive results, surrogate endpoints, approximating the studied drug/procedure effect, are useful in helping in the data analysis and definitive evaluation.

- *Clinical endpoint* directly measures substantial clinical benefit to participants, for example survival or reducing the effect of a disease.
- *Surrogate endpoint* is a laboratory measurement or physical sign used as a substitute for a clinically meaningful endpoint

that measures directly how a participant feels, functions or survives. The main reason for the failure of surrogate endpoints is that the surrogate does not play a crucial role in the pathway of the effect of the intervention.

At least three steps must be registered during the data accrual in a clinical trial:

- *Screening*: Participants are examined before the insertion in the trial in order to evaluate their condition in relation to trial inclusion/exclusion criteria.
- *Baseline*: Once a participant has met the inclusion/exclusion criteria, a baseline value of the trial endpoint measures is recorded. Baseline is fundamental because it represents the time point when a clinical trial starts, just before any treatment administration.
- *End of Trial*: Frequently the research aims to compare the baseline values to those at the end of the trial to see how well the drug/procedure acted.

In planning a clinical trial, especially in emergency surgery and in all those disciplines with a difficult study planning and an equally difficult patients, defining endpoints and sample size is crucial in order to reach a good power of the trial. The "Power of a study" is the adequacy of the number of enrolled patients to confidently achieve or rule out statistically significant results for the principal end point. In estimating the power of a study and in planning the sample size, it should always kept into consideration the estimated dropout rate and the recruitment difficulties. The problems in recruitment and retention of participants until the completion of the study impair power; this could potentially make an investigation hopelessly biased or useless. A subsequent problem in case of an insufficient power is the pursuit of subset analyses under conditions where the main result is negative. The subsets may not have enough power for a sound conclusion. Moreover, the number of participants has to be adequate to allow the study to be completed in a reasonable period of time. In emergency surgery, often the rarity of the disease or the impossibility to enrol many of the potential accruable patients determine the impossibility to obtain sufficient samples to perform reliable studies.

The problem with small trials is that despite indicating a true difference of clinical importance in the treatment effect between trial groups, the difference could not always be proven to be statistically significant. Trials with a small sample size were subject to false negative results, namely, type II error (*type I error*: a *false positive result*; *type II error*: a *false negative result*). The sample size is usually determined based on the primary endpoint of the trial with dedicated formulas.

In emergency surgery, the difficulties in obtaining big numbers of enrolled patients is the main issue that often leads to a study conclusion before the end of the accrual phase. As stated before, the distribution of the patients enrolment on many different centres could help.

3.6 Randomization and Blinding

An open-label trial is a study where both the investigators and participants know which drug/procedure is being administered, with trial participants randomized to one of two treatment groups.

The awareness about the administered drug/procedure could potentially lead to biases that can compromise the definitive data analysis and consequently the results of the trial.

Two of the most important design techniques for avoiding bias are randomization and blinding. The randomization of patients aims to reduce the selection bias, that is the preferential enrolment of patients into one treatment group over another according to even indefinable criteria.

The blinding aims to keep trial participants and/or investigators and/or evaluators uninformed of the assigned intervention. Blinding should be maintained throughout the conduct of a trial; therefore, treatments applied should remain indistinguishable.

There are different levels of blinding:

- *Single blind*: When one of the three categories remains unaware of intervention.
- *Double-blind*: Participants, investigators, and assessors remain unaware of the intervention.
- *Triple blind*: When in a double-blind trial also data analysis is blind.

Blinding and/or masking is intended to reduce the risk of bias in the conduct and interpretation of a clinical trial. In fact, awareness about the drug/procedure may potentially influence on several time points of a trial flow:

- Recruitment of participants
- Treatment group allocation of participants
- Participant care
- Attitudes of participants to the treatment
- Assessment of endpoints
- Handling of withdrawals
- Exclusion of data from analysis
- Statistical analysis

The three most serious biases that could potentially affect a clinical trial are:

- *Investigator bias*: If an investigator either consciously or subconsciously favours one group at the expense of others.
- *Evaluator bias*: If the researcher dedicated to measurements of the endpoints intentionally or unintentionally shades the

measurements to favour one intervention over another; subjective or quality of life endpoints are particularly susceptible to this form of bias.

- *Performance bias* occurs when a participant knows the therapy to which is exposed. A great risk in this case is the higher risk to have a excessive dropout from one of the arms (attrition bias) derived from the research by enrolled patients of an effective therapy if they are for example included in the placebo arm.

3.7 Randomized Controlled Trials in Emergency Surgery

As stated before, the randomization minimizes differences between treatment groups and the optimal strategy to minimize the likelihood of differential treatment or assessments of outcomes is to blind as many individuals as possible in a trial. However, randomized controlled trials (RCTs) of surgical interventions are frequently more difficult to blind than RCTs of medications, which typically achieve blinding with placebos.

So in emergency surgery setting the planning and development of an RCT protocol is hard and exposed to many variables which can potentially include irreversible biases.

Comparing to the clinical scientific activity, the surgical one has a sensible lower number of RCT. Among the surgical disciplines, the emergency surgery has one of the lowest number of completed and published RCTs. This is due to the long list of difficulties explained before and overall to the paucity of sick patients who meet the minimal inclusion criteria, seen by each surgeon in the different centres. In conditions like emergency surgery the use of clinical registries is necessary (www.clinicalregisters.org). This is due on one hand to the impossibility to perform RCT about many different diseases and on the other hand the necessity to enroll a sufficient number of patients to perform statistical analysis and understand the best treatment in common but scattered distributed clinical conditions.

3.8 Clinical Registries

The clinical registries have the power to collect an identical minimum data set from patients treated in multiple hospitals or clinics throughout a country or a continent or the entire world. Dedicated websites exist to allow reasearchers to build up clinical registries (i.e. www.clinicalregisters.org) Data consistency is ensured through the use of identical definitions and data collection procedures. The diffusion and the easiness of access to the different registries is assured by the diffusion of the web. In fact the major part of the registries are placed on the web and has no physical place. Data are maintained into servers that could be potentially located everywhere. Emergency surgeons from any part of the globe can connect and register data at anytime and everywhere without great device-linked necessities. The paucity of patients can in this way be overcome and the numerosity of samples sufficient to evaluate the efficacy of the different treatments to a specific disease can be reached. The main concern about this system to obtain data is that they are not guaranteed from biases, as stated before. As a counterpart this could represent the only way to obtain data about rare or scattered distributed diseases.

References

1. Bortolotti L, Heinrichs B. Delimiting the concept of research: an ethical perspective. Theor Med Bioeth. 2007;28(3):157–79.

2. European Commission, Science, Economy and Society. European text-book on ethics in research. Luxembourg: Publications Office of the European Union; 2010. doi:10.2777/17442. ISBN 978-92-79-17543-5.

3. Hunter D. Bad science equals poor, not necessarily bad, ethics. In: Gunning J, Holm S, editors. Ethics, law and society. 3rd ed. Aldershot: Ashgate Publishing Company; 2007. p. 61–70.

4. Trials of war criminals before the nuremberg military tribunals under Control Council Law. 1949;10(2):181–2. http://ohsr.od.nih.gov/guide-lines/nuremberg.html.

5. World Medical Association. Declaration of Helsinki: ethical principles for research involving human subjects. 2008. http://www.wma.net/en/30publications/10policies/b3/index.html.

6. Council for International Organizations of Medical Sciences. International ethical guidelines for biomedical research involving human subjects. 2002. http://www.cioms.ch/frame_guidelines_nov_2002.htm.

7. European Union. The charter of fundamental rights of the European Union (2000/C 364/01). http://www.europarl.europa.eu/charter/default_en.htm.

8. Convention for the protection of human rights and fundamental free-doms (Rome, 4.XI.1950). http://conventions.coe.int/Treaty/en/Treaties/Html/005.htm.

9. Directive 2005/28/EC of 8 April 2005 laying down principles and detailed guidelines for good clinical practice as regards investigational medicinal products for human use, as well as the requirements for authorisation of the manufacturing or importation of such products. http://ec.europa.eu/enterprise/pharmaceuticals/eudralex/vol1/dir_2005_28/dir_2005_28_en.pdf.

10. Convention for the protection of human rights and dignity of the human being with regard to the application of biology and medicine: conven-tion on human rights and biomedicine (Oviedo, 4.IV.1997). http://con-ventions.coe.int/Treaty/en/Treaties/Html/164.htm.

11. Directive 2001/20/EC of the European Parliament and of the Council of 4 April 2001 on the Approximation of the Laws, Regulations and Administrative Provisions of the Member States Relating to the Implementation of Good Clinical Practice in the Conduct of Clinical Trials on Medicinal Products for Human Use. http://europa.eu/eur-lex/pri/en/oj/dat/2001/l_121/l_12120010501en00340044.pdf.

12. Beecher H. Ethics and clinical research. N Engl J Med. 1966;274(24):1354–60; Maurice Pappworth, "Human guinea pigs: a warning", Twentieth Century 171, (1962): 67–75.

Chapter 4
Organization of an Acute Care Surgery Service and Patient Safety Management

Fredric M. Pieracci and Philip F. Stahel

4.1 Introduction

The term "acute care surgeon" has multiple implications. In general, the designation refers to an in-house, broadly trained general surgeon with expertise in the management of trauma, emergency general surgery, and surgical critical care. Anecdotally, many surgeons argue that this definition represents nothing but a new title reflective of a standard twentieth century general surgery. By contrast, a more rigid approach

F.M. Pieracci, MD, FACS (✉)
Department of Surgery, Denver Health Medical Center, University of Colorado Denver, School of Medicine,
777 Bannock Street, Denver, CO 80204, USA
e-mail: fredric.pieraci@dhha.org

P.F. Stahel, MD, FACS
Department of Orthopaedics, Denver Health Medical Center, University of Colorado Denver, School of Medicine,
777 Bannock Street, Denver, CO 80204, USA
e-mail: philip.stahel@dhha.org

© Springer International Publishing Switzerland 2017
S. Di Saverio et al. (eds.), *Acute Care Surgery Handbook*,
DOI 10.1007/978-3-319-15341-4_4

would restrict the definition of acute care surgeons to those who have completed a dedicated and accredited fellowship (most commonly by the American Association for the surgery of Trauma/AAST). Regardless of the title or training of surgeons who provide acute care, the primary goal of this service is to muster rapidly available, unencumbered, highly skilled surgeons to deal with surgical emergencies. Successfully implementing such a service requires an understanding of several basic principles that are broadly described in this chapter.

4.2   Scope of Coverage

The first task of an institution that considers adoption of a designated acute care surgery service is to define the scope of practice. This scope will be highly dependent upon existing services, and thus a critical analysis of such services and their desire to implement an acute care mode is imperative. Traditional disease processes that fall into the purview of acute care surgery are listed in Table 4.1. Also listed in this table are specialty surgeons who may already be managing these problems. Thus, an initial determination of stakeholders and their desire to abrogate coverage of these issues before implementation of an acute care surgery service will maximize success.

Moreover, coverage of surgical emergencies need not be an "all or nothing" event. For example, it may be decided that, by default, all cases of empyema will be managed by the acute care surgery service. However, the acute care surgeon may exercise his or her judgment to involve a thoracic surgery for complicated cases (e.g., persistent air leak, bronchopleural fistula). In this case, whereas some acute care surgeons may feel comfortable managing complex cases, there exists a "bail

Table 4.1 Typical disorders within the scope of the acute care surgery paradigm, and responsible service lines

Disease process	Specialty service lines
Trauma	General surgery
Surgical critical care	General surgery, pulmonary, anesthesia, emergency medicine
Appendicitis	General surgery, colorectal surgery
Diverticulitis	General surgery, colorectal surgery
Cholelithiasis, choledocholithiasis, cholecystitis	General surgery, hepatobiliary, gastroenterology
Pancreatitis	General surgery, hepatobiliary
Bowel obstruction	General surgery
Acute limb ischemia	General surgery, vascular surgery, interventional radiology, cardiology
Empyema	General surgery, interventional radiology, thoracic surgery

out" option for more complicated cases. In some cases, specialty services may be reluctant to relinquish management of certain disease processes. Such discussion are highly specific to local political environments and should involve, whenever possible, both medical and hospital executive staff. In general, the goal of the acute care surgery service is not to impinge upon the elective volume of either general or specialty services. Rather, it is to provide streamlined, protocolized, 24/7 coverage of surgical emergencies. When this concept is presented in such a way, many busy elective surgeons will be relieved to have dedicated and skilled colleagues in house and available 24/7. Indeed, there is little else more stressful to the surgeon (and unfair to the elective patient) than a distracting call involving a surgical emergency during a complex elective operation.

4.3   Models of Coverage

Once the decision to create an acute care surgery service has been made, key stakeholders identified, and scope of practice delineated, the next step is to specify a model of coverage. Although several successful models exist, the following aspects should be preserved: In general, coverage is split into emergency general surgery, trauma, and surgical critical care. Whenever possible, a separate individual should be "on call" for each of these three aspects of care. This approach will both minimize over-commitment and enhance patient safety. One common model that illustrates this point involves an on call "surgeon of the week." This individual is on emergency general surgery call during the day, performing both new urgent operations and any other urgent operations from prior emergency general surgery call (e.g., open abdomen takebacks, urgent cholecystectomies, tracheostomies). A second surgeon is on call for trauma, and a third covers the surgical intensive care unit. None of these individuals is responsible for either elective clinic or operating during their time on acute care surgery call.

Such a model does not preclude the acute care surgeon from maintaining an elective practice. In fact, it is our contention that a busy elective practice is essential to the development and professional well-being of the acute care surgeon. Specifically, knowledge of anatomy from elective surgery (e.g., hiatal hernia repair) translates readily into the trauma realm (e.g., gunshot to the gastro-esophageal junction) and vice-versa. Table 4.2 illustrates an example of a call schedule for a group of six acute care surgeons. Notice that each has unencumbered call, elective, and academic/teaching time, as well as leave time.

Central to this coverage model is a strong commitment to teamwork. Because both the volume and complexity of surgical emergencies is highly variable, a fair amount of surge capacity must be built into the model. In the aforementioned example,

Table 4.2 Example model of acute care surgery coverage schedule

Surgeon	Week 1	Week 2	Week 3	Week 4	Week 5	Week 6
A	EGS	Trauma	SICU	Elective	Admin	Off
B	Off	EGS	Trauma	SICU	Elective	Admin
C	Elective	Admin	Off	EGS	Trauma	SICU
D	Admin	Off	EGS	Trauma	SICU	Elective
E	SICU	Elective	Admin	Off	EGS	Trauma
F	Trauma	SICU	Elective	Admin	Off	EGS

EGS emergency general surgery call, *SICU* surgical ICU call

the trauma, EGS, and SICU surgeons back each other up, such that when one is inundated with several simultaneous emergencies, the others may "flex up" to provide support. A similar adjustment is made when multiple members of the group are offsite for either academic purposes or personal vacation. Finally, a rotating night and weekend coverage schedule is made among the members of the group.

A second coverage model may prove useful when the average census of acute care surgery patients is too large for one surgeon to manage. This alternative model involves dividing the acute care surgeons into multiple teams, with each team managing their own inpatient census comprised of the patients admitted to their service while on call. Surgical ICU, night, and weekend call remains divided up equally among the group.

4.4   Resource Allocation

Creation of an acute care surgery service requires an initial investment in additional resources. Essential to the profitability of the service line is a dedicated, around-the-clock operating room. In high volume centers, two to three dedicated operating rooms may be required. The existence of a dedicated team that is ready to operate at any given time will prove futile in the absence of operating room availability. Similarly, the operating room must be both staffed and equipped to handle common surgical emergencies.

Adequate, 24/7 coverage must extend beyond the operating room. Dedicated house staff or advanced practice providers must be present and wedded to the acute care surgery team, such that their responsibilities are not split between several services. Ideally, research staff should be hired to create and maintain a data repository of acute care surgery patients, and assist to researching common problems in emergency general surgery. Finally, much in the sense of trauma care, both in-reach and outreach efforts should be made to surrounding facilities to advertise the additional expertise afforded by an acute care surgery service. In general, many surgeons at smaller both rural and community hospitals welcome the opportunity to transfer complex emergency general surgery patients to a "center of excellence." Such outreach efforts have been successful in specific disease processes including chronic enterocutaneous fistulae, chronic pancreatitis, and chronic pain from rib fractures.

4.5   Patient Safety Concerns

There are many intuitive advantages to the acute care surgery paradigm. In-house call will increase attending response time to surgical emergencies and improve the likelihood that urgent operations are performed in a timely fashion, even off hours on nights and weekends. Alleviation of call from primarily elective general and specialty surgeons can improve both efficiency and job satisfaction. Finally, management of most surgical emergencies by a single group of providers can streamline standardized care of these vulnerable patients.

In the past few years, several reports have emerged corroborating these hypothetical advantages. Specifically, time from consultation to operating room, percentage of operations happening at night and weekends, time from operation to discharge, and overall hospital costs have consistently been improved following adoption of an acute care surgery model [1–3]. These findings have been observed in both pre/post study designs, as well as contemporaneous comparisons of two hospitals systems, one with a traditional general surgery call structure and the other with an acute care surgery service. There are, however, disadvantages, risks, and shortcomings of the acute care surgery that require recognition and mitigation.

1. *Surgeon expertise.*

   Most of the aforementioned studies involve relatively common and straightforward surgical diseases, such as acute appendicitis or cholecystitis. Far fewer studies have addressed technically complex emergent operations, such as laparoscopic colectomy for acute diverticulitis, or laparoscopic omental patch for perforated duodenal ulcer. Fundamental to the acute care surgery model is the notion not to compromise the quality of patient care. Acute care surgery fellowships have addressed this concern with standardized case requirements (Table 4.3), which include a wide range of operations of varying frequency and complexity. These case requirements continue to evolve based on the changing scope and complexity of emergency general surgery cases. Furthermore, acute care surgeons should, if needed, maintain competency in advanced techniques through continuing medical education courses, or shadowing specialty surgeons at their own institution. Finally, as mentioned previously, the ideal acute care surgery program involves close collaboration with specialty services such that surgical specialists may be consulted by the acute care surgeon when needed (e.g., ruptured abdominal aortic aneurysm).

Table 4.3 Case requirements of acute care surgery fellowship

Area/procedure	Essential	Desirable	Comment
Airway			
Tracheostomy, open and percutaneous	X		
Cricothyroidotomy	X		
Nasal and oral endotracheal intubation, including rapid sequence induction	X		
Head/face			
Nasal packing	X		For complex facial fracture bleeding
ICP monitor		X	
Ventriculostomy		X	
Lateral canthotomy		X	
Neck			
Exposure and definitive management of vascular and aerodigestive injuries	X		
Thyroidectomy		X	Essential if inadequate prior experience
Parathyroidectomy		X	
Chest			
Exposure and definitive management of cardiac injury, pericardial tamponade	X		
Exposure and definitive management of thoracic vascular injury	X		
Repair blunt thoracic aortic injury: open or endovascular		X	
Partial left heart bypass		X	
Pulmonary resections	X		

Table 4.3   (continued)

Area/procedure	Essential	Desirable	Comment
Exposure and definitive management of tracheo-bronchial and lung injuries	X		
Diaphragm injury, repair	X		
Definitive management of empyema: decortication (open and VATS)	X		
Video-assisted thoracic surgery (VATS) for management of injury and infection	X		
Bronchoscopy: diagnostic and therapeutic for injury, infection, and foreign body removal	X		
Exposure and definitive management of esophageal injuries and perforations	X		
Spine exposure: thoracic and thoraco-abdominal	X		
Advanced thoracoscopic techniques as they pertain to the above conditions	X		
Damage control techniques	X		
Abdomen and pelvis			
Exposure and definitive management of gastric, small intestine, and colon injuries	X		
Exposure and definitive management of gastric, small intestine, and colon inflammation, bleeding, perforation, and obstructions	X		
Gastrostomy (open and percutaneous) and jejunostomy	X		

(continued)

Table 4.3 (continued)

Area/procedure	Essential	Desirable	Comment
Exposure and definitive management of duodenal injury	X		
Management of rectal injury	X		
Management of all grades of liver injury	X		
Hepatic resections	X		
Management of splenic injury, infection, inflammation, or diseases	X		
Management of pancreatic injury, infection, and inflammation	X		
Pancreatic resection and debridement	X		
Management of renal, ureteral, and bladder injury	X		
Management of injuries to the female reproductive tract		X	
Management of acute operative conditions in the pregnant patient		X	
Management of abdominal compartment syndrome	X		
Damage control techniques	X		
Abdominal wall reconstruction following resectional debridement for infection, ischemia	X		

2. *Handovers in patient care*

Shift work and workhour restrictions for surgical trainees represent the clear and present danger for patient safety related to the imminent risk of communication breakdown and errors in patient handover [4]. Ironically, workhour restrictions were originally implemented as a patient safety measure to mitigate the risk of surgical complications originating from overworked and fatigued residents. Contrary to the original intent, years of international experience with resident workhour restrictions revealed that patients are not safer, but rather more susceptible to harm originating from handovers of care, equivocal physician accountability, and breakdowns in communication within the team [5, 6]. These underlying challenges represent a threat to the safety and quality of an acute care surgery service, as in essence most models of acute care surgery involve "shift work." As such, there will be by a necessity for recurring patient handovers. Increased regulation of resident duty hours makes it more likely that house staff will also be relatively unfamiliar with inpatients. As such, a robust and standardized system for patient sign out is imperative to the successful implementation of an acute care surgery service. One of the most widely used and successful systems involves the "morning report," in which the post call and on call team gather for presentation of the new admissions, review of pertinent radiographic studies, and expression of the patient plan. All members of the care team, including the medical students, house staff, and attendings, are present. An open and non-judgmental atmosphere is promoted such that anyone with concerns may raise questions. Patient handovers must also be addressed in the elective practice. Specifically, as shown in Table 4.2, depending on OR availability, surgeons who are scheduling cases in clinic may not necessarily be the ones eventually performing the operations. Mitigation of the risk of breakdown in communication and errors in handovers rely on standardized proformas, proactive and transparent communication, and impeccable documentation [7].

4.6 Verification, Accreditation, and Quality Assurance

Many surgical programs, such as bariatric and transplantation, have the potential for either verification or accreditation by governing bodies. The process of verification typically involves demonstration of organizational delegation, minimum volume requirements, protocolized care, outcomes review, and quality improvement. Recent US data indicate that provision of emergency general surgery coverage at academic hospitals is highly variable, with specific discrepancies in operating room availability, call sharing between general and acute care surgeons, patient hand offs, and data collection [8]. Based on this variability, it is likely that, moving forward, individual acute care surgery services should and will require verification.

4.7 Conclusion

An acute care surgery service is typically charged with care of the sickest surgical patients, including trauma, emergency general surgery, and surgical critical care. The success of such a service begins with identification of key stakeholders to the care of such patients, followed by a clear delineation of the scope of practice. The acute care surgery team must then be organized such that each surgeon is unencumbered, surge capacity is possible, and patients are made aware that transitions in caring surgeons occur frequently. Although additional resources, including dedicated operating room time, 24/7/365 coverage, and data registries, are required initially, the majority of data suggest that the net effect of implementation of an acute care surgery service is to improve patient safety and provide satisfaction.

References

1. Madore JC, Collins CE, Ayturk MD, Santry HP. The impact of acute care surgery on appendicitis outcomes: results from a national sample of university-affiliated hospitals. J Trauma Acute Care Surg. 2015;79:282–8.
2. Kalina M. Implementation of an acute care surgery service in a community hospital: impact on hospital efficiency and patient outcomes. Am Surg. 2016;82:79–84.
3. Murphy PB, Paskar D, Parry NG, Racz J, Vogt KN, Symonette C, Leslie K, Mele TS. Implementation of an acute care surgery service facilitates modern clinical practice guidelines for gallstone pancreatitis. J Am Coll Surg. 2015;221:975–81.
4. Stahel PF, Mauffrey C, Butler N. Current challenges and future perspectives for patient safety in surgery. Patient Saf Surg. 2014;8:9.
5. Businger AP, Laffer U, Kaderli R. Resident work hour restrictions do not improve patient safety in surgery: a critical appraisal based on 7 years of experience in Switzerland. Patient Saf Surg. 2012;6:17.
6. Harris JD, Staheli G, LeClere L, Andersone D, McCormick F. What effects have resident work-hour changes had on education, quality of life, and safety? A systematic review. Clin Orthop Relat Res. 2015;473(5):1600–8.
7. Ferran NA, Metcalfe AJ, O'Doherty D. Standardised proformas improve patient handover: audit of trauma handover practice. Patient Saf Surg. 2008;2:24.
8. Santry HP, Madore JC, Collins CE, Ayturk MD, Velmahos GC, Britt LD, Kiefe CI. Variations in the implementation of acute care surgery: results from a national survey of university-affiliated hospitals. J Trauma Acute Care Surg. 2015;78:60–7; discussion 67–8.

Chapter 5
Safety and the Use of Checklists in Acute Care Surgery

Yasmin Hassen, Maximilian J. Johnston, Emily Barrow, and Ara Darzi

5.1 Introduction

Surgery can often provide complete resolution of a disease state or prevent further injury or disability; however, the processes involved in undertaking these procedures have been shown to be fraught with errors that may instead lead to avoidable patient harm. In this chapter, we explore the development of safety in the context of the surgical patient and consider the interventions that are improving safety both inside and out of the operating theatre. To give an overview of these interventions, we will pay special attention to the surgical checklist. This intervention is one of the most influential changes in surgery of the last decade, which can help minimise error and improve patient safety.

Y. Hassen, MBBS, BSc, MRCS • M.J. Johnston, PhD, MRCS
E. Barrow, MBChB(Hons), BSc(Hons) • A. Darzi, OM, KBE, PC FRS, FREng, FMedSci (✉)
Imperial Patient Safety Translational Research Centre,
Department of Surgery and Cancer,
Imperial College London, UK
e-mail: a.darzi@imperial.ac.uk

© Springer International Publishing Switzerland 2017
S. Di Saverio et al. (eds.), *Acute Care Surgery Handbook*,
DOI 10.1007/978-3-319-15341-4_5

5.2   Patient Safety Before the Era of "Patient Safety"

In 1847, Dr Ignaz Semmelweis of Vienna suggested a controversial new practice of hand decontamination in obstetric clinics, reducing mortality from 18 to 1 % [1]. Meanwhile, Florence Nightingale was pioneering values of strict hygiene and establishing methods of good nursing, which have lasted until today. All doctors around the world subscribe to the notion of '*primum non nocere*' or 'first, do no harm'.

Although healthcare practitioners through the ages have recognised the influence of basic interventions in improving patient outcomes, it is only in the last two decades that patient safety has been addressed as a fundamental concern. Ground-breaking studies revealed adverse events were occurring at an alarming rate and potentially leading to permanent harm or even death. In many cases, the errors were found to be avoidable.

The Institute of Medicine's 1999 report "To Err is Human: Building a Safer Health System" compounded current evidence to produce a damning report of the healthcare system's record of preventable errors and subsequent patient harm [2]. In the report, hospital deaths attributable to preventable error were estimated to be between 44,000 and 98,000 in the United States alone. Around the same time, UK data estimated 1.4 million potential adverse events and 255,000 deaths annually within the NHS [3]. One of the most error-prone areas within a hospital was found to be the operating theatre.

Brennan and Leape's 1991 case record review of 30,000 patients demonstrated high rates of adverse events in surgical specialties – with vascular surgery having the highest rate of 16 %. This compared poorly with general medicine, which had a rate of 3.6 % [4]. Throughout the 1990s, further studies confirmed the propensity for surgical specialties to be troubled with the highest errors of any area of medicine [5, 6]. This has been corroborated by more recent studies: De Vries and colleagues' 2008 systematic review incorporating eight studies from the United Kingdom, United States, New Zealand and Canada revealed an overall operating room adverse event rate of 41 % [7].

In response to findings from these early studies and endeavours to understand and address the phenomenon of avoidable errors and adverse events, patient safety has developed as its own academic field and has also seen the emergence of safety experts. An ever-increasing body of work attempting to identify why safety events occur has helped shape attitudes to safety and led to the development of both small- and large-scale interventions to address these issues.

However, patient safety is still a work in progress. Adverse events still affect 3–16 % of all hospitalised patients, with surgery responsible for at least half; the rate of major complications after surgery is estimated at 3–22 % and the death rate at 0.4–0.8 % [8, 9].

5.3   Causes of Error

With the development of the discipline of patient safety, it became evident that systemic failures had to be addressed in the face of human error being an ubiquitous phenomenon. James Reason describes the combination of active failures (omissions or mistakes) and latent conditions (weakness in the system such as understaffing, faulty equipment, inexperience, etc.) leading to adverse outcomes [10]. He goes on to draw comparison with other high-risk industries such as aviation, which has learnt from past disasters and always expects errors. A combination of openness to discuss errors without apportioning blame and the adoption of specific risk-reducing strategies has improved their outcomes over time.

5.4   The Advent of the Checklist

The aviation industry developed checklists with the aim of standardising tasks and their use ranges from pre-flight to landing. They attempt to eliminate the possibility of accidental omission of critical steps and prompt the user to consider any unexpected events. As part of a greater cultural change, this simple intervention has proven invaluable in minimising aviation disasters.

Checklists also have the advantage of facilitating the user without superseding experience and knowledge; thus, where a checklist can ensure equipment is functioning and the jet is fuelled up, the need for an emergency landing will rely on the skill of the pilot. This can be done with the knowledge that other potential contributory errors have been eliminated from this already critical situation.

These parallels between aviation and surgery mean checklists are readily translatable to the operating theatre. This step-by-step list of tasks and procedures can be adhered to and help resolve any potential for error before the "takeoff" of surgery.

5.5   Safer Surgery Saves Lives: Introducing a Surgical Safety Checklist

The weight of evidence exposing preventable harm in surgery spurred the World Health Organisation (WHO) into action; with an estimated annual volume of major surgery around the world of between 187 and 281 million cases [11], this was recognised as a global crisis. Four key issues were identified by the organisation as challenges to improving surgical safety:

1. It has not been previously recognised as a significant public health concern.
2. There is a lack of basic data about procedures and safety events globally.

3. Existing safety practices (e.g. antibiotic prophylaxis) are not used reliably in any country.
4. Surgical procedures are complex – there are multiple critical steps, each with risk of failure and therefore harm.

One of the results was the development of the surgical safety checklist [12]. The design was undertaken by an international group of operating theatre staff including anaesthetists, surgeons and theatre nurses as well as patients and safety experts. The aim was to produce a checklist that would be relevant to any operating theatre and would "*reinforce accepted safety practices and foster better communication and teamwork among clinical disciplines*" (safe surgery saves lives, 2008).

The checklist outlines critical safety steps broken down into three phases (Fig. 5.1):

1. A "sign-in" before induction of anaesthesia: Confirm patient's identity, the intended surgical procedure and allergy status. Any particular concerns such as airway difficulty or projected blood loss are highlighted to ensure adequate equipment/ intravenous access is in place.
2. A "time out" before the skin incision: Identify each team member's role, re-affirm the patient's identity and declare anticipated critical events. Prophylactic antibiotics and thromboprophylaxis are administered if appropriate at this point.
3. A "sign-out" at the end of the procedure: This allows confirmation of correct swabs and instrument counts and correctly labelled specimens. The team also discusses any key postoperative concerns.

5.6   Implementation of the WHO Surgical Safety Checklist

Just 3 weeks after the initial WHO checklist study was published in 2009, the United Kingdom implemented it on a national scale. In 2011, Nevada in the USA was the first state to mandate the use

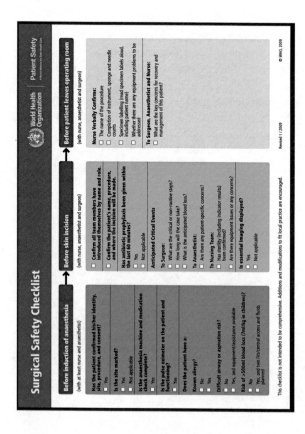

Figure 5.1 The WHO surgical safety checklist published online for universal access along with an implementation manual (http://www.who.int/patientsafety/safesurgery/checklist/en/)

of a surgical checklist in its hospitals. To date, a total of 26 countries have implemented the WHO checklist on a national scale, whilst others are using locally adapted versions.

5.7   The Effect of Checklists on Patient Outcomes

The WHO checklist underwent an international pilot at 8 hospitals in 8 cities across all continents between 2007 and 2008. Its use demonstrated a 36% improvement in the rate of overall complications and decrease in death rates by 47% [13]. Furthermore, the WHO checklist has been associated with significantly improved rates of mortality and complications following implementation in rural and resource-poor settings, which was a documented criticism of the original study [14]. Additional studies exploring surgical checklists have also reported significantly improved mortality though with a smaller overall effect [15, 16].

However, these positive effects have not been universal. In 2014, the statewide mandatory implementation of a surgical safety checklist in Ontario, Canada, was not associated with any improvement in mortality or complication rates [17]. Whilst there have not been any reported direct harms of surgical safety checklists, there are concerns that poor implementation strategies, low rates of compliance and decreased staff vigilance may adversely affect their efficacy [18]. Furthermore, several of the studies have been questioned regarding their pre-post intervention methodology as the inference of causation is not necessarily possible using this study design.

5.8   The Effect of Checklists on Teamwork and Safety Culture

There are multiple theories as to how surgical safety checklists may improve surgical care. As the checklist involves changes in both the system of working and the behaviour of people working within the system, the underlying mechanism of improvement is likely to be multi-factorial. Common theories include the following:

1. The content of the checklist facilitating the detection of unrecognised patient or equipment issues (e.g. blood product availability and clotting abnormalities).
2. The formal pause prior to any direct patient intervention (i.e. knife-to-skin) ensures that patient identification and procedure confirmation are performed correctly.
3. The checklist may lead to an improved culture of safety and greater situational awareness.
4. The checklist encourages greater communication and improved anticipation of likely complications.

In addition to the outcomes reported above, surgical safety checklists have been reported to improve communication within operating theatre teams, through improved teamwork and the use of debriefing [19]. Significantly positive changes in safety culture have been identified after the implementation of surgical safety checklists in Europe [20, 21].

5.9   Checklists and Their Impact on Surgical Care

One of the main controversies over surgical safety checklists is the uncertainty regarding whether the observed improvements in patient outcomes are directly attributable to the content of the checklist or the behaviour changes it may cause. The improved communication and vigilance of surgical staff may play a crucial role in the ongoing success of checklists as they complete their transition from novelty to longstanding tradition in surgery. The signs are encouraging though: checklists have been in use in the aviation since the 1930s and their effectiveness is still enormously valued [22].

A further important issue regarding the efficacy of checklists is compliance. One of the principal criticisms of the Ontario checklist study is that its implementation was mandatory [17, 23]. The method with which a checklist is implemented is thought to be crucial to its future effectiveness. Visible senior leadership and an institutional commitment to quality improvement have been cited as vital factors in ensuring compliance with, and the overall success or failure of, a surgical checklist [24].

5.10   Other Surgical Checklists

Following this, the checklist has been adapted into various forms including wrong-site surgery checklists and anaesthetic equipment checklists. These checklists were implemented in multiple institutions throughout 2009 and 2010.

A "comprehensive surgical safety system" dubbed the SURPASS checklist was also developed to address the other half of adverse events that occur outside the operating room and thus covers the whole patient journey [25]. The SURPASS checklist was also associated with improved outcomes in a controlled pre-post intervention study with its introduction to six hospitals in the Netherlands halving in-hospital mortality [26]. Similarly, when adopted as part of a wider team-training program, checklists have been associated with improved morbidity and mortality [19, 27].

Outside of surgery, checklists have been developed for other interventions that may be prone to adverse events such as endoscopy [28] and regional nerve block administration [29].

5.11   Conclusions

In conclusion, it is extremely likely that surgical safety checklists have a positive impact on surgical teamwork, safety culture and patient outcomes. Whilst the underlying mechanisms of this are not definitively known, the improvements in care mean that implementation of these checklists will continue to spread throughout healthcare globally.

References

1. Best M, Neuhauser D. Ignaz Semmelweis and the birth of infection control. Qual Saf Health Care. 2004;13(3):233–4.
2. Kohn LT, Corrigan J, Donaldson MS. To err is human : building a safer health system. Washington, DC: National Academy Press; 2000.
3. Department of Health An organisation with a memory: report of an expert group on learning from adverse events in the NHS chaired by the Chief Medical Officer; 2000
4. Brennan TA, Leape LL, Laird NM, Hebert L, Localio AR, Lawthers AG, Newhouse JP, Weiler PC, Hiatt HH. Incidence of adverse events and negligence in hospitalized patients. Results of the Harvard Medical Practice study I. N Engl J Med. 1991;324(6):370–6.
5. Baker GR, Norton PG, Flintoft V, Blais R, Brown A, Cox J, Etchells E, Ghali WA, Hebert P, Majumdar SR, O'Beirne M, Palacios-Derflingher L, Reid RJ, Sheps S, Tamblyn R. The Canadian Adverse Events study: the incidence of adverse events among hospital patients in Canada. CMAJ. 2004;170(11):1678–86.
6. Wilson RM, Runciman WB, Gibberd RW, Harrison BT, Newby L, Hamilton JD. The quality in Australian Health Care study. Med J Aust. 1995;163(9):458–71.

7. De Vries EN, Ramrattan MA, Smorenburg SM, Gouma DJ, Boermeester MA. The incidence and nature of in-hospital adverse events: a systematic review. Qual Saf Health Care. 2008;17:216–23.
8. Gawande AA, Thomas EJ, Zinner MJ, Brennan TA. The incidence and nature of surgical adverse events in Colorado and Utah in 1992. Surgery. 1999;126(1):66–75.
9. Kable AK, Gibberd RW, Spigelman AD. Adverse events in surgical patients in Australia. Int J Quality Health Care J Int Soc Quality Health Care/ISQua. 2002;14(4):269–76.
10. Reason J. Human error: models and management. BMJ. 2000;320(7237):768–70.
11. Weiser TG, Regenbogen SE, Thompson KD, Haynes AB, Lipsitz SR, Berry WR, et al. An estimation of the global volume of surgery: a modelling strategy based on available data. Lancet. 2008;372(9633):139–44.
12. WHO guidelines for safe surgery 2009: safe surgery saves lives. WHO Guidelines Approved by the Guidelines Review Committee. Geneva; 2009.
13. Haynes AB, Weiser TG, Lipsitz SR, Breizat AH, Dellinger EP, Herbosa T, Joseph S, Kibatala PL, Lapitan MC, Merry AF, Moorthy K, Reznick RK, Taylor B, Gawande AA, Safe Surgery Saves Lives Study Group. A surgical safety checklist to reduce morbidit and mortality. N Eng J Med. 2009;360(5):491–9.
14. Kwok AC, Funk LM, Baltaga R, et al. Implementation of the World Health Organization surgical safety checklist, including introduction of pulse oximetry, in a resource-limited setting. Ann Surg. 2013;257:633–9.
15. van Klei WA, Hoff RG, van Aarnhem EE, et al. Effects of the introduction of the WHO "Surgical Safety Checklist" on in-hospital mortality: a cohort study. Ann Surg. 2012;255:44–9.
16. Tsai T, Boussard T, Welton M, Morton JM. Does a surgical safety checklist improve patient safety culture and outcomes? J Am Coll Surg. 2010;211:S102–S.
17. Urbach DR, Govindarajan A, Saskin R, Wilton AS, Baxter NN. Introduction of surgical safety checklists in Ontario, Canada. N Engl J Med. 2014;370:1029–38.
18. Treadwell JR, Lucas S, Tsou AY. Surgical checklists: a systematic review of impacts and implementation. BMJ Qual Saf. 2014;23:299–318.
19. Neily J, Mills PD, Young-Xu Y, et al. Association between implementation of a medical team training program and surgical mortality. JAMA. 2010;304:1693–700.

20. Haugen AS, Softeland E, Eide GE, et al. Impact of the World Health Organization's Surgical Safety Checklist on safety culture in the operating theatre: a controlled intervention study. Br J Anaesth. 2013;110:807–15.
21. Nugent E, Hseino H, Ryan K, Traynor O, Neary P, Keane FB. The surgical safety checklist survey: a national perspective on patient safety. Ir J Med Sci. 2013;182:171–6.
22. Mastracci TM, Greenberg CC, Kortbeek JB, Grp EBRS. What are the effects of introducing the WHO "Surgical Safety Checklist" on in-hospital mortality? J Am Coll Surg. 2013;217:1151–3.
23. Leape LL. The checklist conundrum. N Engl J Med. 2014;370:1063–4.
24. Russ SJ, Sevdalis N, Moorthy K, et al. A qualitative evaluation of the barriers and facilitators toward implementation of the WHO surgical safety checklist across hospitals in England: lessons from the "Surgical Checklist Implementation Project". Ann Surg. 2014;261:81–91.
25. de Vries EN, Hollmann MW, Smorenburg SM, Gouma DJ, Boermeester MA. Development and validation of the SURgical PAtient Safety System (SURPASS) checklist. Qual Saf Health Care. 2009;18:121–6.
26. de Vries EN, Prins HA, Crolla RM, et al. Effect of a comprehensive surgical safety system on patient outcomes. N Engl J Med. 2010;363:1928–37.
27. Young-Xu Y, Neily J, Mills PD, et al. Association between implementation of a medical team training program and surgical morbidity. Arch Surg. 2011;146:1368–73.
28. Matharoo M, Thomas-Gibson S, Haycock A, Sevdalis N. Implementation of an endoscopy safety checklist. Frontline Gastronenterol. 2014;5(4):260–5.
29. Mulroy MF, Weller RS, Liguori GA. A checklist for performing regional nerve blocks. Reg Anesth Pain Med. 2014;39(3):195–9.

Chapter 6
Emergencies in Otolaryngology: Head and Neck Surgery

Pierre Guarino, Matteo Alicandri-Ciufelli, and Livio Presutti

Emergencies in otorhinolaryngology may be focused on two major issues: acute respiratory distress secondary to the upper respiratory way obstructions and intractable epistaxis.

6.1 Epistaxis

Epistaxis is the most common otorhinolaryngology emergency that accounts for emergency room consultations [1]. The nosebleeds can be a paraphysiological manifestation like vicarious or premenstrual epistaxis in young girls, or be in the form of slight bleeding in children with lymphatic "habitus." These are defined as essential epistaxis. In most cases, however, it underlies a local or systemic disease or follows nasal surgery (iatrogenic epistaxis) [2].

P. Guarino, MD (✉) • M. Alicandri-Ciufelli, MD • L. Presutti, MD
University Hospital of Modena, Modena, Italy
e-mail: pierreguarino@hotmail.com

© Springer International Publishing Switzerland 2017   81
S. Di Saverio et al. (eds.), *Acute Care Surgery Handbook*,
DOI 10.1007/978-3-319-15341-4_6

Epistaxis	
Systemic causes	Vascular disorders (hypertension, Rendu-Osler-Weber disease)
	Congenital or acquired heart diseases
	Diabetes
	Liver failure
	Kidney diseases
	Viral and bacterial infectious diseases
	Antiplatelet and anticoagulant therapies
	Vitamin deficiencies (vit. C, vit. K)
	Hemopathies (von Willebrand disease, hemophilia)
	Endocrine disorders
	Autoimmune disorders (Wegener disease, etc.)
	Barotraumatisms
	Paraneoplastic syndromes
Local causes	Nasal surgery (FESS, septoplasty, etc.)
	Traumatisms
	Neoplasms
	Nasal foreign bodies
	Nasal septum varicose veins
	Acute rhinitis

Although epistaxis usually represents a benign symptom, it can quickly turn into a life-threatening condition. As a matter of fact, the majority of cases are controlled with common first-line intervention such as electrical cautery, the application of hemostatic agents, or anterior nasal packing, but there is a subset of patients who continue to bleed and require more aggressive therapy. It is therefore important to distinguish anterior nosebleeds from posterior ones.

The majority of epistaxis originates from the anterior nasal septum (*locus Valsalvae*) and is classified as anterior epistaxis. The minority of cases bleeds beyond a classic anterior rhinoscopy, mainly from the posterior lateral nasal wall and the posterior nasal septum, and is so classified as posterior epistaxis.

The aim of this chapter is to focus on the intractable epistaxis, whose origin is most commonly the *sphenopalatine artery* (SPA). Epistaxis from the AEA more rarely occurs in association with midface trauma or iatrogenic injury during endoscopic sinus surgery [1].

A thorough knowledge of the anatomy is necessary to optimize the surgical treatment, so we will follow a brief but comprehensive description of the vascular and surgical anatomy of the nasal cavity.

6.2   Nasal Vascular Anatomy

The frequency of nosebleeds is linked to the richness of the nasal vascular supply, which is provided from the *external carotid artery system* through *maxillary* and *facial arteries* and from the *internal carotid artery system* through the *ophtalmic artery* with its *anterior and posterior ethmoidal branches* [3].

6.2.1   External Carotid Artery System (ECA)

6.2.1.1   Maxillary Artery (Internal Maxillary Artery: IMA)

The *maxillary artery*, a terminal branch of the *external carotid artery* along with the *superficial temporal artery*, enters the pterygopalatine fossa through the pterygomaxillary fissure, where it gives life to the *descending palatine artery* and the *pterygopalatine artery* that supplies the mucosa of nasopharynx and choanae. Once passing through the sphenopalatine foramen, it takes the name of *sphenopalatine artery* (Fig. 6.1), its terminal branch, and then it splits into medial and lateral branches. The medial one, or *posteroseptal nasal artery* (Fig. 6.2), emerges from upper portion of the sphenopalatine foramen and gives rise to a branching for the upper turbinate, and then it goes inward to reach the septum. Then it flows by a groove excavated along the ethmoid-chondral-vomerian suture

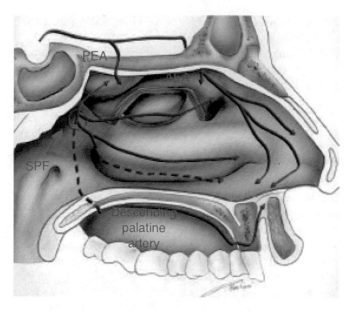

Fig. 6.1 Sphenopalatine foramen (*thick arrow*) and the lateral nasal wall supply by the sphenopalatine artery

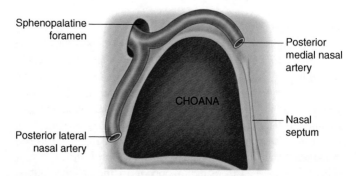

Fig. 6.2 SPA splitting into the posteroseptal nasal artery and the posterior lateral nasal artery

to enter the anterior palatine canal and join the *septal branch of the superior labial artery*. Along its course, it also provides some septal branches.

The lateral one, or *posterolateral nasal artery*, emerges from the lower portion of the sphenopalatine foramen to provide the *middle nasal artery* for the region of the middle meatus and the *inferior nasal artery* that goes to the inferior turbinate.

6.2.1.2 Facial Artery

The *facial artery* provides the *superior labial artery* at the level of the upper lip and then it anastomoses with the contralateral one to form the *superior coronary arcade* and becomes *angular artery* rising up along the nasolabial fold. From the superior coronary arcade arises the *septal branch of the superior labial artery* that flows along the anterior-inferior portion of the septum to provide septal and vestibular branches. The angular artery supplies the lateral face of the pyramid.

6.2.1.3 Internal Carotid Artery System (ICA)

The *ophthalmic artery* originates from the *internal carotid artery* at the level of the anterior clinoid process of the sphenoid bone and enters the orbit through the optic canal along with the *optic nerve*. It provides nasal vascular supply through *anterior and posterior ethmoidal arteries*. Its other collateral branches are the *central retinal artery*, *ciliary arteries*, *lateral palpebral arteries*, and the *supraorbital artery*.

6.2.1.4 Anterior Ethmoidal Artery (AEA)

The *anterior ethmoidal artery* reaches the *anterior ethmoid foramen* whose orbital orifice is located approximately 15 mm from the orbital edge. The insertion of the anterior superior ethmoid bulla is an important landmark both for the frontal recess and the AEA, which runs on the ethmoid roof and is separated from the frontal recess by the first ethmoid foveola (Fig. 6.3); the artery is present on its dorsal edge [4]. After crossing the ethmoid roof passing through the *ethmoidal lateral lamella*, AEA enters the cranial cavity giving rise to a nasal branching that reaches the anterior superior part of the nasal cavity through the cribriform plate.

From this nasal branching originate the lateral and medial branches. The lateral ones supply the anterosuperior part of the lateral nasal wall, the anterior ethmoid, and the frontal sinus. The medial ones supply the anterior superior portion of the septum. The terminal tract of the anterior ethmoid artery then gives rise to a meningeal branch in front of the olfactory shower level [3, 5].

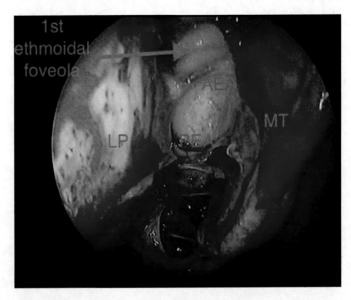

Fig. 6.3 Right nasal fossa: *LP* lamina papiracea, first ethmoidal foveola, *MT* middle turbinate, *AEA* anterior ethmoidal artery and *PEA* posterior ethmoidal artery

6.2.1.5 Posterior Ethmoidal Artery (PEA)

The *posterior ethmoidal artery* is much smaller than the anterior one, it runs on the posterior ethmoid roof in a very thick bony canal, so its dehiscence or injury is very rare [5]. PEA reaches the *posterior ethmoid foramen* in order to supply *posterior ethmoidal cells*, the posterior-superior portion of the lateral nasal wall, and the septum at the level of the olfactory shower. The relatively high frequency of posterior ethmoidal artery agenesia (12.5 % of cases) should be also emphasized.

These two arterious systems are abundantly anastomosed, as briefly described below [3]:

- At the level of the septum:

  - Anastomosis on the anterior nasal septum where the *locus Valsalvae* (or Little's area), which is supplied by Kiesselbach's plexus, is formed by the confluence of the *sphenopalatine artery* (SPA – terminal branch of the *maxillary artery*), the *greater palatine artery* (from the *maxillary artery*), medial branches of *anterior* and *posterior ethmoidal arteries* (from the *ophthalmic artery*), and the *septal branch of the superior labial artery* (from the *facial artery*).
  - Anastomosis between *posterior ethmoidal artery* and branches from the *sphenopalatine artery*.

- On the superior lateral wall: anastomosis between *ethmoidal arteries* and *upper turbinate artery*.

6.2.2 Venous System

Particularly represented at the level of the turbinates as cavernous tissue, it is formed by two different routes of drainage, communicating with each other, that refer to the *internal jugular vein* and the *cavernous sinus*, as follows [2–4]:

- Superiorly, the blood is drained from the *superior ophthalmic vein*, tributary of the *cavernous sinus*, through the *ethmoidal veins*; some venous branches can perforate the cribriform plate to flow into the veins of the frontal lobe of the brain.
- On the posterior side, after passing through the *sphenopalatine foramen*, veins flow into the *pterygoid plexus* surrounding the pterygoid muscles and from which *maxillary veins* arise; at first they flow into the *posterior facial vein* (or retromandibular vein) and then into the *internal jugular vein*. The most important connection between *pterygoid plexus* and *cavernous sinus*, mainly through the *oval foramen*, is the "*Vesalius vein*"; *pterygoid plexus* is also connected with the *facial vein* (via the *deep facial vein*) and the *pharyngeal plexus*.
- There is a rich venous vascular network called "*Woodruff plexus*" at the level of the rhinopharynx, on the posterior side of middle and inferior meati.
- Some veins flows anteriorly into the *facial vein*.

6.2.3   Surgical Anatomy of the SPA

Just as described above, the SPA is a terminal branch of the IMA and enters the nasal cavity at the level of the posterior attachment of the middle turbinate through the *sphenoplatanine foramen* (SPF). The SPF sets a communication between the *pterygopalatine space*, laterally, and the nasal cavity, medially. It is formed by the sphenoid bone body that closes superiorly the *sphenopalatine incisure* of the *palatine bone*. This portion is in relationship anteriorly with the palatine orbital process, posteriorly with the palatine sphenoidal process, and inferiorly with the superior border of the palatine perpendicular lamina.

Three classes of anatomical variability of the SPF localization have been identified. Class I SPF (35 % of cases) is identified completely above the posterior projection of the middle turbinate. Class II SPF (56 % of cases) has its lower border below the *crista ethmoidalis*. *Crista ethmoidalis* or ethmoidal process of the palatine bone is a slight relief of the medial face of its perpendicular lamina.

Class III SPF (9 % of cases) is characterized by two distinct foramina: the superior one in the upper meatus and the inferior one in the middle meatus.

But according to Lee et al. [6], SPF in located in 90 % of cases in the upper meatus, superiorly to the *crista ethmoidalis*.

In all cases, crista ethmoidalis can be considered as an important surgical landmark for its relationship with the SPF.

Furthermore it has been founded that in most cases, the SPA splitting in three or four branches occurs in the infratemporal fossa before its entrance in the nasal cavity. This situation has important clinical and surgical consequences such as the possibility of a selective ligation of the only bleeding vessel, so sparing the rest of the vascular supply but also the vitality of turbinates. Indeed some cases of necrosis of the turbinates after SPA ligation are well described in literature.

Although several anatomic variations are described in the literature, all studies indicate that the SPF is usually located posteriorly at the junction of the middle and superior meati. The ethmoid crest (or crista ethmoidalis) is an important surgical landmark, because it is always present and is located anteriorly to the SPF in 98 % of cases [4].

6.2.4   Surgical Anatomy of the AEA and PEA

To sum up, the AEA branches off medially the orbital cavity and supplies the superior lateral nasal wall and septum after reaching the ethmoid skull base. Externally, the AEA can be identified about 2 cm posterior to the lacrimal crest, in the space between

P. Guarino et al.

the *orbital periosteum* and *lamina papyracea*. Endonasally, it can be located either at the ethmoid skull base attachment of the *ethmoid bulla lamella* or just posterior to this site, along the posterior wall of the frontal recess.

Critical aspects of the surgical anatomy of the ethmoidal arteries concern the location variability on the coronal plane, related to the ethmoidal roof and to lateral lamella, and on the sagittal plane, because of the relationship with the *ethmoidal lamellae*.

On the sagittal plane, the AEA is located in most cases between the *ethmoid bulla lamella* and middle turbinate lamella. Simmen et al. have identified the AEA at the average distance of 11 mm from the posterior wall of the frontal recess.

On the coronal plane, another key element is the relationship between the AEA and the *ethmoidal roof*. Recent cadaver studies indicate that AEA runs in a bony arterial mesentery in 35.5 % of cases, with an average distance of 3.5 mm from the skull base, while it is amenable to surgical ligation in about 20 % of cases. Patients with an AEA located in a mesentery can be identified on preoperative CT and they tend to have longer *lateral lamella* (Keros type 2 or 3) and a high ethmoid skull base [1].

Other aspects concern the possibilities of dehiscence of their bony canals and the different spatial orientation of their pathways.

Some authors have identified real spatial coordinates to reach the AEA: the optical endoscopic stretched between the *dome of the alar cartilage* and the *axilla of the middle turbinate* is a real "pointer" oriented toward the AEA in the *fovea ethmoidalis* [4].

6.2.5   General Management of Epistaxis

The first priority during intractable epistaxis is to slow or trying to control the active hemorrhage with temporizing packing in order to occlude the posterior choanae and avoid the blood inhalation through the upper airway. In the past few years, the classic posterior nasal packing has been giving the way to anterior-posterior balloon combo packs such as *Bivona*® or a *Foley*® catheter combined with anterior packing.

Once the active bleeding is controlled, a meticulous medical history investigation is necessary to identify critical medical factors and correct them if possible.

Recurrent episodes of epistaxis in elderly patients in anticoagulant-antiplatelet therapy often pose the challenging question whether to suspend, reduce, or not to change the treatment because they tend to have more severe epistaxis and bleed from several sites. All patients should have a CBC (complete blood count) and an INR (International normalized ratio) evaluated at the time of presentation. During warfarin-related epistaxis, about 80 % of patients were outside their disease-specific INR range [1].

A multidisciplinary team to optimize safe therapy is often required. A protocol to manage the anticoagulation-antiplatelet related epistaxis is showed below [7]:

Management protocol for anticoagulation-related epistaxis	
All anticoagulated epistaxis	Order labs: CBC and INR
Warfarin-related epistaxis	INR in therapeutic range: continue Warfarin INR outside therapeutic range: hold and consult with cardiology or hematology
Aspirin- or clopidogrel-related epistaxis	Continue medications, but for life-threatening hemorrhage consult cardiology for role of platelet transfusion

If the hemorrhage is not well managed with the classic anterior-posterior nasal packing, it is often necessary to perform an endoscopic look under general anesthesia or an angiographic study.

6.3 Surgery for Intractable Epistaxis

In the clinical evaluation of epistaxis, posterior bleeding, hematocrit less than 38 % and necessity of blood transfusions seem to be significant predictors of the need for surgical treatment [8].

It has been demonstrated that an early surgical intervention compared to prolonged posterior nasal packing results in a significantly shorter hospital stay and reduced health care costs [1, 9].

Since the mid-1960s, surgical control of posterior epistaxis involved a Caldwell-Luc approach with transantral ligation of the IMA [10]. This external intervention was associated with high patient morbidity and often failed to control the epistaxis because of collateral circulation supplying the SPA distal to the IMA ligation site.

Over the years there has been a progressive refinement of techniques and an increasingly shift toward the distal point of ligation of the vessel. So the external carotid artery ligation (ECAL) has been progressively replaced by the ligation of the IMA, while in the 1970s, the first endoscopic occlusion of the SPA was described [4].

The following text will mainly focus on two endoscopic surgical approaches for intractable epistaxis, both performed under general anesthesia, comparing them to the selective arterial embolization:

1. TESPAL – Transnasal endoscopic sphenopalatine artery ligation
2. TEAEAL – Transnasal endoscopic anterior ethmoid artery ligation

But it is important not to forget a very rare but life-threatening cause of epistaxis: internal carotid artery (ICA) injury during endonasal approaches to the sphenoid sinus.

6.3.1 Transnasal Endoscopic Sphenopalatine Artery Ligation

TESPAL begins with thorough nasal preparation, such as nasal packing removal, nasal cavity cleaning of all blood clots, and decongesting through pledgets soaked with 1 % xylocaine, in order to perform a detailed endoscopic evaluation with a 4 mm 0° optics and define the site of bleeding.

After medializing the middle turbinate, it follows lateral nasal wall incision posterior to the maxillary sinus and a subperiosteal elevation of the mucosa. The ethmoid crest is so identified, then SPA tented up at the level of the SPF and subsequently cauterized (bipolar or Dessi clamp) or clipped. The elevated nasal mucosa is then redraped. In some cases, patients do not need nasal packing and can be discharged in the first postoperative day. Some authors indicate that SPA cauterization, rather than clipping, provides a higher success rate [11, 12].

6.3.2 Transnasal Endoscopic Anterior Ethmoid Artery Ligation

AEA-related epistaxis is less common than the SPA. Its ligation was traditionally performed with an external Lynch incision and clipping between the lamina papyracea and periorbita.

As already described above, a preoperative CT scan of the sinuses is essential to review the AEA anatomy to determine whether it is amenable to endoscopic ligation.

TEAEAL starts with a maxillary antrostomy and anterior ethmoidectomy, then the ethmoid roof and the lamina papyracea are defined. A small opening in the lamina papyracea using a small curette is made below the AEA canal after its identification (image-guidance navigation may be helpful).

After unshelling the bony fragments off the AEA adjacent to the lamina papyracea and their posterior and anterior elevation, small clips are placed across the AEA next to the orbital periosteum [13].

Before choosing to perform TEAEAL, it is important for the surgeon to weigh the potential benefits of avoiding an external scar from the traditional external approach, with the potential for serious complication complications such as cerebral spinal fluid leak, orbital injury, or failure to control epistaxis.

The role of isolated TEAEAL still has to be entirely defined and it is difficult to determine its success rate, because it is typically combined with SPA ligation.

6.3.3   Internal Carotid Artery Rupture

During sphenoid sinus approach, it is important to consider anatomy variations of the ethmoid sinus: an Onodi cell is a posterior ethmoid cell that develops laterally and superiorly to the sphenoid sinus and this could be problematic for the possible presence of the optic nerve and of the ICA inside it. The preoperative CT scan evaluation is necessary to not putting these noble structures in jeopardy. However, in case of ICA lesion a prompt and massive nasal packaging with a manual compression of common carotid artery on the neck is mandatory. Right after the patient must be immediately transferred to an Interventional Neuroradiology Center in attempt to perform a monitored endovascular occlusion [14].

Postoperative belated massive hemorrhage (on average between 7 days and 8 weeks) can be due to a microtraumatism of the ICA through the formation of a pseudoaneurysm whose rupture is a rare cause of potentially deadly epistaxis [15, 16].

6.3.4   Selective Arterial Embolization

The role of percutaneous endovascular embolization in the management of intractable epistaxis was first described by Sokoloff in 1974 [17] and over the years has become a well-accepted therapeutic option.

It can be employed as a gold standard or like an emergency bridge treatment to elective surgery procedures. It presents the following indications:

- The patient's impossibility to undergo a surgical intervention for a severe cardiopathy
- The recurrence of epistaxis after surgical ligation of the IMA and its branches
- Spontaneous hemorrhage or uncontrollable epistaxis after nasal cavity hypervascularized tumors biopsy

- More rarely hemorrhages secondary to maxillofacial trauma
- ICA injury during or following FESS

  The contraindications are represented by:

- Impossibility to perform a selective arterial catheterization of the epiaortic region (severe atherosclerotic plaques, especially at the level of the carotid bulb)
- Hemorrhage in areas supplied by ICA branches (e.g., ethmoid arteries)
- Contrast medium allergy

6.3.5   Basic Technique

This section will underline the only basic technique, while for a more detailed explanation, it is suggested to refer to specialized interventional radiology texts.

The procedure is performed under local anesthesia with a previous femoral access. The first step consists of a preembolization angiogram of the ICA and ECA systems in order to localize the site of bleeding or identify rare causes of epistaxis, such as tumors, vascular malformation, or pseudoaneurysm. It can also identify dangerous anastomoses between the ECA and ICA that can predispose to stroke and blindness.

The selective catheterization of the ECA should be performed the most distally as possible, at least until the IMA, after excluding the presence of plaques and the involvement of the ICA.

The next choice of the embolization materials, absorbable or nonabsorbable, occurs on the basis of the caliber and extension of the lesion.

Absorbable material consists in Gelfoam fragments mixed with contrast medium and it is indicated in cases of acute bleeding like a bridge treatment to the surgical intervention.

Nonabsorbable material consists of solid particles of polyvinyl alcohol diluted in contrast medium and it is more indicated in case of massive epistaxis.

The procedure continues under careful radioscopic control. In the end, an angiographic control is made in order to demonstrate the pathologic circle exclusion.

The decision to perform a bilateral IMA embolization is controversial and may increase the soft tissue ischemia-related complication [18].

6.3.6 Complications

Complications associated with arterial embolization can be categorized into three classes: minor transient, major transient, and persistent. Minor transient complications, including headache, facial or jaw pain, trismus, facial edema and numbness, mild palatal ulceration, groin hematoma, and fever, occur between 25 and 50 % of cases.

Major transient and persistent complications, such as temporary visual loss until blindness, TIA and stroke, temporary hemiparesis until facial nerve paralysis, and mucosal necrosis, are rare, but they must be carefully discussed with the patient, because they can result in substantial morbidity [1, 19].

6.4 Surgery Versus Embolization

Both TESPAL and selective arterial embolization for intractable epistaxis have similar high success rate (about 85–90 %) and there is no definitive evidence indicating when one treatment modality is superior to the other. So the choice of treatment represents a challenging dilemma and needs to be tailored to the patient conditions and to the institution resources (surgical and interventional radiology expertise, patient comorbidity and preference, health care costs).

Surgical ligation (TESPAL ± AEAL) may be the preferable option over the arterial embolization because of the lower risk of major complications and the reduced economic impact.

Although embolization prcedure has high costs [20–22], it has become a standard procedure for intractable epistaxis and may be a better option in patients unfit for general anesthesia or under anticoagulation therapy and in surgical failures.

6.5 Emergency Tracheotomy

6.5.1 Introduction

The acute respiratory distress secondary to the upper respiratory ways obstruction is a really life-threatening condition that often involves ENT specialists and requires an emergency tracheotomy.

The term tracheotomy indicates the surgical opening of the tracheal wall and skin, with consequent communication between the cervical trachea and the external environment, in order to ensure a sufficient air passage for an efficient breathing. The conservation of this pathway requires the use of a tracheal tube to avoid the soft tissues collapse.

Tracheostomy instead is the creation of a permanent opening of the trachea through the connection of the tracheotomy borders with the cervical skin and a consequent direct contact between tracheal lumen and external environment [23].

It cannot be considered only as an emergency intervention, since sometimes it has typically elective indications (as complement in several surgical procedures to protect the tracheobronchial tree or to limit the prolonged intubation decubitus damage in hospitalized patients in intensive care units).

Despite no significant modifications in the surgical procedure, in the last decades there have been other significant improvements:

- In the field of both adult and pediatric intensive care and resuscitation
- In the endoscopic techniques of the pharyngo-laryngotracheal structures visualization with the consequent ability to intubate even the so-called difficult cases
- Availability of increasingly effective drugs such as corticosteroids and antibiotics that allows to reduce several clinical scenarios which led to a tracheotomy in the past

It is relatively easy to perform, but sometimes execution errors are not so uncommon, as well as in the choice of the cannula, or in the management after the operation, and the occurrence of various kinds of complications.

Emergency tracheotomy is different from the elective one in terms of anesthesia, methods, difficulty of execution, and kind of complications.

So a thorough knowledge of the anatomy and physiology, during the execution and maintenance of the tracheotomy, as well as the decannulation of the patient and the restoration of the natural airways, is absolutely necessary and may allow to minimize adverse events [24].

6.5.2   Indications

- Acute massive laryngeal obstruction secondary to edema, phlegmons, foreign body and neoplasms
- Severe trauma of head and neck and pharyngo-laryngotracheal tract
- Bilateral vocal fold paralysis (BVFP) in abduction
- Severe burns of the upper airway
- Major laryngeal or proximal tracheal tract malformations

The major indication to perform a tracheotomy is the acute respiratory distress during acute massive laryngeal obstruction that makes these patients impossible to intubate for phlegmons, edema, neoplasm, or foreign body.

Although the neoplastic obstruction has a slow evolution and patients achieve a sort of adaptation even for very important stenosis, emergency tracheotomy is sometimes required for the sudden overlap of oedematigenous inflammatory phenomena or the carelessness in delaying the emergency room access. It would be appropriate to limit as much as possible the temporal gap between the emergency tracheotomy and treatment (surgery, radiotherapy, etc.) in order to reduce the risk of peristomal recurrence.

Severe trauma with fractures of the pharyngo-laryngotracheal tract requires a tracheotomy because intubation may increase the risk of further osteo-cartilaginous and bony fragments displacement.

More rarely bilateral vocal fold paralysis (BVFP) in abduction may occur after a total thyroidectomy or during important pharyngo-laryngeal phlogosis. In these cases, emergency tracheotomy is a bridge intervention to surgical glottic space improvements (LASER posterior cordotomy or aritenoidectomy).

Tracheotomy also plays a role in severe burns of the upper airways and major laryngotracheal malformations, situations that could be worsened by intubation and lead to cicatricial stenosis.

6.5.3 Anatomy

The trachea is a fibrocartilaginous conduit, which begins at the lower border of the cricoid cartilage, at the level of the VI cervical vertebra, and ends in the chest splitting into two main bronchi at the level of the V thoracic vertebra. Its position varies with age. In the newborn, the upper end is higher (between IV and V cervical vertebrae), while in the elderly the lower end may be up to the VI thoracic vertebra in reason of the general ptosis of viscera and cervicodorsal stiffness.

The trachea descends obliquely in the midline from front to back gradually moving away from the skin surface. It is placed at 18 mm from the skin at the level of the cricoid, 40–45 mm at the entrance in the chest, 70 mm at the level of the tracheal carina. Therefore, the access to the trachea is easier in its superior cervical segment than to the lower one.

It consists of 15–20 posteriorly incomplete cartilaginous rings, where the membranous tracheal muscle of Reisseinen separates the trachea from the esophagus. The contraction of these muscle fibers approaches the ends of the cartilaginous rings by varying the transverse tracheal diameter.

The trachea is conventionally divided into two segments (Fig. 6.4):

- The cervical segment, extending from the lower border of the cricoid (C6) to a horizontal plane passing through the upper edge of the sternum (D2) and composed of the first 6–7 tracheal rings.
- The thoracic segment, which extends from the jugular notch of the sternum (D2) to the tracheal bifurcation (D5). The carina is a useful landmark for the terminal end of the trachea, being clearly definable both endoscopically and radiologically.

It is important to remember that in the young subject, especially if not obese, the hyperextension of the neck pulls up more than 50 % of the trachea in cervical position. In elderly and kyphotic subjects, particularly if obese, the cricoid cartilage may be situated at the level of the sternal notch, and even an extreme hyperextension is not able to pull up the trachea in the neck.

The average length of the trachea is 12 cm in adult men and 11 cm in women. However, it is very variable, even in the same subject, depending on whether the larynx is at rest or in

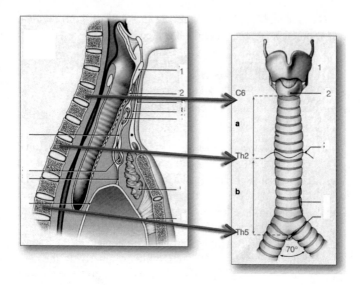

Fig. 6.4 *1* thyroid cartilage, *2* cricoid cartilage, trachea and corresponding vertebral levels

motion and depending on the position of the head, with maximum variations of 3–4 cm. The trachea, in fact, is a very mobile structure in both horizontal and vertical planes and follows the mechanical movements of neighboring organs during swallowing and phonation. The fixation is guaranteed by its continuity at the top with the larynx, down with the main bronchi and pulmonary pedicles, posteriorly with esophageal and spinal plans. There seems to be no correlation between the length of the trachea and height or body weight.

The cartilaginous rings determine the shape (circular, triangular, etc.) and the caliber of the lumen of the trachea, which varies according to age and gender; this explains the need to have tracheostomy tubes and endotracheal tubes of different sizes.

The tracheal diameter is uniform in height in both cervical and thoracic segments, and is on average:

- 6 mm in children (1–4 years)
- 8 mm in children (4–8 years)
- 10 mm in children (8–10 years)
- From 13 to 15 mm in the adolescent
- From 16 to 18 mm in adults

Diameter also varies for the simple tracheal muscle tone, which can cause almost the contact between the two ends of the cartilaginous rings reducing the diameter of the lumen. The length and diameter of the trachea increase during inspiration and decrease during expiration. Moreover, the tracheal diameter increases during closed glottis exertions.

It seems to have a higher growth percentage in the first 4 years of life compared to the uterine life or puberty. In the neonatal period, trachea is funnel shaped, with the upper end wider than the bottom, and during the first 5 years of life, it becomes almost cylindrical.

During childhood, the tracheal cartilages progressively increase in length, but the cartilage at the upper end remains longer than those at the lower end.

The relationship between cartilage and muscle length remains unchanged during growth, thus allowing the maintenance of the rigidity of the tracheal wall [25].

6.5.3.1 Vascular Supply

The tracheal vascular supply in its upper portion is provided mainly by branches of the inferior thyroid artery. The lower portion, however, is vascularized by branches of the bronchial artery and collateral arteries from subclavian, supreme inter-

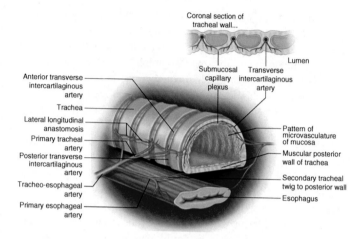

Fig. 6.5 Tracheal vascular supply

costal, internal thoracic, and innominate arteries. These vessels, coming through lateral stalks, provide branches back to the esophagus and to the trachea anteriorly. The tracheal vascular supply comes from longitudinal pedicles interconnected along its lateral walls through the intercartilaginous transverse arteries, which anastomose with the contralateral ones and ends in a submucosal capillary plexus (Fig. 6.5). Excessive lateral tissues dissection from the trachea can easily destroy these sources of blood supply, even leading to serious complications [25].

6.5.3.2   Cervical Trachea

Cervical trachea is 2–4 cm long and its lower limit is marked by the jugular notch of the sternum. The first three rings are covered anteriorly by the thyroid isthmus that adheres very closely to them. Anteriorly and below the thyroid isthmus, the trachea is covered by adipose connective tissue, which becomes more abundant near the jugular notch and continues to the mediastinum inferiorly. This connective tissue contains the pretracheal lymph nodes, the inferior thyroid veins, and sometimes there is also the thyroid ima artery of Neubauer; in the early childhood, there are also the horns of cervical thymic lobes. More superficially the cervical part of the trachea corresponds to the cervical sheets of the neck, the infrahyoid muscles, and the suprasternal space formed by the splitting of the superficial cervical fascia that attaches to the two lips (anterior and posterior) of the jugular notch. The trachea is embraced laterally and superiorly by the thyroid lobes that adhere closely with their medial faces; this would explain the tracheal deviation in some goiters. Its lateral face is also in relationship with the terminal tract of the inferior thyroid artery, with the parathyroid glands and the neurovascular bundle of the neck (common carotid artery, internal jugular vein, and vagus nerve). Between the tracheal axis and the neurovascular bundle there is an adipose tissue space full of lymph nodes, particularly along the recurrent layngeal nerves pathways. The posterior surface of the trachea, the so-called *pars membranacea*, is in close relationship with the anterior surface of the esophagus, which is separated by a loose connective allowing their reciprocal movements. The esophagus has a S-shaped pathway that makes its anterior face protrude from the trachea to the left side. The left inferior laryngeal nerve runs in the resulting dihedral angle, while the right inferior laryngeal one corresponds to the posterior tracheal face. The rear faces of the thyroid lobes, on which the parathyroid glands are placed, may send prolongations between the trachea and the anterior face of the esophagus, especially if the lobes are hypertrophied (retrotracheal goiter). In the same way a parathyroid gland can migrate in the tracheo-esophageal space and a parathyroid adenoma can be found in that position [25].

6.5.3.3   Thoracic Trachea

Thoracic trachea is 6–9 cm long and its shape varies depending on the level even in the same subject. The thoracic tract is surrounded by loose connective tissue that contains the tracheal lymph nodes and runs to the limits between the anterior and posterior mediastinum. It is crossed by the left innominate vein anteriorly and more forward corresponds to the thymus. More superficially there are the sternohyoid muscles and sternum. The lower portion of its anterior face is related to the aortic arch, to the brachiocephalic artery (also named innominate artery), which crosses it obliquely taking up and to the right between sixth and 13th tracheal ring, and to the left common carotid artery, which runs obliquely upwards and to the left. On the right side, the thoracic trachea is related to the right vagus nerve and the azygos vein; on the left side, it is related to the left recurrent nerve and to the aortic arch. The mediastinal fat typically separates the trachea from the left lung, which only occasionally comes into contact with the tracheal wall. However, on the right side, 1–2 cm below the entrance in the chest, lung comes in contact with a part of the posterior tracheal wall. Posteriorly the trachea maintains the relationship with the esophagus that separates it from the spine. At the level of the bifurcation, the trachea comes in connection with the pericardium and the atria of the heart. At this level the right anterolateral face is related to the superior vena cava, while on the left one there is the ascending aorta imprint ("Nicaise-Lejers" imprint). Anteriorly to the tracheal bifurcation, and on a level just below, there is the bifurcation of the pulmonary artery trunk, whose right branch is more directly related to the trachea [25].

6.5.3.4   Telescoping of the First Tracheal Ring and Cricoid Cartilage

The external cross-sectional area of the first tracheal ring is about 1.5 times greater than the cross-sectional area of the lower portion of the cricoid ring. The contraction of the trachealis muscle results in a lowering of the first tracheal ring cross-sectional area. Thus in physiological conditions (swallowing, normal coughing), there is an intermittent telescoping of the first tracheal ring into the cricoid cartilage ring that is very important to preserve in order to avoid posttracheotomy subglottic stenosis [26].

6.5.4 Surgical Technique

The surgical technique may widely vary depending on the urgency severity.

Sometimes the patient is still able to ventilate stably during a respiratory crisis, even in a nonoptimal way, thanks to an adequate anesthesiologic support. In these cases the surgical steps are substantially similar to the elective tracheotomy.

So the more serious the state of hypoxia and the quicker you will reach and open the tracheal lumen.

In extreme cases, unless it is a laryngeal malignancy, a quick opening of the cricothyroid membrane is necessary: cricothyrotomy (also called crike, intercricothyrotomy, coniotomy, or emergency airway puncture).

It can be performed using the currently trading coniotomy sets (figura) but also through traditional instruments [24].

Cricothyroidotomy is difficult in young children and is not recommended in children under the age of 5 years. Indeed a caver dissection study has demonstrated that the neonatal cricothyroid membrane has a mean height of 2.61 mm and width of 3.03 mm and therefore too small to allow a tracheal tube passage. This could fracture the cartilages of the larynx [27].

Traditional surgical cricothyrotomy steps:

- Head hyperextension and quick palpatory identification of the cricothyroid membrane, which is just inferior to thyroid prominence and superior to cricoid cartilage

- Stabilization of the larynx with the nondominant first three finger hand
- 3 cm vertical skin incision
- Tissues divarication with the first two fingers of nondominant hand and quick dissection of them, also with digital technique, until cricothyroid membrane identification
- Horizontal inter-cricothyroid space incision as close as possible to the top edge of the cricoid cartilage
- Divarication through a Killian speculum and introduction of the tube

Cricothyrotomy set technique steps:

- The first two steps are the same of traditional technique.
- Perforation through the needle of the soft tissues of the neck at right angle (sometimes preliminary skin incision is unnecessary).
- Introduction into the trachea and check the correct lumen perforation through the aspiration of air with an empty syringe.
- Inclination of the cricothyrotomy unit of 45° and further advancement in trachea until the removable stopper meets the skin.
- Removal of the stopper and needle advancing only the plastic cannula into the trachea until its fixation flange lies on the skin; then it is secured to the patient neck with padded straps.
- To ventilate the patient, the connecting tube is connected to 15 mm connector on the plastic cannula.

It is mandatory to convert as soon as possible this approach to a classical tracheotomy performed in quiet conditions, in order to avoid the potential scarring stenotic complications (Fig. 6.6).

When it is supposed to have a little more time (2–3 min) despite a severe hypoxia and it is considered preferable not to open the cricothyroid membrane, a similar technique could be employed:

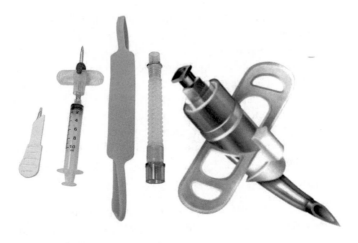

Fig. 6.6 Plastic cannula with fixation flange; removable cricothyrotomy needle; removable stopper; 10 cc syringe; connecting tube with 15 mm adapter

- Vertical median skin incision extended down to the jugular notch
- Blunt or digital dissection until cricotracheal junction identification
- Horizontal incision of the pretracheal fascia immediately below the cricoid in order to unstick the thyroid isthmus far enough to expose the first 2–3 tracheal rings where the opening will be practiced

When ENT surgeons are faced with a relative urgency, tracheotomy surgical steps may be similar to the elective one.

The patient is placed supine with a roll under the shoulders and neck hyperextended. Not always this position can be kept for the possible sudden worsening of the degree of hypoxia. So the surgeon is sometimes forced to operate in uncomfortable conditions.

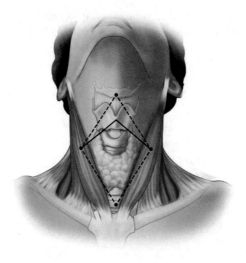

Fig. 6.7 Anesthetic infiltration area

Anesthesia is always performed by local infiltration (1 or 2 % xylocaine without adrenaline), trying to cover up a diamond-shaped area including vertically the portion between the bottom of the thyroid cartilage and the jugular notch, horizontally between the medial borders of sternocleidomastoid muscles at the height of the cricoid and the first tracheal rings [25] (Fig. 6.7).

The skin incision is usually a 5–6 cm horizontal incision with slight inferior convexity. In case of severe urgencies, a midline incision can be performed in order to improve the surgical field exposure and prevent damage to the anterior jugular veins.

Pretracheal dissection must be performed on the midline. The middle cervical aponeurosis is cut and prelaryngeal strap muscles separated and pulled laterally until the pretracheal plan exposure. A careful hemostasis through thyroid veins ligation is very important to prevent dangerous postoperative bleeding.

It is good palpate the position of the laryngeal cartilages and trachea to each maneuver since it is possible that the retractors cause a laryngotracheal axis lateralization.

When the thyroid isthmus is little it can be simply displaced upward or down. Some authors agree to dissect it (trans-isthmus tracheotomy) both for the risk of bleeding related to the postoperatively decubitus of the cannula concavity and for a possible obstacle to the emergency repositioning of an accidentally displaced tracheal cannula [24].

After a previous horizontal incision of the pretracheal fascia just below to its lower border and a retro-capsular blunt dissection in cephalad-caudal direction, thyroid isthmus is sectioned between two Kocher or Klemmer forceps placed laterally to the midline. Subsequently the two stumps are sutured with slow resorption sutures.

In doubtful cases, it is desirable to verify that you are in the presence of the trachea through an empty syringe.

The anterior tracheal wall incision and opening is a very important step. It is always advisable to cut between second and third or between third and fourth tracheal ring for two reasons:

1. A too "high" tracheotomy raises the risk of meeting a possible malignancy or a subsequent tracheal stenosis.
2. A too "low" tracheotomy at fourth–fifth ring, that is always recommended in severe laryngeal trauma, raises the risk of leakage of the cannula during neck movement and eventual recumbency on vessels such as the innominate artery, especially in children.

It is recommended to respect as much as possible the anatomy and physiology of the tracheal wall. Therefore the incision should be horizontal between two adjacent rings, not too laterally extended in order to not compromise the blood supply and to avoid the cephalad-caudal disconnection of the two lateral stumps. In case of a "low" tracheotomy or when a long stay is predictable it is possible to prepare a cartilaginous bottom hinge flap with subsequent anchoring to the bottom edge of the skin incision in order to facilitate the subsequent changes of the cannula and protect the underlying cervical vessels. Once the asphyxial emergency is resolved with the tracheal opening, a careful hemostasis is necessary. Then it proceeds with the placement of a cuffed tracheal cannula (No. 8 or 6 normally in adults) to protect the bronchial tree. If too wide, it proceeds to the possible reduction of the skin incision, which must not be excessive to avoid the risk of subcutaneous emphysema. Subsequently, the cervical fixing of the cannula has to be safe to facilitate the correct skin-tracheal route consolidation and so avoid the urgency difficult repositioning and the risk of false routes or injury.

6.5.5 Early Postoperative Management

In the early postoperative days is important to keep the tracheal tube patency and cleanliness by aspirating secretions with flexible probes, frequent cleaning of the inner cannula and instilling a few drops of mucolytics regularly. The wound must be cleaned and disinfected daily. The cannula should be decuffed in the first postoperative day and then replaced with a fenestrated one around the second or third postoperative day [24].

6.5.6 Complications

Complications occur in 5–40 % of tracheotomies. The mortality rate of tracheotomy is less than 2 %. Numerous studies demonstrate a greater complication and mortality rate in emergency situations, in severely ill patients, and in small children [28]. They can be classified according to the onset time and severity, but above all, it is necessary not to forget the variables that come into play during an urgency and/or emergency tracheotomy.

There are several variables related to the patient type, such as his general conditions and underlying disease, the hypoxia degree, the presence of a "short" fatty neck, massive thyroid goiters, or malignant neoplasms that make difficult and slower dissection and tracheal axis reaching or severe osteoarthritis and cervical kyphosis that does not allow hyperextension of the head and therefore a low enough tracheotomy execution. Variables related to the environmental conditions and surgical and anesthesiological team are very important as well [24].

Complications of tracheotomy (onset time)		
Intraoperative	Early postoperative	Late postoperative
Hemorrhage	Hemorrhage	Hemorrhage – granulations, tracheoinnominate artery blowout
Air emobolism	Tube dislodgement or obstruction	
Apnea		Tracheal stenosis
Damage to adjacent structures	Subcutaneous emphysema, pneumothorax, etc.	Tracheocutaneous fistula
Intraoperative fire [29]		Tracheoesophageal fistula
	Infection	

Complications of tracheotomy (severity)		
Major	Intermediate	Minor
Cardiopulmonary arrest	Ab ingestis	Subcutaneous emphysema
Massive hemorrhage (tracheoinnominate artery blowout)	Posterior tracheal wall injury	Wound infections
	Intraoperative desaturation	Difficult tube change
Tracheal stenosis	Pneumonia	Keloid
Tube dislodgement/obstruction	Atelectasia	Dysphonia
Tracheoesophageal fistula	Tracheal ring lesions	Peristomal granulations
Infections		Small bleedings
Pneumothorax		
Pneumomediastinum		

The most life-threatening, but fortunately rare, complication is the tracheoinnominate artery blowout, whose onset usually occurs in the first seven postoperative days because of a decubitus by dislodged cannula on the anonymous trunk, false routes, or infections.

Tracheal stenosis is the most common complication [28]. While it may reflect the tracheal damage originally caused by prolonged intubation before the tracheotomy, all other complications of tracheotomy may be prevented or minimized by careful surgical technique and postoperative tracheotomy care [30].

References

Epistaxis

1. Rudmik L, Smith TL. Management of intractable spontaneous epistaxis. Am J Rhinol Allergy. 2012;26(1):55–60. doi:10.2500/ajra.2012.26.3696.
2. Rossi G. Manuale di otorinolaringoiatria. Torino: Minerva Medica; 1992.
3. Gicquel P e Fontanel JP. Epistassi. Encycl Méd Chir (Editions Scientifiques et Médicales Elsevier SAS, Paris, tutti i diritti riservati), Otorinolaringoiatria, 20-310-A-10, 2002, 9 p.
4. Presutti, Le tecniche endoscopiche nel controllo delle epistassi severe, in la chirurgia endoscopica dei seni paranasali e della base cranica, Quaderni Monografici di Aggiornamento A.O.O.I., p. 189–198.
5. E. Cunsolo, R. Consalici, in L'anatomia vascolare clinica del distretto naso-sinusale, Epistassi, San Felice Circeo, 2006, p. 45–71.
6. LLee HY, Kim HU, Kim SS, Son EJ, Kim JW, Cho NH, et al. Surgical anatomy of the sphenopalatine artery in lateral nasal wall. Laryngoscope. 2002;112:1813–8.
7. Melia L, McGarry GW. Epistaxis: update on management. Curr Opin Otolaryngol Head Neck Surg. 2011;19:30–5.
8. Koh E, et al. Epistaxis, vascular anatomy, origins and endovascular treatment. Am J Roentgenol. 2000;174:845–51.
9. Leung RM, Smith TL, Rudmik L. Developing a laddered algorithm for the management of intractable epistaxis: a risk analysis. JAMA Otolaryngol Head Neck Surg. 2015;141:405–9. doi:10.1001/jamaoto.2015.106.
10. Chandler JR, Serrins AJ. Transantral Ligation of the internal maxillary artery for epistaxis. Laryngoscope. 1965;75:1151–9.
11. Kumar S, Shetty A, Rockey J, Nilssen E. Contemporary surgical management of epistaxis. What is the evidence for sphenopalatine artery ligation ? Clin Otolaryngol. 2003;28:360–3.

12. Nouraei SA, Maani T, Hajioff D, Saleh HA, Mackay IS. Outcome of endoscopic sphenopalatine artery occlusion for intractable epistaxis: a 10-year experience. Laryngoscope. 2007;117(8):1452–6.

13. Pletcher SD, Metson R. Endoscopic ligation of the anterior ethmoid artery. Laryngoscope. 2007;117:378–81.

14. Citardi MJ, et al. Management of carotid artery rupture by monitored endovascular therapeutic occlusion. Laryngoscope. 1995;105:1086–9.

15. Chen D, et al. Epistaxis originating from traumatic pseudoaneurysm of the internal carotid artery : diagnosis and endovascular therapy. Laryngoscope. 1998;108:326–31.

16. Celil G, et al. Intractable epistaxis related to cavernous carotid artery pseudoaneurysm: treatment of a case with covered stent. Auris Nasus Larynx. 2004;31:275–8.

17. Sokoloff J, Wickbom I, McDonald D, et al. Therapeutic percutaneous embolization in intractable epistaxis. Radiology. 1974;111:285–7.

18. Guss J, Cohen MA, Mirza N. Hard palate necrosis after bilateral internal maxillary artery embolization for epistaxis. Laryngoscope. 2007;117:1683–4.

19. Willems PW, Farb RI, Agid R. Endovascular treatment of epistaxis. AJNR Am Neuroradiol. 2009;30:1637–45.

20. Moshaver A, Harris JR, Liu R, et al. Early operative intervention versus conventional treatment in epistaxis: randomized prospective trial. J Otolaryngol. 2004;33:185–8.

21. Christensen NP, Smith DS, Barnwell SL, et al. Arterial embolization in the management of posterior epistaxis. Otolaryngol Head Neck Surg. 2005;133:748–53.

22. Miller TR, Stevens ES, Orlandi RR. Economic analysis of the treatment of posterior epistaxis. Am J Rhinol. 2005;19:79–82.

Emergency Tracheotomy

23. De Leyn P, Bedert L, Delcroix M, Depuydt P, Lauwers G, Sokolov Y, Van Meerhaeghe A, Van Schil P, Belgian Association of Pneumology and Belgian Association of Cardiothoracic Surgery. Tracheotomy: clinical review and guidelines. Eur J Cardiothorac Surg. 2007;32(3):412–21. Epub 2007 Jun 27.

24. Fois V. La tracheotomia d'urgenza, in le urgenze ed emergenze in orl, Quaderni di aggiornamento A.O.O.I., 2003.

25. E. Colombo, La tracheotomia: principi e conseguenze sul piano anatomico e funzionale, in le tracheotomie, Quaderni monografici di aggiornamento A.O.O.I., p. 23–30.
26. Damrose EJ. On the development of idiopathic subglottic stenosis. Med Hypotheses. 2008;71(1):122–5. doi:10.1016/j.mehy.2007.12.017. Epub 2008 Mar 4.
27. Navsa N, Tossel G, Boon JM. Dimensions of the neonatal cricothyroid membrane – how feasible is a surgical cricothyroidotomy? Paediatr Anaesth. 2005;15(5):402–6.
28. Goldenberg D, Ari EG, Golz A, Danino J, Netzer A, Joachims HZ. Tracheotomy complications: a retrospective study of 1130 cases. Otolaryngol Head Neck Surg. 2000;123(4):495–500.
29. Rogers ML, Nickalls RW, Brackenbury ET, Salama FD, Beattie MG, Perks AG. Airway fire during tracheostomy: prevention strategies for surgeons and anaesthetists. Ann R Coll Surg Engl. 2001;83(6): 376–80.
30. Sarper A, Ayten A, Eser I, Ozbudak O, Demircan A. Tracheal stenosis aftertracheostomy or intubation: review with special regard to cause and management. Tex Heart Inst J. 2005;32(2):154–8.

Chapter 7
Hemothorax, Pneumothorax, and Chest Empyema

Pantelis Vassiliu and Elias Degiannis

7.1 Pneumothorax

7.1.1 Definition and Classification

Pneumothorax is defined as the accumulation of air in the pleural space, secondary to a lacerated or punctured lung or loss of the integrity of the thoracic wall. This can be *open* or *closed* pneumothorax, depending on the presence or absence of pleural cavity communication with the atmosphere through a thoracic wall defect. The presence of a pneumothorax results to lung collapse with the corresponding ventilation-perfusion

P. Vassiliu, MD, PhD, FACS (✉)
4th Surgical Clinic, "Attikon" University Hospital, Athens, Greece
e-mail: pant_greek@hotmail.com

E. Degiannis, MD, PhD, FRCS (Glasg), FACS
Department of Surgery, Faculty of Health Sciences, University of the
Witwatersrand, Milpark Trauma Centre, Johannesburg, South Africa

© Springer International Publishing Switzerland 2017
S. Di Saverio et al. (eds.), *Acute Care Surgery Handbook*,
DOI 10.1007/978-3-319-15341-4_7

117

mismatch, acute and excessive hypoxia as well as hypercarbia. Penetrating or blunt thoracic injury, locally advanced lung cancer, rupture of pulmonary bullae (Fig. 7.1), and advanced pulmonary disease, such as cystic fibrosis, are the most common causes of pneumothorax. Less frequently, this can be related with disruption of the tracheobronchial tree or the esophagus.

Spontaneous nontraumatic pneumothorax is a clinical entity, usually associated with underlying pulmonary pathology (Table. 7.1). Primary spontaneous pneumothorax is due to rupture of pulmonary bullae (Fig. 7.1), and risk factors include tobacco smoking, tall stature, and age between 15 and 35 or over 55 years [3]. Secondary spontaneous pneumothorax is associated with chronic obstructive pulmonary disease (COPD), cystic fibrosis, asthma, and lung cancer.

7.1.2 Simple (Nontension) Pneumothorax

Simple pneumothorax results in decreased breath sounds on the affected side as well as hyper-resonance on percussion. Depending on the size of the pneumothorax, as well as on the noise in the examination environment, a simple pneumothorax can be difficult to be clinically detected [4]. In this case, an erect chest X-ray in expiration can establish the diagnosis. It is important to be alert of the fact that general anesthesia and positive pressure ventilation can result in the increase of the size of the pneumothorax, even leading to the creation of a tension pneumothorax, making the insertion of an intercostal drain obligatory as a preemptive step. Small closed pneumothoraces (less than 15 %) can be treated by oxygen administration and clinical observation, coupled with follow-up X-rays, as there is a good chance that this will lead to its resolution. Generally speaking, apart from the previous case, all pneumothoraces are dealt with by intercostal drain insertion.

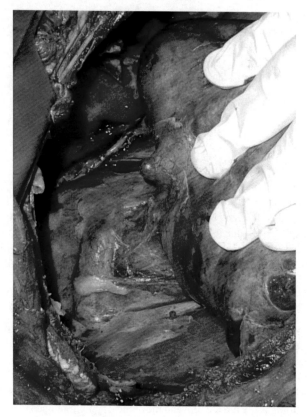

Figure 7.1 Pulmonary bullae

7.1.3 *Tension Pneumothorax*

Tension pneumothorax is a life-threatening condition and develops when a "one-way valve" air leak results in accumulation of air under tension in the pleural cavity, the air originating from the lung, or through a chest wall defect. Particularly in the case of the latter, if its size is approximately the 2/3 of the diameter

Table 7.1 Main causes of spontaneous nontraumatic hemothorax

Neoplasia (primary or metastatic)
Bullous emphysema
Tuberculosis
Anticoagulation complications
Necrotizing infections
Pulmonary arteriovenous fistula
Pulmonary embolism with infarction
Hereditary hemorrhagic telangiectasia

of trachea, the air will preferentially pass through the chest wall defect with each respiratory effort, as the air tends to follow the path of least resistance [5].

As the air is entrapped in the pleural cavity without means of escape, it results in intrapleural pressure increase with every breath, leading to collapse of the ipsilateral lung. There is displacement of the mediastinum to the opposite side with ipsilateral increase of the intercostal spaces and depression of the diaphragm. The combination of the above leads to marked decrease in venous return, causing reduction of cardiac output. Any simple pneumothorax can be converted to tension pneumothorax irrespective of its cause; therefore, the clinician must be vigorously alert. This can occur particularly if a patient with a simple pneumothorax is on positive pressure ventilation.

The diagnosis of tension pneumothorax should be clinical as the condition is life threatening and the clinical symptoms and signs are profoundly obvious. The patient presents with chest pain – frequently related to concomitant rib fractures – air hunger and respiratory distress. There is deviation of the trachea to the opposite side, distention of the neck veins, tympanic sound on percussion, and absence of breath sounds on auscultation. There is tachycardia, sometimes related with hypotension. Cyanosis is a late sign.

The treatment is rapid insertion of a large caliber needle into the second intercostal space in the midclavicular line of the affected side. This should be followed by the insertion of an intercostal drain and the simultaneous occlusion on the thoracic wall opening usually with stitches [6]. In the presence of an open pneumothorax, secondary to a large defect of the chest wall, this defect must be managed by the application of a "three side dressing." This should be square shaped, sterile occlusive dressing, large enough to overlap the edges of the wound, and should be taped on the three of its four sides in order to provide a flutter-type valve effect. On inspiration, the dressing occludes the wound preventing air from entering, while on expiration, the nontaped side of the dressing allows air to escape from the pleural cavity [2]. "Bubbling" at the intercostal drain collecting canister is an indication of air leak related to bronchial injury (Fig. 7.2) [7]. This may require an operative management of the pneumothorax.

7.2 Hemothorax

7.2.1 Simple Hemothorax

This is characterized by collection of less than 1500 ml of blood in the pleural cavity, and in most cases, it is related to lung laceration or injury of an intercostal vessel. It may infrequently take place in nontraumatic cases, particularly in pleural infiltration by malignancy, complication of infectious disease (e.g., tuberculosis), erosion of a vessel, or rupture of an aneurysm.

Clinical examination will reveal decreased breath sound on auscultation, and dullness on percussion particularly on the examination of the posterior lower hemithorax, with the patient in the sitting-up position. An erect chest X-ray will show obliteration of the costophrenic angle, formed by the accumulation of blood (if it is less than 500 cc, it could well not show in the erect X-ray), or by an air-fluid level in the presence of a

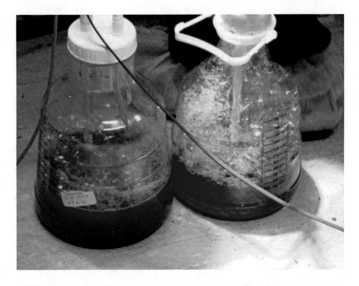

Figure 7.2 "Bubbling" inside the intercostal drain collection canister: indication of major air leak probably related to bronchial injury

concomitant pneumothorax. The supine chest X-ray will show a homogeneous haziness of the hemithorax that is caused by the creation of a film of blood of variable "thickness" (relevant to the volume of the blood retained) that lies at the posterior aspect of the affected pleural cavity. The treatment is the insertion of an intercostal drain, which should be directed downwards and backwards (Fig. 7.3a proper positioning, Fig. 7.3b improper positioning) so that the drainage of the hemothorax would be effective irrespective if the patient is sitting up or lies flat in his bed [8]. Taking into consideration the fact that many times hemothorax coincides with pneumothorax, this is the ideal positioning of the intercostal drain, as the pneumothorax will, in any case, be drained from the pleural cavity irrespective of the positioning of the intercostal drain as the air will be pumped out the pleural cavity by the lung expansion during inspiration. In contradiction, this is not always happening with a hemothorax,

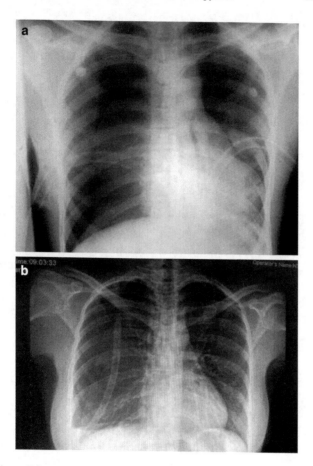

Figure 7.3 (**a**) Right-sided tension pneumothorax despite proper intercostal drain position. (**b**) Right-sided simple pneumothorax. Ineffective intercostal drain positioning. A potentially co-existing hemothorax will residue in the posterior lower pleural cavity

which is usually retained at the lower posterior part of the pleural cavity, where due to gravity, it is mostly accumulated [9]. Insertion of another drain in the presence of retained hemothorax is acceptable. It is important to make sure that there is no retained hemothorax after the drains stop working or after they get removed. A chest X-ray at those cases is imperative. If there is retained hemothorax that cannot be drained with a further insertion with an intercostal drain, a video-assisted thoracoscopy (VATS) should be considered. If a retained hemothorax is not drained, there is a possibility of development of an empyema. It is recommended that VATS should take place at an early stage preferably after the fifth post injury day. Otherwise, evacuation of the retained clot can be technically difficult. Instillation of streptokinase for liquidification has been suggested but has not found wide application.

Nontraumatic hemothoraces are dealt with in the same principles. Management of the underline disease process should also be undertaken. This may include repair of vascular abnormalities (aortic aneurysms), stapling or resection of bullous disease, removal of necrotic tissue, and pleurodesis of persistent malignant fluid collection.

7.2.2 Massive Hemothorax

As with tension and open pneumothorax, massive hemothorax is a life-threatening condition that must be diagnosed and treated at a very early stage, in case of trauma, during the primary survey. Massive hemothorax is defined as the rapid accumulation of more than 1500 cc of blood or 1/3 or more of the patient's blood volume in the chest cavity. It is most frequently related with the injury of the heart, mediastinal vessels, hilar vessels, or intercostal arteries. These are usually secondary to penetrating trauma; blunt trauma can also well be the cause.

The *clinical picture* is that of hypovolemia with the neck veins being collapsed except if there is accumulated air in the pleural cavity that could develop a tension pneumothorax, in which case the neck veins could be distended. On percussion, there is dullness, and absence of breath sounds on auscultation. The clinical picture could well be related with hypoxia. A chest X-ray will show a "whipped-out" lung – an intense opacity of the affected pleural space – or a very high sited air-fluid level in the presence of a concomitant pneumothorax in an erect chest X-ray (Fig. 7.4). The management of a massive hemothorax has to do with simultaneous replacement of the lost blood volume and drainage of the blood by insertion of an underwater sealed intercostal drain. It is always advisable to use 200–500 ml of N/S as fluid in the underwater sealed container and add in to that 1000 IU of heparin. When the container gets filled with blood, a blood-administration-set can be applied at the container and the patient can be transfused with his own blood (autotransfusion) [10]. If after the initial drainage of 1500 ml of blood, the hemorrhage continues to the rate of more than 200 cc of blood for every 4 h, post intercostal drain insertion, a thoracotomy for control of bleeding is required. Of course, we should not be dogmatic about it, as the patients' physiological status should also be considered [11]. It is important in all cases with massive pneumothorax to repeat the chest X-ray after insertion of the intercostal drain if unexpected pause of drainage occurs, to exclude continued hemorrhage, which does not show because of blockage of the drain or formation of clot in the pleural space [4].

7.3 Chest Empyema

Empyema is a collection of pus in the pleural cavity, following infection of a retained hemothorax most frequently secondary to trauma, or infective pathology of the lung parenchyma. Identification of patients at greater risk for empyema is contributing to establishing the correct diagnosis. Patients usually present with subtle symptoms, such as anorexia, weight loss, and poor energy.

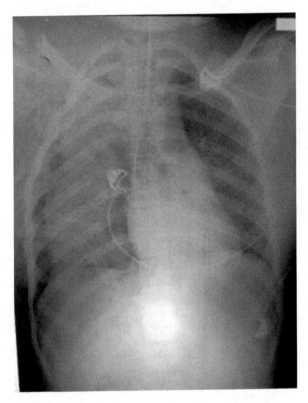

Figure 7.4 Massive right-sided traumatic hemothorax and lung contusion

On clinical examination, there will be evidences of collection of fluid in the pleural cavity. A chest X-ray or a CT scan will show pleural fluid accumulation with possible concomitant lung pathology. The stage of the empyema is associated with the length of the infectious process (Table 7.2) [12]. Fluid sample analysis verifies the final diagnosis.

An optimal treatment for posttraumatic chest empyema is yet to be determined. Removal of the purulent fluid and re-expansion of the lung are critical as well as managing the causative pathology. In early stage empyema, drainage with thoracocentesis may be adequate treatment. Administration of antibiotics is not recommended, unless there are indications for underlying lung pathology or specific bacteria identified in the drained fluid. If the patient becomes septic, antibiotics are administered for the interval between the sepsis presentation and the definitive drainage of the empyema. Larger fluid collections that appear single and homogeneous at imaging are drained with placement of a chest tube. A CT scan must be obtained to assess possible presence of residual pleural fluid after drainage. Utilization of intrapleural fibrinolytics (i.e., streptokinase) to decrease the need for operative intervention has been reported with mixed outcomes [13].

In patients who do not respond to treatment with antibiotics and chest tube drainage, VATS or an open surgical intervention is required. VATS decortication has been utilized widely as a minimally invasive approach for treatment of posttraumatic empyema with reduced morbidity as VATS proves more effective for stage I and II empyema (Table 7.2) [12]. In more advanced stages, an open surgical approach via a posterior lateral thoracotomy may be necessary for evacuation of the empyema, decortication of the lung (Fig. 7.5) and possible

Table 7.2   Stages of posttraumatic thoracic empyema

	Early (I)	Intermediate (II)	Late (III)
Fluid characteristics (≥1 of the following)	pH <7.2 Glucose <40 mg/dL Lactate dehydrogenase >1000 IU/dL Protein >2.5 g/dL White blood cell count >500/μL Specific gravity >1.018	Thick opaque fluid Positive culture	Organizing peel with lung entrapment

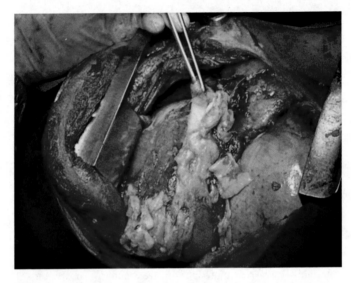

Figure 7.5 Surgical management of empyema: lung decortication (cortex: white tissue grasped with forceps). Special attention should be given to avoid lung perforation during the procedure

section of a pulmonary causative pathology. Pleurectomy can be indicated in certain cases. Given the increased rate of early diagnosis and the abundance of therapeutic modalities, the role of surgery in empyema is declining, alongside with the related surgical skill [14].

7.4   Intercostal Drain Insertion Technique

The site and technique of intercostal drain insertion [2] apply to all three pneumothorax, hemothorax, and empyema. The patient is in supine position, and the ipsilateral arm is abducted at 90°. At the fifth intercostal space between anterior and mid axillary lines, the skin, subcutaneous tissue, *and muscle* are infiltrated with local anesthetic [15]. The patient should also be loaded with morphine (in adults, initial IV dose 0.1 mg/kg and then titrate with 0.3 mg/kg if pain persists) [16], as if not he is going to have excruciating pain with the insertion of the intercostal drain and its friction with the visceral and parietal pleura. The pleural cavity is inserted by using a pair of closed Kelly forceps, and then enlarging the entry point by opening the limbs of the forceps. This is followed by insertion of the index finger and accessing the possibility of the lung being adherent to the thoracic wall, in which case this is freed by whipping it off with the tip of the finger. Then, one limb of the Kelly forceps is inserted in the most proximal hole of the intercostal tube, grasped firmly, and the distal open end of the tube is occluded with another heavy clamp. The tip of the intercostal drain in then guided with the Kelly forceps inside the pleural cavity, and it is directed posteriorly and inferiorly. The posterior inferior positioning of the tip of the drain (Fig. 7.3a, b) [8, 9] – in contrast to other suggestions to be directed to the apex of the thoracic cavity – reduces the incidence of undrained hemothorax. When this posterior – inferior direction is secured usually after insertion of approximately 5 cm of the intercostal drain, the Kelly forceps is removed, and the intercostal drain forwarded insight the pleural cavity for 10–15 cm. The distal part (of the intercostal drain) is connected to the tube of the underwater sealed bottle. Then the intercostal drain is secured at the thoracic wall. The patient is encouraged to cough several times immediately after the completion of the procedure and a chest X-ray is ordered.

References

1. Schoell SL, Doud AN, Weaver AA, Barnard RT, Meredith JW, Stitzel JD, et al. Predicting patients that require care at a trauma center: analysis of injuries and other factors. Injury. 2015;46:558–63.
2. Advanced trauma life support for doctors: student course manual. Chicago: American College of Surgeons; 2012.
3. Bobbio A, Dechartres A, Bouam S, Damotte D, Rabbat A, Régnard J-F, et al. Epidemiology of spontaneous pneumothorax: gender-related differences. Thorax. 2015;70:653–8.
4. Degiannis E, Zinn RJ. Pitfalls in penetrating thoracic trauma (lessons we learned the hard way…). Ulus Travma Acil Cerrahi Derg. 2008;14(4):261–7.
5. Zigiriadis E, Smith MD, Yilmaz TH, Degiannis E. Thoracic trauma. In: Velmahos G, Degiannis E, Doll D, editors. Penetrating trauma, 2nd ed. Springer: Berlin, Heidelberg; 2016 (In press).
6. Mayberry JC. Loss of chest wall. In: Velmahos G, Degiannis E, Doll D, editors. Penetrating trauma. Springer: Berlin, Heidelberg; 2012, p. 293–8.
7. Zigiriadis E, Loogna P, Yilmaz TH. Pulmonary and bronchotracheal trauma. In: Velmahos G, Degiannis E, Doll D, editors. Penetrating trauma. Springer: Berlin, Heidelberg; 2012, p. 259–66.
8. Scott AJ, Davies SJ, Vassiliu P. Development of a tension pneumothorax despite intercostal drain insertion. BMJ Case Rep. 2012, p. 1–2. doi:10.1136/bcr-2012-006358.
9. Degiannis E, Smith MD. Pot pouri of heuristics in penetrating trauma to the chest. ANZ J Surg. 2008;78(12):1103–5. doi:10.1111/j.1445-2197.2008.04759.x.
10. Loogna P, Bonanno F, Bowley DM, Doll D, Girgensohn R, Smith MD, Glapa M, Degiannis E. Emergency thoracic surgery for penetrating, non-mediastinal trauma. ANZ J Surg. 2007;77(3):142–5.
11. The chest. In: Boffard K, editor. Manual of definitive surgical trauma care. CRC Press: Berlin, Heidelberg; 2016, p. 75–97.
12. Billeter AT, Druen D, Franklin GA, Smith JW, Wrightson W, Richardson JD. Video-assisted thoracoscopy as an important tool for trauma surgeons: a systematic review. Langenbecks Arch Surg. 2013;398:515–23.
13. Stiles PJ, Drake RM, Helmer SD, Bjordahl PM, Haan JM. Evaluation of chest tube administration of tissue plasminogen activator to treat retained hemothorax. Am J Surg. 2014;207:960–3.

14. DuBose J, Inaba K, Okoye O, Demetriades D, Scalea T, O'Connor J, et al. Development of posttraumatic empyema in patients with retained hemothorax: results of a prospective, observational AAST study. J Trauma Acute Care Surg. 2012;73:752–7.
15. Vassiliu P. ABC heuristics. In: Velmahos G, Degiannis E, Doll DP, editors. Penetrating trauma. Springer: Boca-Raton, FL, USA; 2012, p. 53–60.
16. Soukup E, Masiakos P. Pediatric trauma rescuscitation. In: Velmahos G, Degiannis E, Doll D, editors. Penetrating trauma. Springer: Berlin, Heidelberg; 2012, p. 53–60.

Chapter 8
Anorectal Emergencies

Korhan Taviloglu

When a patient presents with swelling, pain, tenderness, itching, and bleeding symptoms of the anal region, the initial step should be to maintain a thorough history of the patient. Following this step, the patient is usually examined with the left lateral or the Sims position, and rarely in prone jackknife position. Rectal examination can be a great burden for many patients; therefore, the patient should be informed of pressure to the anal canal during inspection. External hemorrhoids, external fistula orifice, anal carcinoma, anal condylomas, anorectal abscess, sexually transmitted diseases (STD), and anal discharge can be detected. Anorectal examination may reveal anal pain, anal stenosis, anal sphincter problems, manifest blood, and anorectal abscess.

K. Taviloglu
Taviloglu Proctology Center, Abdi Ipekci Cad, No 59,
Kizilkaya ap, Kat 4, Nisantasi, 34365 Sisli, Istanbul, Turkey
e-mail: korhan@taviloglu.com; http://www.taviloglu.com

© Springer International Publishing Switzerland 2017
S. Di Saverio et al. (eds.), *Acute Care Surgery Handbook*,
DOI 10.1007/978-3-319-15341-4_8

133

8.1 Lower Gastrointestinal Bleeding

Lower gastrointestinal (GI) bleeding is defined as bleeding from the bowel distal to the ligament of Treitz, and usually manifests with maroon stools or bright red blood per rectum. The incidence of lower gastrointestinal bleeding is not exactly known but is assumed to be 20/100.000, and constitutes 25 % of all gastrointestinal bleedings with a male predominance. Bright red blood per rectum strongly suggests a lower gastrointestinal (GI) source of bleeding unless the patient is hemodynamically unstable, in which case, the hemorrhage may originate from a source proximal to the ligament of Treitz. Initially, a digital rectal examination is performed, and then an upper GI source of bleeding should be ruled out by placing a nasogastric tube. It is recommended to carry out colonoscopy immediately in patients with third- and fourth-degree hypovolemia and within 12–24 h in patients with first- and second-degree hypovolemia. It is strongly recommended to carry out an upper gastrointestinal endoscopy if a bleeding site cannot be detected during colonoscopy. Zuckerman and Prakash showed in a meta-analysis that colonoscopy identified the source of bleeding in 69 % (48–90 %) of the patients. Elderly (older than 65 years) and the patients with co-morbidities warrant hospitalization because of high morbidity and mortality rates (10–20 %).

8.2 Anal Pain

Anal pain is an embarrassing problem for many patients. Acute anal fissures, thrombosed hemorrhoids, anorectal abscess, herpesvirus infection, anal condylomas, anal trauma (sexual, etc.), obstructive defecation syndrome (ODS), anal dyssynergia, anal cryptitis, and proctalgia fugax may cause severe anal or rectal pain. Warms sitz baths, topical ice application, diltiazem, Glyceryl trinitrate ointment, and nonsteroidal antiinflammatory drugs (NSAIDs) are helpful in 60–70 % of cases.

8.3 Acute Anal Fissure

Acute anal fissures may present with severe anal pain and rectal bleeding with defecation (Fig. 8.1). The initial treatment should consist of pain relief, anal hygiene, and warm sitz baths. Topical application of anesthetic jelly, % 0.2–0.4 nitroglycerin ointment or glyceryl trinitrate, diltiazem, nifedipine or L-arginine, bulking and softening the stool with psyllium seed is useful in acute conditions.

8.4 Acute Hemorrhoidal Disease

Hemorrhoids are not masses of dilated venules. The anal cushions are composed of blood vessels, smooth muscle (Treitz's muscle), and elastic connective tissue in the submucosa. Three cushions lie in left lateral, right anterolateral, and right posterolateral positions. The prolapse of these anal cushions is defined as hemorrhoids. In the presence of irreducible prolapse or thrombosis of hemorrhoids, generally present with severe edema and severe pain as main symptoms where surgery may be required.

8.5 Grading of Hemorrhoids

Degree	Description
I	Hemorrhoids prolapse beyond the dentate line on straining
II	Hemorrhoids prolapse through the anus on straining but reduce spontaneously
III	Hemorrhoids prolapse through the anus which require manual reduction
IV	Prolapsed hemorrhoids cannot be manually reduced

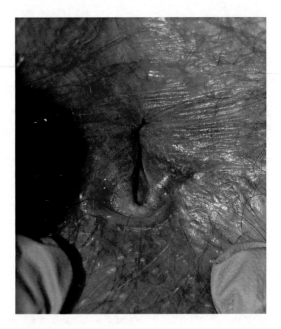

Fig. 8.1 A chronic anal fissure

Prolapsed third-degree or fourth-degree hemorrhoids may cause strangulation. On examination, edema is obvious, and if untreated, prolapsed hemorrhoids may end up with ulceration and necrosis. Thrombosed or strangulated hemorrhoids due to hormonal changes and the pressure of the fetus on pelvic veins can cause a serious problem in pregnant and postpartum women.

8.6 Thrombosed External Hemorrhoids

Thrombosis of external hemorrhoids (Fig. 8.2) occurs with an unknown cause, and follows an abrupt onset of anal mass and pain within 48 h. The pain diminishes after the fourth day and if left alone dissolves spontaneously in a few weeks. The treatment should consist of pain relief, prevention of recurrent thromboses, and residual skin tags. The thrombus is excised with local or general anesthesia. Greenspon et al. detected on a case series of 231 patients with thrombosed hemorrhoids that with conservative treatment, symptoms resolved in 24 days and with surgery in 4 days. The recurrence rate was 25 % in the conservative group and 6 % in the surgery group.

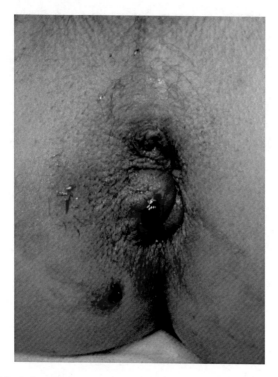

Fig. 8.2 A thrombosed external hemorrhoid

8.7 Strangulated Hemorrhoids

Strangulated hemorrhoids (Fig. 8.3) arise from prolapsed Grade 3 or 4 hemorrhoids that cannot be reduced due to excessive swelling. The edema may progress to ulceration or necrosis if not treated with urgent three quadrant hemorrhoidectomy. If the procedure is performed with stapled hemorrhoidopexy without decompressing the edematous tissue, pain is more compared to the hemorrhoidectomy technique in the immediate postoperative period, but less in 6 weeks.

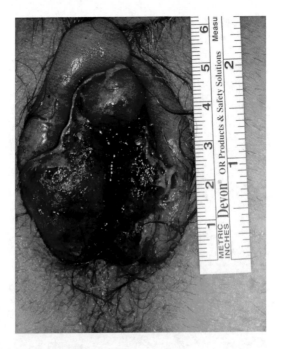

Fig. 8.3 A strangulated hemorrhoid

8.8   Hemorrhoids in Pregnancy

Acute prolapse and thrombosis during pregnancy require hemorrhoidectomy and should be treated under local anesthesia. Immediate postpartum period is the best term for hemorrhoidectomy. Mild laxatives are proven to be helpful in the last 3 months of pregnancy. Traumatic deliveries, such as perineal tear and heavy babies, were associated with thrombosed external hemorrhoids.

8.9   Hemorrhoids and Portal Hypertension

Hemorrhoid are quite common (almost 60 %) in portal hypertension. Patients with large esophageal varices have more frequent anorectal varices. Anorectal varices rarely bleed compared to esophageal varices. Bleeding hemorrhoids in patients with portal hypertension must be distinguished from anorectal varices, true consequence of portal hypertension. Bleeding from anorectal varices can be controlled with absorbable running sutures.

8.10   Hemorrhoids in Inflammatory Bowel Disease

The treatment of hemorrhoids is accepted as safe in patients with ulcerative colitis, whereas it is relatively contraindicated in patients with Crohn's disease and only recommended in a quiescent stage.

8.11 Hemorrhoids in Leukemia

Surgical treatment of patients with leukemia or lymphoma presenting with hemorrhoidal disease is quite difficult, since abscesses are common and wound healing is rather poor. Surgery does not increase the mortality in these high-risk patients, but is performed to relieve pain and sepsis usually caused by *Escherichia coli* and *Pseudomonas aeruginosa*.

8.12 Proctitis

Proctitis is an inflammation limited to the rectum. Inflammation leads to bleeding and mucous secretion. Although constipation may be encountered, diarrhea is more frequent. Irritation of the rectum may cause an urgency to defecate. There is a tendency to spread proximally during the course, which is defined as proctocolitis.

8.13 Acute Cryptoglandular Infection

The majority of anorectal suppurative disease results from obstruction and infection of the ducts of mucous-secreting anal glands (cryptoglandular infection) found in the intersphincteric plane. Their ducts traverse the internal sphincter and empty into the anal crypts at the level of the dentate line. Infection of an anal gland results in the formation of an abscess that enlarges and spreads along one of several planes in the perianal and perirectal spaces, which are unable to resist the spread of infection and lead to various clinical presentations at the perineum.

8.14   Hidradenitis Suppurativa

Hidradenitis suppurativa (Fig. 8.4) is an infection of the cutaneous apocrine sweat glands. The infection may mimic and is often misdiagnosed as cryptoglandular abscesses. Chronically infected glands may rupture and form subcutaneous sinus tracts. This infection is differentiated from cryptoglandular perianal septic disease by the lack of communication to the anal canal, due to the absence of apocrine glands there, and by microbiologic criteria as will be detailed below.

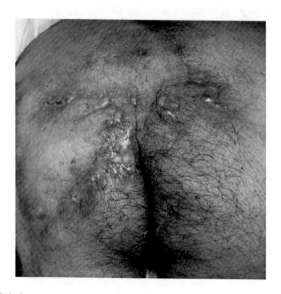

Fig. 8.4 Presentation of anal hidradenitis suppurativa

8.15   Anorectal Abscess

Anorectal abscesses (Fig. 8.5) are more common in men than in women, with a ratio of 2:1–5:1. The most common cause of fistulous abscess is the infection of anal glands and anal crypts. Obstruction of these ducts, whether secondary to fecal material foreign bodies, or trauma, results in stasis and infection. Predominant organisms are *Escherichia coli*, *Enterococcus*, and *Bacteroides fragilis*. The initial signs are usually severe anal pain, swelling, and tenderness. Sometimes, pus may be seen exuding from a crypt. Anal canal involvement is present in 30–70 % of patients with Crohn's disease; however, only 3–5 % require surgical intervention. Abscess locations are perianal, intersphincteric, ischioanal, intersphincteric, and supralevator.

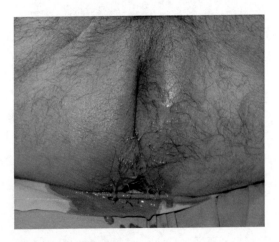

Fig. 8.5 Ruptured anorectal abscess

In suspected cases, intrarectal ultrasound (IRUS), endoscopic rectal ultrasound (ERUS), and pelvic magnetic resonance imaging (MRI) are useful.

In terms of an anorectal abscess, prompt drainage is favored. The abscess may be drained under local or general anesthesia according to conditions. Detailed rectal examination under general anesthesia may reveal the problem. Neglect only allows extension of the abscess and may lead to ischioanal and supra-levator abscesses and possibly to horseshoe extensions, with each of these conditions more difficult to manage than the simple intersphincteric abscess. If an abscess is detected, preferably it is drained via the anal canal or by removing a skin anal region or placing a mushroom catheter (Thompson-Fawcet). Lay-open technique may end up with several complications. Antibiotics are not generally necessary if the abscess is drained adequately; however in patients with Crohn's disease, immune deficiency, and cardiac valve abnormalities, antibiotics should be administered. In general, mixed aerobic and anaerobic organisms are isolated in 7–80 % of patients; aerobic organisms in 10–12.5 %; and anaerobic organisms in 5–7.5 %. The most common bacterial isolates are *Bacteroides fragilis*, *Peptostreptococcus* spp., *Prevotella* spp., *Staphylococcus aureus*, *Streptococcus* spp., and *Escherichia coli*. More recently, however, a larger percentage of these abscesses (23 %) contained methicillin-resistant *S. aureus*. These abscesses are also less likely to be of cryptoglandular origin and manifest greater inflammatory response. Identifying the bacterial etiology of perianal sepsis is important not only in the tailoring antibiotic treatment in patients that fail to respond to incision and drainage alone but also in deciding whether these patients should be submitted to further anorectal examination to rule out a fistula as an underlying factor.

8.16 Fournier's Gangrene

Necrotizing fasciitis of the perineal area (Fournier's gangrene–Fig. 8.6) is a rare soft-tissue infection, primarily
involving the superficial fascia and resulting in extensive
undermining of the surrounding tissues. The incidence of
such extensive infection has been estimated as less than 1 %
of all anorectal sepsis. If untreated, it is invariably fatal, and
thus a high index of suspicion for the diagnosis is required.
Mortality remains still high in necrotizing fasciitis despite use
of modern powerful antimicrobial drug regimens and advances
in the care of the critically ill patients. Overall mortality
ranges from 25 to 73 % in the published literature. The disease's manifestation can range from a fulminant presentation

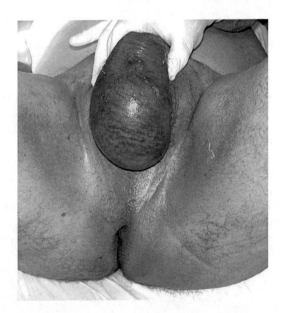

Fig. 8.6 Fournier's gangrene

to a subtle and insidious development. After initial fluid and electrolyte corrections and administration of broad-spectrum antibiotics, radical debridement involving extensive excision of all involved skin, fascia, and muscles is performed. Extension may reach the abdominal wall, thighs, chest wall, and axilla. Testicular involvement is rare, and the only indication for orchiectomy is testicular gangrene. Repeat exploration should be conducted as necessary until the necrotizing process has been interrupted.

8.17 Perianal Sepsis in Immunocompromised Patients

Perianal infection in patients with acute leukemia has been associated with mortality rates of 45 to 78 %. If the granulocyte counts are increased above 1,000 cell/mm^3, the postoperative course was uncomplicated; otherwise, if surgery is performed with severe granulocytopenia (<500 polymorphonuclear leukocytes/mm^3), the survival rate does not increase.

8.18 Acute Pilonidal Abscess

Pilonidal disease refers to a hair-containing sinus, cyst, or abscess occurring mainly in the sacrococcygeal region. The etiology is unknown, but it is speculated that the intergluteal cleft draws hair into the midline pits when a patients sits. An inflammatory process surrounding these ingrown hairs results in a cyst or a sinus tract. If this in turn becomes infected, the patient will present with an acute abscess (Fig. 8.7) in the sacrococcygeal region, which generally requires surgical drainage and/or antibiotic therapy.

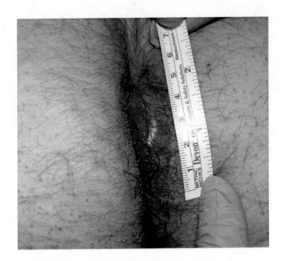

Fig. 8.7 Acute abscess in the sacrococcygeal region

Bibliography

1. Zuckerman GR, Prakash C. Acute lower gastrointestinal bleeding. Part II: etiology, therapy and outcomes. Gastrontest Endosc. 1999;49:228–38.
2. Greenspon J, Williams SB, Ha Y, et al. Thrombosed external hemorrhoids: outcome after conservative surgical treatment. Dis Colon Rectum. 2004;47:1493–8.
3. Nivatvongs S. Hemorrhoids. In: Gordon PH, Nivatvongs S, editors. Principles and practice of surgery for the colon, rectum and anus. 3rd ed. New York: Informa Healthcare; 2007. p. 143–66.
4. Gordon PH. Anorectal abscesses and fistula-in-ano. In: Gordon PH, Nivatvongs S, editors. Principles and practice of surgery for the colon, rectum and anus. 3rd ed. New York: Informa Healthcare; 2007. p. 191–233.
5. Taviloglu K, Yanar H. Necrotizing fasciitis: strategies for diagnosis and management. World J Emerg Surg. 2007;7(2):19.
6. Yanar H, Taviloglu K, Ertekin C, et al. Fournier's gangrene: risk factors and strategies for management. World J Surg. 2006;30(9):1750–4.

7. Eke N. Fournier's gangrene: a review of 1726 cases. Br J Surg. 2000;87:718–28.
8. Cason FD, Duwayri Y. Perirectal and perineal sepsis. In: Rabinovici R, Frankel HL, Kirton OC, editors. Trauma, Critical Care and Surgical Emergencies: a case and evidence-based textbook. London: Informa; 2010. p. 479–89.
9. Gebbensleben O, Hilger Y, Rohde H. Do we at all need surgery to treat thrombosed external hemorrhoids? Results of a prospective cohort study. Clin Exp Gastroenterol. 2009;2:69–74.
10. Henderson PK, Cash BD. Common anorectal conditions: evaluation and treatment. Curr Gastroenterol Rep. 2014;16(10):408.
11. Klein JW. Common anal problems. Med Clin North Am. 2014;98(3):609–23.
12. Steele SR, Madoff RD. Systematic review: the treatment of anal fissure. Aliment Pharmacol Ther. 2006;24(2):247–57.
13. de Parades V, Bouchard D, Janier M, et al. Pilonidal sinus disease. J Visc Surg. 2013;150(4):237–47.
14. Lamb CA, Lamb EI, Mansfield JC, et al. Sexually transmitted infections manifesting as proctitis. Frontline Gastroenterol. 2013;4(1):32–40.
15. Kim WB, Sibbald RG, Hu H, et al. Clinical features and patient outcomes of hidradenitis suppurativa: a cross-sectional retrospective study. J Cutan Med Surg. 2015; pii: 1203475415602840.

Chapter 9
Skin and Soft Tissue Infections

Massimo Sartelli and Fikri M. Abu-Zidan

9.1 Introduction

Skin and soft tissue infections (SSTIs) include many pathological conditions involving the skin and the underlying subcutaneous tissue, fascia, or muscle. They may range from simple superficial infections to severe necrotizing infections.

M. Sartelli, MD (✉)
Department of Surgery, Macerata Hospital, Macerata, Italy
e-mail: massimosartelli@gmail.com

F.M. Abu-Zidan, MD, FACS, FRCS, PhD, DAST
Department of Surgery, College of Medicine and Health Sciences, UAE University, Al-Ain, Abu Dhabi, UAE
e-mail: fabuzidan@uaeu.ac.ae

© Springer International Publishing Switzerland 2017   149
S. Di Saverio et al. (eds.), *Acute Care Surgery Handbook*,
DOI 10.1007/978-3-319-15341-4_9

9.2   Classification

Various systems of classification have been used to describe SSTIs based on the severity of infections, the anatomical tissue layers involved, and the presence of necrotizing component.

WSES classified soft tissue infections by the classification illustrated in Table 9.1 [1].

The first group includes surgical site infections (SSIs) of the soft tissues. They are considered a separate category of soft tissue infections. They are infections that occur after surgery within the surgical site at any depth from the skin itself and extend to the deepest cavity that remains after resection of an organ [2].

SSIs are classified into incisional and organ/space infections. Organ/space infections are not soft tissue infections. The incisional SSIs are further classified into superficial (skin and subcutaneous tissue) and deep infections (deep soft tissue–muscle and fascia).

Table 9.1 WSES classification for soft tissue infections

| **Surgical site infections** |
| Incisional |
| *Superficial* |
| *Deep* |
| **Non-necrotizing SSTIs** |
| *Superficial infections (Impetigo, erysipelas, cellulitis)* |
| *Simple abscess, boils, and carbuncles* |
| *Complex abscesses* |
| **Necrotizing SSTIs (NSTIs)** |
| *Necrotizing cellulitis* |
| *Necrotizing fasciitis* |
| *Fournier's gangrene* |
| *Necrotizing myositis* |

Soft tissue non-surgical site infections are divided into non-necrotizing and necrotizing soft tissue infections. Non-necrotizing soft tissue infections include superficial infections, complex abscesses, and infections developing in damaged skin.

Necrotizing soft tissue infections (NSTIs) are life-threatening, invasive, soft tissue infections associated with widespread necrosis and systemic toxicity. They may involve dermal and subcutaneous components (necrotizing cellulitis), fascial component (necrotizing fasciitis (NF)), and muscular components (necrotizing myositis). Fournier's gangrene is a progressive variant of necrotizing fasciitis involving the external genitalia and perineum.

NSTIs are also usually classified into three groups based on their bacterial pathogens initiating the infection: type 1 – poly-microbial, type 2 – mono-microbial pathogenic β-hemolytic *Streptococci* or community acquired methicillin-resistant *Staphylococcus aureus* CA-MRSA, and type 3 – mono-microbial secondary to a virulent gram-positive or gram-negative bacilli such as *Clostridia*, *Vibrio*, *Aeromonas*, *Eikenella*, and *Bacillus* species.

9.3   Principles of Treatment

9.3.1   Antimicrobial Therapy

The majority of SSTIs are caused by aerobic gram-positive cocci, such as *Staphylococcus aureus* and *Streptococci*. Aerobic gram-negative bacteria and anaerobes may occur in surgical site infections following surgery on the gastrointestinal, or genito-urinary tract or soft tissue infections in the perineum or the genitourinary tract.

Among gram-positive bacteria, some strains of *S. aureus* and β-hemolytic *Streptococci* can produce toxins that may affect the severity of the soft tissue infection [1].

In the last years, emergence of *Staphylococcus aureus* resistant to penicillin has complicated antimicrobial therapy for SSTIs. Methicillin-resistant *Staphylococcus aureus* (MRSA) are usually acquired during exposure to healthcare facilities. However, in the last years, there has been an increase in MRSA infections presenting in the community (CA-MRSA) [3].

CA-MRSA strains are genetically and phenotypically distinct from hospital-acquired MRSA (HA-MRSA). They may be susceptible to a wider range of antistaphylococcal antimicrobials, and may produce the pathogenic Panton–Valentine leukocidin (PVL) toxin, a toxin that destroys white blood cells. The staphylococcal virulence factor [3] aggravates the severity of infection. Staphylococcal resistance to glycopeptides remains rare [4].

For empirical coverage of CA-MRSA in outpatients having SSTI, oral antibiotic options include clindamycin, trimethoprim-sulfamethoxazole (TMP-SMX), a tetracycline (doxycycline or minocycline), and linezolid. If coverage for both β-hemolytic *Streptococci* and CA-MRSA is required, options include clindamycin alone or TMP-SMX or a tetracycline in association with a β-lactam (e.g., amoxicillin) or linezolid alone [5].

For hospitalized patients with severe SSTI, in addition to surgical debridement and broad-spectrum antibiotics, empirical therapy for MRSA should be considered, pending culture data. Options include intravenous (IV) vancomycin 15–20 mg/kg/dose IV every 8–12 h, orally or IV linezolid 600 mg twice daily, daptomycin 4/6 mg/kg/dose IV once daily, IV or orally clindamycin 600 mg 3 times every day [5], tigecycline 100 mg IV loading dose, then 50 mg twice daily.

Staphylococcal resistance to glycopeptides remains rare, although rising minimal inhibitory concentrations (MICs) of glycopeptides may affect the efficacy of these antibiotics [1].

New antibiotics, such as dalbavancin and tedizolid, are extremely valuable additions to treatment options due to the convenient dosing regimen and the fact that there are fewer resistant organisms to these therapies at this time [6]. Telizolid is a second-generation oxazolidinone approved for the treatment of acute bacterial skin and skin structure infections (ABSSSIs). In a randomized, double-blind, phase 3, non-inferiority trial (ESTABLISH-2), once-daily tedizolid 200 mg for 6 days was non-inferior to twice-daily linezolid 600 mg for 10 days for treatment of patients with ABSSSIs [7].

9.3.2   Source Control

Source control represents a key component of success in the management of soft tissue infections [1]. Source control for SSTIs includes drainage of infected fluids, debridement of infected soft tissues, and removal of infected devices or foreign bodies.

In the setting of necrotizing infections, it must be prompt and aggressive in order to halt the progression of the infectious process.

9.4   Surgical Site Infections (SSIs)

The development of the SSIs depends on the contamination of the wound site during the surgical procedure. Surgical site infections may be caused by a variety of micro-organisms. In patients who have undergone clean operations, they are frequently caused by gram-positive organisms. In contrast, they may be caused by both gram-positive and gram-negative organisms in patients who had gastrointestinal or genitourinary surgery.

Treatment includes opening the incision. Antimicrobial therapy is required if source control is not complete or in immunocompromised patients. Broad-spectrum empiric antimicrobial therapy should be initially administered to cover potentially resistant pathogens [1].

9.5 Non-necrotizing SSTIs

Superficial infections are spread within the epidermis, dermis, and the subcutaneous tissue. They may be managed either by antibiotics alone or, in the case of a well-circumscribed abscess, by drainage alone.

Superficial infections present as impetigo, erysipelas, and cellulitis. They are usually caused by gram-positive bacteria, particularly *Streptococci* and *S. aureus*. Cellulitis is an acute bacterial infection of the dermis and the subcutaneous tissue that may cause local signs of inflammation, such as warmth, erythema, pain, lymphangitis, and systemic effects like fever and leukocytosis [1].

Therapy for these infections should include antibiotics active against *Streptococci* and *S. aureus*. A penicillinase-resistant penicillin is the drug of choice, although first-generation cephalosporin is an alternative. In the case of allergy to beta lactams, a fluoroquinolone regimen with either levofloxacin or moxifloxacin can be used.

Lack of clinical response could be due to resistant strains, or deeper active processes, such as necrotizing fasciitis or myonecrosis. In patients who become increasingly ill, deeper infections should be always suspected [1].

Incision and drainage is the primary treatment for a simple superficial abscess or a boil without the need for antibiotics [1].

Complicated abscesses can be caused by perineal or perianal infections, perirectal abscesses, diabetic foot or lower-extremity ulcerations, traumatic injuries, chronic cutaneous cysts, intravenous drug injection sites, gastrointestinal pathology with perforation, genitourinary pathology, animal bites, and pressure ulcers. Complicated skin and subcutaneous abscesses are typically well circumscribed and respond to incision and drainage with adjuvant antibiotic therapy.

Antimicrobial therapy is required in immunocompromised patients, if source control is incomplete, and for abscesses associated with significant cellulitis. The initiating pathogens differ according to the originating site. Aerobic gram-positive pathogens are isolated in most complicated abscesses. Depending on the origin, anaerobes, *Enterobacteriaceae*, and *Clostridium* spp. can be isolated.

9.6   Necrotizing Soft Tissue Infections (NSTIs)

NSTIs include necrotizing cellulitis, necrotizing fasciitis, necrotizing myositis, and Fournier's gangrene. They are life-threatening aggressive soft tissue infections. Delay in treating these infections increases the risk of mortality.

NSTI can involve any part of the body but primarily the extremities, abdomen, and perineum [8].

NSTIs can be precipitated by various conditions like blunt or penetrating trauma, surgical site infection, burns, ulcers, abscess, improperly treated superficial infections, body piercing and tattooing, and even minor injury such as abrasions and insect bites. Occasionally, NSTI occurs without an identifiable cause [9].

Predisposing factors for necrotizing fasciitis include diabetes mellitus, immunosuppression, HIV, tuberculosis, and chickenpox. It is important to look for an underlying cause of immunosuppression, although it may not always be found [10, 11].

The mortality associated with NSTI is high ranging from 6 to 76 % [8]. Necrotizing cellulitis is usually similar to non-necrotizing cellulitis in bacterial etiology and pathogenesis but may be rapidly progressive and accompanied by significant systemic inflammatory changes (toxic shock syndrome). Necrotizing fasciitis (NF) involves the fascial planes overlying the muscle (Fig. 9.1). It is characterized by extensive, rapidly progressive necrosis involving the fascia and perifascial planes [1]. Fournier's gangrene is a rapidly progressive, variant of necrotizing fasciitis involving the external genitalia and perineum. Because of the complexity of fascial planes, this infection may extend up to the abdominal wall, down into the perirectal and gluteal spaces, and, occasionally, into the retroperitoneum [1]. Necrotizing myositis is a rare infection of the muscle with local and systemic complications [1].

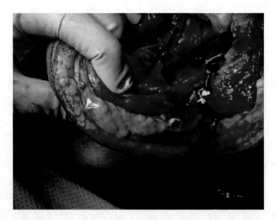

Fig. 9.1 The clinical presentation of necrotizing fasciitis is very deceiving. The skin looks normal while the necrosis of the fascia spreads swiftly under the skin. This spread may be dramatic within few hours, and the general condition of the patient may deteriorate quickly. The most important clinical finding is severe tenderness disproportionate with the appearance of the skin (Courtesy of Professor Fikri Abu-Zidan, Al-Ain Hospital, Al-Ain, UAE)

9.6.1   Diagnosis

It may be initially difficult to distinguish cellulitis from necrotizing soft tissue infection. Most cases of necrotizing soft tissue infections are originally diagnosed as cellulitis. However, early diagnosis and surgery improve the outcome of NSTIs. Patients with necrotizing soft tissue infections usually have severe pain that is out of proportion to the physical findings [12].

Physical findings of necrotizing soft tissue infections include tenderness beyond the area of erythema, crepitus, and cellulitis that is refractory to antimicrobial therapy. Crepitus is usually caused by gas within tissues. The presence of crepitus and gas within tissues is suggestive of NSTI. Nevertheless, its absence does not rule out its presence.

A rapidly progressive soft tissue infection should be always treated as a necrotizing infection until proven otherwise. The clinical picture may worsen very quickly during few hours.

In order to predict the presence of necrotizing soft tissue infection, a Laboratory Risk Indicator for Necrotizing infection (LRINEC) score was reported [13]. This scoring system assigned points for abnormalities in six independent variables: serum C-reactive protein level (>150 mg/L), WBC count (> 15,000/μL), hemoglobin level (< 13.5 g/dL), serum sodium level (< 135 mmol/L), serum creatinine level (> 1.6 mg/dL), and serum glucose level (> 180 mg/dL). With a score of 8 or higher, there is a 75 % risk of having necrotizing soft tissue infection.

The diagnosis of NSTIs is primarily clinical. However, plain radiographs, ultrasound, computed tomography (CT), and magnetic resonance imaging (MRI) may help the diagnosis of necrotizing infection when uncertain [1].

Ultrasound has the advantage of being rapidly performed at bedside in critically-ill patients who are unable to perform CT or MRI and may be helpful in differentiating simple cellulitis from necrotizing fasciitis in the emergency setting [14].

Subcutaneous air will show as shiny white dots in the facial plane while edema will show as hypoechoic areas (Fig. 9.2)

Computed tomography (CT) has higher sensitivity in identifying early NSTI. CT findings of patients with NF include fat stranding, fluid and gas collections that dissect along fascial planes [15], and gas in the involved soft tissues (Fig. 9.3). Additionally, fascial thickening and non-enhancing fascia on contrast CT suggest fascial necrosis [16, 17].

Although MRI can be difficult to perform under emergency situations, it may be useful in diagnosing NSTI [18, 19]. The MRI findings of patients with necrotizing fasciitis include thick (≥3 mm) abnormal signal intensity on fat-suppressed T2-weighted images, low signal intensity in the deep fascia on

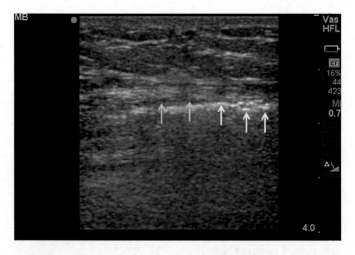

Fig. 9.2 Surgeon performed point-of-care ultrasound of the thigh of a 56-year-old diabetic male having necrotizing fasciitis using a linear probe. The B mode image shows hypoechoic areas representing edema (*yellow arrows*) and hyperechoic white spots (*white arrows*) representing gas in the subcutaneous tissue (Courtesy of Professor Fikri Abu-Zidan, Al-Ain Hospital, Al-Ain, UAE)

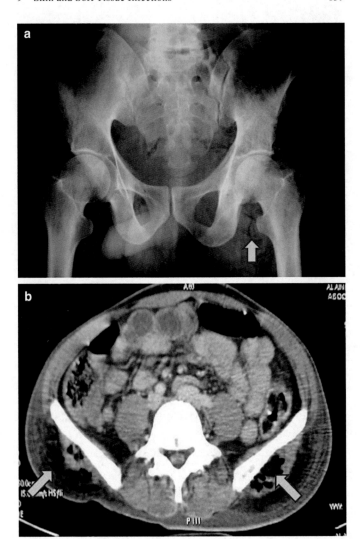

Fig. 9.3 A 45-year-old diabetic man presented to the Emergency Department, Al-Ain Hospital complaining of severe gluteal pain following a needle injection. Plain X-ray (**a**) and CT scan of the pelvis (**b**) showed extensive subcutaneous air in both gluteal regions (*yellow arrows*) (Courtesy of Professor Fikri Abu-Zidan, Al-Ain Hospital, Al-Ain, UAE)

fat-suppressed T2-weighted images, a focal or diffuse non-enhancing portion in the area of abnormal signal intensity in the deep fascia, extensive involvement of the deep fascia, and involvement of three or more compartments in one extremity.

9.6.2 Management of NSTI

Patients with severe sepsis or septic shock caused by NSTI require early source control, antimicrobial therapy, and supportive treatment. Early admission to ICU and aggressive resuscitation is advised for septic patients [10].

9.6.3 Source Control

The management of necrotizing fasciitis is mainly surgical by removing the necrotic tissue which is the cause of organ failure. Antibiotic treatment is only supportive and would not help if all necrotic tissues were not excised (Fig. 9.4). The most important factor for reducing mortality of patients with NSTI is early recognition and urgent operative debridement [20]. Surgical debridement should be aggressive to control the progression of infection. Any patient with diffuse necrosis or who has not been adequately debrided should be returned to the operating room in

---

Fig. 9.4 A 52-year-old diabetic man presented with perianal pain of 10 days duration. Clinical examination showed a normal skin but severe tenderness around the anus ((**a**), hashed area). Exploration under general anesthesia showed extensive necrotizing fasciitis in the same area (**b**). The patient has been taken repeatedly to the theater till the wound became clear 1 week later (**c**). The wound became healthy with nice granulation tissue within 2 weeks (**d**) (Courtesy of Professor Fikri Abu-Zidan, Al-Ain Hospital, Al-Ain, UAE)

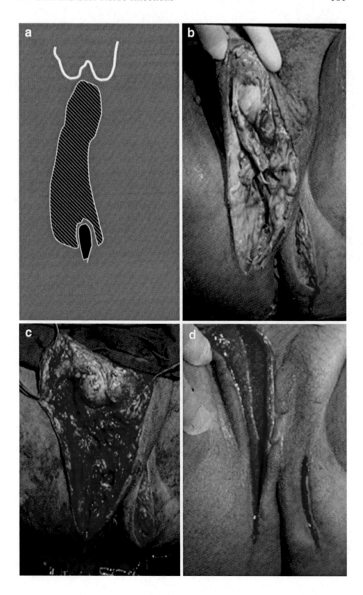

24–48 h for a second look [1]. Further debridement should be repeated until the infection is controlled.

9.6.4   Antimicrobial Therapy

Early empiric coverage against suspected pathogens should be started, based upon the clinical setting for patients with NSTI. Since it is impossible to exclude with certainty a poly-microbial infection, an aggressive empiric broad-spectrum antimicrobial therapy toward gram-positive, gram-negative, and anaerobic organisms should be started as soon as possible in patients with suspected NSTI. Subsequent modification (de-escalation) of the initial regimen becomes possible later, when culture results are available and clinical status can be better assessed

An acceptable empiric antimicrobial regimen should always include antibiotics covering MRSA with the additional benefit of inhibiting invasive group A *Streptococcus* virulence proteins. Selection of antibiotics that inhibit toxin production such as clindamycin or linezolid may be helpful, particularly in those patients who have evidence of toxic shock syndrome. This potentially occurs in patients having streptococcal and staphylococcal infections [1].

9.6.5   Supportive Treatment

Early detection of severe sepsis and prompt aggressive treatment of the underlying organ dysfunction are essential components for improving outcome of critically ill patients.

Deep soft tissue infections may have a fulminant course and may be associated with high morbidity and mortality, especially when they occur in conjunction with toxic shock syndrome [1].

9.6.6 Intravenous Immunoglobulin

The use of intravenous immunoglobulin for treating necrotizing soft tissue infections remains controversial [21]. There is little evidence supporting its benefits in treating necrotizing soft tissue infections. It is based on a potential benefit related to neutralizing circulating exotoxins produced by gram-positive organisms and modulating the systemic inflammatory response induced by cytokine stimulation [22]. Early immunoglobulins should be limited to patients having NSTI and presenting organ dysfunction.

9.6.7 Hyperbaric Oxygen Therapy

The role of Hyperbaric oxygen therapy in the treatment of patients with NSTI is still controversial, because there is little evidence supporting its value [23].

Important Learning Points
- Various classification systems have been used to describe skin and soft tissue infections based on the severity of infection, the anatomical tissue layers involved, and the presence of a necrotizing component.
- Necrotizing soft tissue infections (NSTIs) are life-threatening, aggressive infections. Delay in treating these infections increases mortality.
- Distinguishing cellulitis from necrotizing soft tissue infection may be difficult. Most cases of necrotizing soft tissue infections are originally diagnosed as cellulitis.

- The diagnosis of NSTIs is primarily a clinical diagnosis. However, ultrasound, computed tomography, and magnetic resonance imaging may help this diagnosis when uncertain.
- The management of NSTIs is mainly surgical by removing the necrotic tissue which is the cause of organ failure. Antibiotic treatment is only supportive and would not help if all necrotic tissues were not removed.
- Since it is impossible to exclude with certainty a polymicrobial infection, an aggressive empiric broad-spectrum antimicrobial therapy toward gram-positive, gram-negative, and anaerobic organisms should be started as soon as possible in patients with suspected NSTIs.

References

1. Sartelli M, Malangoni MA, May AK, Viale P, Kao LS, Catena F, Ansaloni L, Moore EE, Moore FA, Peitzman AB, Coimbra R, Leppaniemi A, Kluger Y, Biffl W, Koike K, Girardis M, Ordonez CA, Tavola M, Cainzos M, Di Saverio S, Fraga GP, Gerych I, Kelly MD, Taviloglu K, Wani I, Marwah S, Bala M, Ghnnam W, Shaikh N, Chiara O, Faro Jr MP, Pereira Jr GA, Gomes CA, Coccolini F, Tranà C, Corbella D, Brambillasca P, Cui Y, Segovia Lohse HA, Khokha V, Kok KY, Hong SK, Yuan KC. World Society of Emergency Surgery (WSES) guidelines for management of skin and soft tissue infections. World J Emerg Surg. 2014;9(1):57.
2. Barie PS, Eachempati SR. Surgical site infections. Surg Clin North Am. 2005;85(6):1115–35.
3. Nathwani D, Morgan M, Masterton RG, Dryden M, Cookson BD, French G, Lewis D, British Society for Antimicrobial Chemotherapy Working Party on Community-onset MRSA Infections. Guidelines for UK practice for the diagnosis and management of methicillin-resistant Staphylococcus aureus (MRSA) infections presenting in the community. J Antimicrob Chemother. 2008;61(5):976–94.
4. Awad SS, Elhabash SI, Lee L, Farrow B, Berger DH. Increasing incidence of methicillin-resistant Staphylococcus aureus skin and soft-

tissue infections: reconsideration of empiric antimicrobial therapy. Am J Surg. 2007;194:606–10.

5. Liu C, Bayer A, Cosgrove SE, Daum RS, Fridkin SK, Gorwitz RJ, Kaplan SL, Karchmer AW, Levine DP, Murray BE, J Rybak M, Talan DA, Chambers HF, Infectious Diseases Society of America. . Clinical practice guidelines by the infectious diseases society of America for the treatment of Methicillin-resistant Staphylococcus Aureus infections in adults and children. Clin Infect Dis. 2011;52(3):e18–55.

6. Gleghorn K, Grimshaw E, Kelly EK. New antibiotics in the management of acute bacterial skin and skin structure infections. Skin Therapy Lett. 2015;20(5):7–9.

7. Moran GJ, Fang E, Corey GR, Das AF, De Anda C, Prokocimer P. Tedizolid for 6 days versus linezolid for 10 days for acute bacterial skin and skin-structure infections (ESTABLISH-2): a randomised, double-blind, phase 3, non-inferiority trial. Lancet Infect Dis. 2014;14(8):696–705.

8. Anaya DA, McMahon K, Nathens AB, Sullivan SR, Foy H, Bulger E. Predictors of mortality and limb loss in necrotizing soft tissue infections. Arch Surg. 2005;140(2):151–7.

9. Taviloglu K, Cabioglu N, Cagatay A, Yanar H, Ertekin C, Baspinar I, Ozsut H, Guloglu R. Idiopathic necrotizing fasciitis: risk factors and strategies for management. Am Surg. 2005;71(4):315–20.

10. Hefny AF, Eid HO, Al-Hussona M, Idris KM, Abu-Zidan FM. Necrotizing fasciitis: a challenging diagnosis. Eur J Emerg Med. 2007;14:50–2.

11. Hefny AF, Abu-Zidan FM. Necrotizing fasciitis as an early manifestation of tuberculosis: report of two cases. Ulus Travma Acil Cerrahi Derg. 2010;16:174–6.

12. Benjelloun el B, Souiki T, Yakla N, Ousadden A, Mazaz K, Louchi A, Kanjaa N, Taleb KA. Fournier's gangrene: our experience with 50 patients and analysis of factors affecting mortality. World J Emerg Surg. 2013;8:13.

13. Wong CH, Khin LW, Heng KS, Tan KC, Low CO. The LRINEC (Laboratory Risk Indicator for Necrotizing Fasciitis) score: a tool for distinguishing necrotizing fasciitis from other soft tissue infections. Crit Care Med. 2004;32:1535.

14. Yen ZS, Wang HP, Ma HM, Chen SC, Chen WJ. Ultrasonographic screening of clinically-suspected necrotizing fasciitis. Acad Emerg Med. 2002;9(12):1448–51.

15. Abu-Zidan FM, Al-Hussona M, Eid HO, Czechowski J. Massive necrotizing fasciitis. J Trauma. 2008;64:241.

16. Walshaw CF, Deans H. CT findings in necrotising fasciitis—a report of four cases. Clin Radiol. 1996;51(6):429–32.

17. Zacharias N, Velmahos GC, Salama A, Alam HB, de Moya M, King DR, Novelline RA. Diagnosis of necrotizing soft tissue infections by computed tomography. Arch Surg. 2010;145(5):452–5.
18. Kim KT, Kim YJ, Won Lee J, Kim YJ, Park SW, Lim MK, Suh CH. Can necrotizing infectious fasciitis be differentiated from nonnecrotizing infectious fasciitis with MR imaging? Radiology. 2011;259(3):816–24.
19. Schmid MR, Kossmann T, Duewell S. Differentiation of necrotizing fasciitis and cellulitis using MR imaging. Am J Roentgenol. 1998;170(3):615–20.
20. McHenry CR, Piotrowski JJ, Petrinic D, Malangoni MA. Determinants of mortality for necrotizing soft tissue infections. Ann Surg. 1995;221:558.
21. Darenberg J, Ihendyane N, Sjölin J, Aufwerber E, Haidl S, Follin P, Andersson J, Norrby-Teglund A, StreptIg Study Group. Intravenous immunoglobulin G therapy in streptococcal toxic shock syndrome: a European randomized, double-blind, placebo-controlled trial. Clin Infect Dis. 2003;37(3):333–40.
22. Koch C, Hecker A, Grau V, Padberg W, Wolff M, Henrich M. Intravenous immunoglobulin in necrotizing fasciitis - a case report and review of recent literature. Ann Med Surg (Lond). 2015;4(3):260–3.
23. Eskes A, Vermeulen H, Lucas C, Ubbink DT. Hyperbaric oxygen therapy for treating acute surgical and traumatic wounds. Cochrane Database Syst Rev. 2013;(12):CD008059.

Chapter 10
Surgical Site Infections and Their Management

Mark A. Malangoni

10.1 Background

Surgical site infections (SSIs) is a common postoperative complication and accounts for 15–17 % of all nosocomial infections. Surgical site infections occur following 2–5 % of all inpatient operations and in up to 20 % of patients undergoing emergency intra-abdominal procedures [1]. Their incidence is less among patients having ambulatory surgery. The mortality of SSIs is estimated at about 2 %, with most deaths related to deep and organ/space infections. Importantly, 75 % of deaths among these patients are directly attributable to the SSI. Surgical site infections also result in substantial short- and long-term morbidity, prolonged hospital stays, excessive readmissions, and additional home healthcare. They are estimated to increase healthcare

M.A. Malangoni, MD

American Board of Surgery, University of Pennsylvania Perelman School of Medicine, 1617 John F. Kennedy Blvd., Suite 860, Philadelphia, PA 19103, USA

e-mail: mmalangoni@absurgery.org

© Springer International Publishing Switzerland 2017
S. Di Saverio et al. (eds.), *Acute Care Surgery Handbook*,
DOI 10.1007/978-3-319-15341-4_10

costs by $10 billion annually. Most importantly, they are a source of patient dissatisfaction related to associated pain and discomfort, inconvenience, long-term disability, and expense.

Potential complications associated with SSIs include impaired wound healing, incisional hernias, and excessive scarring. Importantly, it has been estimated that 40–50 % of these infections are preventable. Minimizing SSIs should be a high priority for surgeons and healthcare institutions to ensure a safer environment for surgical care.

10.2 Definition

There is controversy among surgeons and other interested parties about what actually constitutes an SSI. This is particularly true when there is evidence of cellulitis around an incision in the absence of systemic perturbations or other local signs of concern.

Surgical site infections can occur at any depth from the skin to the deepest organ or cavity involved in the operation. A superficial infection involves only the skin and subcutaneous tissues while a deep SSI involves the fascia and muscular tissue (Fig. 10.1). Organ/space infections are below the fascia and either involve a solid organ or are intracavitary. The National Health Safety Network (NHSN) of the Centers for Disease Control and Prevention (CDC) has developed criteria for defining an SSI (Table 10.1).

10.3 Epidemiology and Pathogenesis

We are constantly exposed regularly to microorganisms in our environment; yet, infection is uncommon in healthy individuals with intact host defenses. These microbes populate our skin and

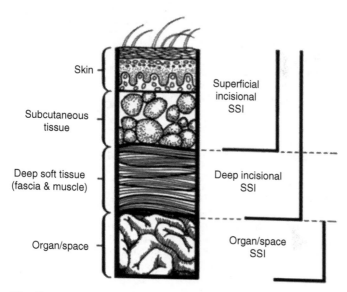

Fig. 10.1 Cross section of abdominal wall depicting the CDC classification of surgical site infection (Adapted from Horan et al. [2])

mucous membranes as well as some organs but usually exist in a commensal relationship with humans as their hosts.

Microbial contamination of the surgical site is a necessary precursor for SSI. This happens most commonly when an incision is exposed to the patient's exogenous or endogenous bacterial flora. Exposure can also occur from healthcare personnel, the operating environment, or from contaminated equipment or instruments. Less commonly, the surgical site can be contaminated by hematogenous seeding from a remote site of infection.

Infection occurs when there is an imbalance among the degree of contamination, host defenses, and the environment. Contamination is influenced by inoculum size and virulence of the involved organisms. Examples of local host factors include desiccation or tissue damage at the incision, and a hematoma or seroma at the surgical site. There also are a variety of systemic,

Table 10.1 Criteria for defining a surgical site infection (NHSN, 2008)

Superficial incisional SSI

Infection occurs within 30 days after the operation and infection involves only skin or subcutaneous tissue of the incision and at least one of the following:

1. Purulent drainage from the superficial incision.
2. Organisms isolated from an aseptically obtained culture of fluid or tissue from the superficial incision.
3. At least one of the following signs or symptoms of infection (pain or tenderness, localized swelling, redness, or heat) and superficial incision is deliberately opened by surgeon, and is culture-positive or is not cultured.
4. Diagnosis of superficial incisional SSI is made by the surgeon or attending physician.

Deep incisional SSI

Infection occurs within 30 days after the operation if no implant is left in place or within 1 year if an implant is in place and the infection appears to be related to the operative procedure, involves deep soft tissues (e.g., fascial and muscle layers) of the incision, and the patient has at least one of the following:

1. Purulent drainage from the deep incision but not from the organ/space component of the surgical site.
2. A deep incision spontaneously dehisces or is deliberately opened by a surgeon and is culture-positive or not cultured and the patient has at least one of the following signs or symptoms: temperature >38 °C or localized pain or tenderness (a culture-negative finding does not meet this criterion).
3. An abscess or other evidence of infection involving the deep incision is found on direct examination, during reoperation, or by histopathologic or radiologic examination.
4. Diagnosis of a deep incisional SSI is made by a surgeon or attending physician.

Note:

An infection that involves both superficial and deep incision sites should be reported as a deep incisional SSI

An organ/space SSI that drains through the incision should be reported as a deep incisional SSI

Table 10.1 (continued)

Organ/Space SSI

Infection involves any part of the body, excluding the skin incision, fascia, or muscle layers, that is opened or manipulated during the operative procedure. Specific sites are assigned to organ/space SSI to further identify the location of the infection (e.g., endocarditis, endometritis, mediastinitis, vaginal cuff, and osteomyelitis). Organ/space SSI must meet the following criteria:

1. Infection occurs within 30 days after the operative procedure if no implant is in place or within 1 year if implant is in place and the infection appears to be related to the operative procedure.

2. Infection involves any part of the body, excluding the skin incision, fascia, or muscle layers, that is opened or manipulated during the operative procedure, and the patient has at least one of the following: purulent drainage from a drain that is placed through a stab wound into the organ/space, organisms isolated from an aseptically obtained culture of fluid or tissue in the organ/space, an abscess or other evidence of infection involving the organ/space that is found on direct examination, during reoperation, or by histopathologic or radiologic examination, and diagnosis of an organ/space SSI by a surgeon or attending physician

---

Adapted from Horan et al. [3]

environmental, and treatment-related factors associated with an increased propensity to develop an SSI (Table 10.2).

The risk of SSI is highly dependent on the degree of contamination and is markedly increased when the inoculum is $>10^7$ microorganisms per gram of tissue. However, a much lower dose of contaminating microorganisms can produce infection when foreign material is present or if the host or local environment is compromised by other factors or conditions [4].

10.4 Risk Factors

There are a number of risk factors that have been identified to influence the occurrence of SSI (Table 10.2). Understanding the

Table 10.2 Risk factors for the development of surgical site infection

Local factors
Damage from electrocautery
Degree of contamination
Duration of expose to contamination
Hematoma or seroma
Poor operative technique
Prior irradiation of the site
Skin disease at or near the incision
Tissue desiccation
Tissue hypoxemia
Systemic factors
Abnormalities of coagulation
Advanced age
Altered immune response
Anemia
Chronic liver disease
Chronic inflammation
Chronic renal disease
Corticosteroid therapy
Diabetes mellitus
Hypoalbuminemia
Hypovolemic shock
Hypoxemia
Infection at a remote body site
Malnutrition
Obesity
Organ dysfunction
Peripheral vascular disease
Smoking
Environmental factors
Contamination from personnel
Inadequate disinfection/sterilization
Inadequate skin antisepsis
Preoperative hair removal
Preoperative skin preparation
Substandard operating room ventilation

Table 10.2 (Continued)

Treatment factors
Drains
Hypothermia
Prolonged operative time
Prolonged preoperative hospitalization

contribution of each of these elements to the occurrence of SSI encourages targeted interventions aimed at reducing the incidence of infection. It is useful to explore some of the risk factors that are potentially controllable in some detail.

Increased serum glucose (>200 mg/dL) in the postoperative period has been associated with a greater incidence of SSI, particularly among patients undergoing cardiac surgery [5]. It has also been suggested that chronic glucose control as assessed by serum hemoglobin A1c levels may influence infection risk [6]. The independent contribution of diabetes mellitus to SSI risk is difficult to discern, since most studies do not control for confounding factors.

Nicotine use delays primary wound healing and may increase the risk of SSI via this mechanism. In a large prospective study, current smoking of cigarettes was an independent risk factor for sternal and/or mediastinal deep SSI following cardiac surgery [7]. Others have corroborated cigarette smoking as an important risk factor [8].

Although individual comorbid conditions may have some impact on infection risk, results from the NNIS have demonstrated that the overall predictive risk of SSI can be assessed by using the American Society of Anesthesiologists (ASA) physical status score, duration of operation, and incision classification (Tables 10.3 and 10.4). Assigning one point each when the ASA physical status score is ≥3, duration of operation exceeds the 75th percentile for the particular operation, and incision site (wound) class is contaminated or dirty, provides a reasonably accurate prediction for the risk of SSI [9]. This model is most accurate to predict the occurrence of superficial SSI. There may be different risk factors for deep and organ/space SSI [10].

Table 10.3 American Society of Anesthesiology (ASA) physical status score

ASA 1- A normal healthy patient
ASA 2- A patient with mild to moderate systemic disturbance that does not result in functional limitations. Examples: Hypertension, diabetes mellitus, chronic bronchitis, morbid obesity, and extremes of age
ASA 3- A patient with severe systemic disturbance that may result in functional limitations but is not incapacitating. Examples: Poorly controlled hypertension, diabetes mellitus with vascular complications, angina pectoris, prior myocardial infarction, and pulmonary disease that limits activity
ASA 4- A patient with a severe systemic disturbance that is life threatening with or without the planned procedure. Examples: Congestive heart failure, unstable angina pectoris, advanced pulmonary, and renal or hepatic dysfunction
ASA 5- A moribund patient who is not expected to survive with or without the operative procedure. Examples: Ruptured abdominal aortic aneurysm, pulmonary embolism, and head injury with increased intracranial pressure

Since development of the NNIS risk model, it has been recognized that the method by which an operation is done also affects SSI risk. For example, laparoscopic cholecystectomy, the predominant method of gallbladder removal, is associated with a lesser risk of SSI than an open cholecystectomy even when adjusted for other risk factors. It has been postulated that the reasons for this phenomenon include a smaller incision, less exposure of the incision site to bacterial contamination, reduced local trauma at the incision site, and a diminished stress response induced by laparoscopic operations. In order to adjust for this phenomenon, it has been suggested that the NNIS risk score should be reduced by one factor when an operation is done laparoscopically [2].

Every patient should be assessed for risk factors that can be corrected in the preoperative period before elective surgery. In addition, any open skin lesions should be healed and the patient should be free of other bacterial infections of any kind. The

Table 10.4 Surgical wound classification

Clean: An operative wound in which no inflammation or infection is encountered and the respiratory, alimentary, genital, or uninfected urinary tracts are not entered. In addition, clean wounds are primarily closed with or without closed drainage. Operative incisional wounds that follow nonpenetrating (blunt) trauma should be included in this category if they otherwise meet the criteria

Clean-contaminated: An operative wound in which the respiratory, alimentary, genital, or urinary tracts are entered under controlled conditions and without unusual contamination. Specifically, operations involving the biliary tract, appendix, vagina, and oropharynx are included in this category, provided no evidence of infection or major break in technique is encountered

Contaminated: Open, fresh, accidental wounds. In addition, operations with major breaks in aseptic technique (e.g., open cardiac massage) or gross spillage from the gastrointestinal tract, and incisions in which acute, nonpurulent inflammation is encountered are included in this category

Dirty-infected: Old traumatic wounds with retained devitalized tissue and those that involve existing clinical infection or perforated viscera. This definition suggests that the organisms causing postoperative infection were present in the operative field before the operation

---

patient should cease smoking, preferably at least 1 month before the operation. Patients should bathe or shower with an antibacterial soap such as chlorhexidine the night before – and some say the morning of – the operation [11]. If hair removal is necessary, it should be clipped rather than shaved immediately prior to operation, since the use of a razor for hair removal increases the likelihood of SSI. Depilatories are another option but sometimes produce a hypersensitivity reaction.

Several antiseptic agents are commonly available for preoperative skin preparation of the operative site (Table 10.5). Alcohol-containing products, chlorhexidine gluconate, and iodophors (e.g., povidone-iodine) are the most commonly used agents. No well-controlled, operation-specific studies have determined the superiority of any of these skin antiseptics to

Table 10.5 Antiseptic agents commonly used for preoperative skin preparation

Agent	Mechanism of action	Rapidity of effect	Residual activity	Toxicity	Comments
Alcohol	Denatures proteins	Immediate	None	Volatile; drying	Most effective against gram-positive and gram-negative bacteria, mycobacteria, fungi, and viruses
Chlorhexidine	Disrupts cell membranes	Intermediate	Excellent	Ototoxicity; keratitis	Most effective against gram-positive and gram-negative bacteria
Iodophors	Oxidation	Intermediate	Minimal	Skin irritation	Most effective against gram-positive and gram-negative bacteria, mycobacteria, fungi, and viruses

prevent SSI. Alcohol-based products are readily available, inexpensive, and are the most rapid-acting skin antiseptic. Aqueous alcohol solutions have germicidal activity against bacteria, fungi, and viruses; however, many spores are resistant to these agents. One potential disadvantage of using alcohol solutions is their flammability. Both chlorhexidine gluconate and iodophors have a broad spectrum of antimicrobial activity (Table 10.5). In some comparisons of these antiseptics used as preoperative hand scrubs, chlorhexidine gluconate achieved greater reductions in skin microflora than povidone-iodine and also had greater residual activity after a single application. Chlorhexidine gluconate has the advantage of being resistant to inactivation by blood or serum proteins. Although iodophors can be inactivated by these proteins, they have the advantage of exerting a bacteriostatic effect as long as they are present on the skin. In certain situations, skin preparation may need to be modified, depending on the condition of the skin (e.g., burns) or the location of the incision (e.g., face).

Antiseptic agents appropriate for preoperative skin scrub by the surgical team that are commercially available in the United States include alcohol, chlorhexidine, iodophors, or parachloro-meta-xylenol (PCMX). There have not been controlled clinical trials assessing the utility of these agents on SSI risk. Some of these agents have an irritative effect when used repeatedly; this may lead operative team members to prefer one agent to another. This also emphasizes the importance of proper skin care and moisturization. There are other regulations about proper nail care and the avoidance of artificial nails. Double-gloving may also lower the risk of SSI by providing an extra barrier between the patient and skin of the operating room team members. Operating room personnel who have an active infection should avoid patient contact. Personnel who are carriers of *Staphylococcus aureus* should be evaluated by their institutional infection control practitioner to determine if decontamination is warranted.

10.5 Microbiology

The microbiology of SSI will usually vary depending on the operation being performed and the incision site. Most SSIs are caused by gram-positive cocci that are primarily skin or environmental contaminants, including *Staphylococcus aureus*, coagulase-negative staphylococci and *Enterococcus* species (Table 10.6). There is an increased likelihood of infection due to gram-negative bacilli following operations on the gastrointestinal, gynecologic, urologic, or respiratory tracts.

The microbiology of SSI has been remarkably consistent over time. Besides the prominence of gram-positive bacteria, there has been an increase in the frequency of antimicrobial-resistant bacteria and fungal organisms as causative of SSI. It is important to understand the microbial profile and antibiotic resistance patterns in your hospital in order to anticipate which organisms may be encountered in SSIs that are unique to the local environment.

Table 10.6 Microbiology of surgical site infection

Pathogen	Prevalence (% of isolates)
Staphylococcus aureus	20
Coagulase-negative staphylococci	14
Enterococcus sp.	12
Escherichia coli	8
Pseudomonas aeruginosa	8
Enterobacter sp.	7
Klebsiella pneumoniae	3
Proteus mirabilis	3
Miscellaneous streptococci	3
Candida	3

10.5.1   *Perioperative Antimicrobial Prophylaxis*

Perioperative antimicrobial prophylaxis (PAP) was determined to be effective in randomized clinical trials more than 45 years ago. Since then PAP has been repeatedly demonstrated to reduce the incidence of SSI when used properly and in the appropriate circumstances. The need for PAP is based in general on the wound class as anticipated preoperatively (Table 10.4). Prophylaxis is indicated for some clean operations, most clean-contaminated, and all contaminated (or potentially contaminated) operations. The administration of antibiotics in the course of operations where the wound class is dirty represents treatment for an established infection rather than prophylaxis.

There are some clean operations where PAP is indicated. Two well-recognized indications are when intravascular prosthetic material or a prosthetic device will be inserted, and for any operation in which an incisional or organ/space SSI would pose catastrophic risk. Examples include cardiac operations including cardiac pacemaker placement, vascular operations involving prosthetic graft placement at any site or revascularization of the lower extremities, and most neurosurgical operations (Table 10.4). Although some have advocated use of PAP during all operations on the breast and in hernia repairs when prosthetic materials are used, the data remain controversial [12].

Elective colon resections require additional consideration. Despite some recent controversy over whether mechanical bowel preparation is necessary, it has become apparent that mechanical bowel preparation on the day prior to operation is effective in reducing the SSI rate. Also, the administration of oral antimicrobials on the day prior to operation effectively reduces the incidence of SSI [13].

Table 10.7 Principles of antimicrobial prophylaxis

Select an antimicrobial agent that is safe, inexpensive, and has been demonstrated to be effective in preventing SSI in a prospective, randomized clinical trial for the operation in question. When this evidence is not available, an agent should be selected based on information about the microorganisms most likely to be involved in contamination at the incision site

Administer the drug intravenously within 30 min prior to making the skin incision. Some alternative agents (e.g., vancomycin, fluoroquinolones) must be given over a longer period and should be given within 60 min

Select an appropriate dose to assure an adequate drug concentration at the incision site when exposure to contamination first occurs. Dosage should be adjusted based on the patient's weight

Maintain a therapeutic concentration of the agent in the serum and exposed tissues during the entire operation. This may require redosing of agents based on their pattern of elimination and excretion. In general, antimicrobials should be redosed every two half-lives

Stop prophylaxis within 24 h of initiation. There is no benefit to a longer duration. In many procedures, a single dose is sufficient

The principles of PAP have been firmly established in prospective, randomized clinical trials (Table 10.7). These principles include selection of the appropriate antimicrobial, giving the appropriate dose, maintaining an adequate drug concentration at the surgical site throughout the operation, and stopping prophylaxis within 24 h after the operation. Exceptions to these standards include patients undergoing cesarean section in whom the initial dose is administered immediately following clamping of the umbilical cord, and patients undergoing cardiac surgery in which case PAP can be continued for up to 48 h [14].

The ideal properties of a prophylactic antimicrobial are listed in Table 10.8. There is little evidence suggesting that broad-spectrum antimicrobial agents are more effective in the prevention of postoperative SSI compared with older agents that have a narrower spectrum of activity. Cephalosporins are the most

Table 10.8 Ideal properties of an antimicrobial agent for prophylaxis

Has been demonstrated to prevent surgical site infection (SSI) based on prospective randomized clinical trials
Has no adverse effects for the patient
Does not affect the microbial flora for the institution or the community
Reduces the cost of healthcare
Can be administered in a single dose

thoroughly studied and commonly used agents for PAP. These drugs are effective across a broad spectrum of both gram-positive and gram-negative bacteria. Cephalosporins also have a demonstrated safety profile, acceptable pharmacokinetics, and are relatively inexpensive. These agents possess time-dependent bactericidal action.

The routine use of vancomycin for PAP is not recommended. However, vancomycin may be used in circumstances when the incidence of SSI due to methicillin-resistant *S. aureus* or methicillin-resistant coagulase-negative staphylococci is high. Fluoroqunolones are alternative agents for PAP and are useful in patients who are allergic to cephalosporins.

Traumatic injury poses an entirely different scenario. Severe injury can induce profound immunosuppression, and these patients are at high risk for infections of all types. Certain circumstances, including hemorrhagic shock, the need for blood transfusion, substantial contamination, and a high degree of injury severity, are independently associated with morbidity from infection [15]. Despite these unique characteristics and the fact that initiation of PAP often follows the time of contamination, the basic principles of PAP still apply. Although severe injury increases the risk of infection, this is not a justification for prolonged prophylaxis.

"On-call" prophylaxis regimens have been shown to be ineffective, since delays in transport or schedule changes can interfere with appropriate timely drug administration as outlined above. Most institutions initiate infusion of the prophylactic agent in the operating room or preoperative holding area in order to achieve optimal results.

Bratzler and colleagues conducted a retrospective study of 34,133 Medicare inpatients from 2,965 acute-care hospitals and evaluated patients undergoing cardiac surgery, vascular surgery, colorectal surgery, hip and knee total-joint arthroplasty, and abdominal and vaginal hysterectomy in 2001 that served as the basis for a sea change in PAP [16]. They found that only 55.7 % of patients received PAP within 1 h of surgery, although the agents selected were consistent with published guidelines in more than 90 % of cases. It was disconcerting that PAP was discontinued within 24 h of operation in only 41 % of cases, and within 12 h only 14.5 % of the time. These disturbing results affirmed the results of other studies and provided the basis for initiation of the Surgical Improvement Project by the Center for Medicare and Medicaid Services (CMS), which was done in conjunction with the Joint Commission (JC). In 2006, this initiative became the Surgical Care Improvement Project (SCIP) and incorporated six process measures designed to reduce the incidence of SSI (Table 10.9).

10.5.2 Treatment of SSI

Once an SSI is identified, the next step is to open the incision and drain the site of infection. Superficial SSIs can be treated by removing sutures or staples, taking care to expose an area sufficient to evacuate any pus or other fluid and to assess the underlying tissue for necrosis as well as involvement of the fascia. When there is necrosis, all necrotic tissues should be debrided and the fascial closure should be inspected for possible dehiscence and possibility of evisceration. Drainage emanating from beneath the fascia should prompt additional diagnostic study or return to the operating room to assess and control any cavitary infection.

Table 10.9 Surgical care improvement project core measure set effective January 1, 2014

Prophylactic antibiotic received within 1 h prior to surgical incision
Prophylactic antibiotic selection is appropriate in surgical patients
Prophylactic antibiotics discontinued within 24 h after surgery end time
Cardiac surgery patients with controlled postoperative blood glucose
Appropriate hair removal (Joint Commission only)

Once the involved area has been properly drained and the fascial closure is intact, the incision should be packed with gauze material moistened with a physiologic saline solution (usually 0.9 % normal saline). Dressings should be changed regularly; however, there are no studies that have definitively identified a superior regimen for dressing changes. They should then be allowed to heal by secondary intention. Once local and systemic signs of infection are controlled, debridement completed, and granulation tissue has appeared, healing time can sometimes be shortened and the patient made more comfortable by using a negative pressure therapy device.

If the fascia needs debridement, the fascial incision should be reclosed without tension. Intracavitary and organ infections are generally treated by evacuation of all infected materials and closed suction drainage. It may be necessary to perform a temporary closure and reevaluate the condition of the fascia within 48–72 h.

Cultures of pus and infected tissue are useful to identify the involved organisms. They can be particularly helpful in identifying unusual pathogens or antibiotic-resistant organisms, information that may alter treatment. Cultures are also helpful when there is an outbreak of infection due to nosocomial colonization or contaminated instruments or other materials. Obtaining an aliquot of pus or infected material for culture is preferable to swabbing the area, the results of which may be falsely influenced by contaminants from the skin.

Antimicrobial therapy is usually unnecessary for most superficial SSIs. Antimicrobials are indicated when cellulitis, fever, leukocytosis, or other signs of the systemic inflammatory response syndrome (SIRS) are present. Antimicrobial agents are also indicated when a prosthetic device remains in place or for patients with a compromised immune response. The empiric choice of agents should be based on the likely pathogens. Treatment should be adjusted based on culture results and sensitivities to antibiotics.

References

1. Barie PS. Surgical site infections: epidemiology and prevention. Surg Infect (Larchmt). 2002;3 Suppl 1:S9–21.
2. Horan TC, Gaynes RP, Martone WJ, et al. CDC definitions of nosocomial surgical site infections, 1992: a modification of CDC definitions of surgical wound infections. Infect Control Hosp Epidemiol. 1992;13:606–8.
3. Horan TC, Andrus M, Dudeck MA. CDC/NHSN surveillance definition of health care-associated infection and criteria for specific types of infections in the acute care setting. Am J Infect Control. 2008;36:309–32.
4. Livingston DH, Malangoni MA. An experimental study of susceptibility to infection after hemorrhagic shock. Surg Gynecol Obstet. 1989;168:138–42.
5. Latham R, Lancaster AD, Covington JF, et al. The association of diabetes and glucose control with surgical-site infections among cardiothoracic surgery patients. Infect Control Hosp Epidemiol. 2001;22:607–12.
6. Zerr KJ, Furnary AP, Grunkemeier GL, et al. Glucose control lowers the risk of wound infection in diabetics after open heart operations. Ann Thorac Surg. 1997;63:356–61.

7. Nagachinta T, Stephens M, Reitz B, et al. Risk factors for surgical wound infection following cardiac surgery. J Infect Dis. 1987;156:967–73.

8. Vinton AL, Traverso LW, Jolly PC. Wound complications after modified radical mastectomy compared with tylectomy with axillary lymph node dissection. Am J Surg. 1991;161:584–8.

9. National Nosocomial Infections Surveillance System (NNIS) System Report, Data summary from January 1992–June 2001, issued August 2001. Am J Infect Control. 2001;29:404–21.

10. Haridas M, Malangoni MA. Predictive factors for surgical site infection in general surgery. Surgery. 2008;144:496–503.

11. Edmiston Jr CE, Lee CJ, Krepel CJ, et al. Evidence for a standardized preadmission showering regimen to achieve maximal antiseptic skin surface concentrations of chlorhexidine gluconate, 4%, in surgical patients. JAMA Surg. 2015;150:1027–33.

12. Bratzler DW, Dellinger EP, Olsen KM, et al. Clinical practice guidelines for antimicrobial prophylaxis in surgery. Surg Infect (Larchmt). 2013;14:73–156.

13. Kiran RP, Murray AC, Chiuzan C, et al. Combined preoperative mechanical bowel preparation with oral antibiotics significantly reduces surgical site infection, anastomotic leak, and ileus after colorectal surgery. Ann Surg. 2015;262:416–25.

14. Harbarth S, Samore MH, Lichtenberg D, et al. Prolonged antibiotic prophylaxis after cardiovascular surgery and its effect on surgical site infections and antimicrobial resistance. Circulation. 2000;101:2916–21.

15. Bozorgzadeh A, Pizzi WF, Barie PS, et al. The duration of antibiotic administration for penetrating abdominal trauma. Am J Surg. 1999;177:125–31.

16. Bratzler DW, Houck PM, Richards C, et al. Use of antimicrobial prophylaxis for major surgery. Baseline results from the National Surgical Infection Prevention Project. Arch Surg. 2005;140:174–82.

Chapter 11
Nontraumatic Peripheral Vascular Emergencies

Venu Bhamidipaty, Anastasia Dean, and Ian Civil

11.1 Introduction

Managing a patient with a vascular surgical emergency can be challenging. Often a patient will have multiple comorbidities, an extensive surgical history, and a lengthy medication list including novel anticoagulation and antiplatelet agents. Even if managed in a timely fashion, vascular emergencies can lead to significant and long-term morbidity or mortality.

Nontraumatic peripheral vascular emergencies can be either hemorrhagic or ischemic, but the vast majority are associated with impaired blood flow from either embolism or thrombosis.

V. Bhamidipaty • A. Dean • I. Civil (✉)
Department of Vascular Surgery, Auckland City Hospital,
Auckland, NZ
e-mail: icivil@xtra.co.nz

© Springer International Publishing Switzerland 2017   187
S. Di Saverio et al. (eds.), *Acute Care Surgery Handbook*,
DOI 10.1007/978-3-319-15341-4_11

11.2 Aetiology

Embolism	Thrombosis
1. Atrial fibrillation	1. Atherosclerotic occlusion
2. Mural thrombus	2. Thrombosed aneurysm
3. LV aneurysm	3. Bypass or stent graft occlusion
4. Paradoxical	4. Hypercoagulable states
5. Endocarditis	5. Dissection
6. Atrial myxoma	6. Vasospasm
7. Aortic/large vessel atheroma	7. Iatrogenic

Emboli can arise from the heart (80–90 %) or diseased proximal arteries (10–20 %). Common cardiac causes include atrial thrombus with atrial fibrillation and mural thrombus in acute coronary syndrome and left ventricular dysfunction, to septic emboli in infective endocarditis, thrombus with prosthetic valves and myxoma much less frequently. Also, atherosclerotic plaque or mural thrombus can embolize from a diseased proximal artery.

Acute thrombosis most often occurs at a site of atherosclerotic plaque in peripheral arteries either the plaque hemorrhages, exposing the hypercoaguable subendothelial collagen, which leads to thrombus formation or the plaque causes a critical stenosis, which reduces the blood flow, promoting thrombus formation. Vein bypass grafts can thrombose in the context of an anastomotic stenosis, a kink in the graft or if there is a retained valve cusp, all of which result in a flow disturbance or low-flow state. Thrombosed vein grafts are often preceeded by clinical symptoms or arterial compromise (e.g. claudication) prior to thrombosing. A prosthetic graft can thrombose at any point often without any prodrome or warning signs. Large vessel aneurysms – most commonly aortic, popliteal, and femoral – cause turbulent flow, which is prothrombotic. Some prothrombotic states can result in arterial thrombosis, for example, antiphospholipid syndrome, heparin-induced thrombocytopenia, or malignancy, as can systemic low flow (hypotension) in an unwell patient. Rare causes of an acute ischemic limb include compartment syndrome, dissection, external compression, cystic adventitial disease, and popliteal entrapment.

11.3   Diagnosis

The history and examination in the diagnosis of acute limb ischemia revolves around the "six P's" – pulselessness, pain, pallor, paralysis, paresthesia, and poikilothermia. Patients with embolic limb ischemia often report the sudden onset of limb pain and paresthesia (often able to pinpoint their exact action/movements at the time of onset), followed shortly by pallor and varying degree of paralysis depending on the arterial bed involved.

Unlike lower limb ischemia, upper limb ischemia is almost exclusively due to embolic causes. Atherosclerotic occlusive disease is extremely unusual in the upper limb with numerous collateral pathways providing adequate flow to ensure ischemia is rarely limb threatening, and thus treatment can be approached in a less urgent fashion.

The contralateral limb and abdomen should always be examined carefully as they provide vital clues as to the underlying etiology. One must strongly suspect an embolic cause, particularly if the asymptomatic limb has a full complement of palpable pulses. A prominent pulse in the abdomen or in the popliteal fossa of the contralateral leg suggests an aortic or popliteal aneurysm respectively, particularly if a mass can be felt in the popliteal fossa of the affected leg (Fig. 11.1). Lack of pulses in the contralateral extremity may be a sign of chronic underlying stenotic disease as arterial disease often affects both limbs in a mirror pattern.

In patients with thrombotic occlusion, there is often a history of low-grade ischemia, most often presenting as intermittent

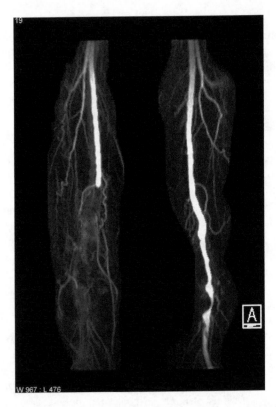

Fig. 11.1 MRA showing occluded popliteal aneurysm on the right and patent but aneurysmal popliteal artery on the left

claudication, suggesting an underlying impairment of normal arterial flow prior to the acute presentation.

Other nonatherosclerotic and nonembolic causes should be suspected in those patients who are relatively young, without the typical risk factor profile or with another diagnosis that predisposes them to a thrombotic condition (e.g., thrombocytosis, polycythemia rubra vera, malignancy).

On examination, the ischemic limb is initially cool, pale, with delayed capillary refill and with or without changes associated with chronic ischemia (atrophic skin, loss of hair, and nail thickening). After 6–12 h, the limb can turn red due to vasodilation, after which it becomes mottled and blanches, and finally mottled with fixed skin staining. Pulses must be examined bilaterally from the femoral to the popliteal, dorsalis pedis, and posterior tibial. If pulses are absent, a handheld continuous Doppler should be used to assess for an audible signal, suggesting residual blood flow. Finally, it is important to examine for motor-sensory deficits. Based on the examination findings, the limb can be classified in terms of viability and urgency of revascularization (see table below).

Critical limb ischemia occurs when a decrease in perfusion threatens the viability of the limb, manifesting in rest pain, tissue loss, and/or gangrene.

11.4   Investigations

Urgent blood tests should include a full blood count, renal function, and coagulation profile to assist the choice of imaging modality and preparation for surgery. An electrocardiogram (ECG) should also be done routinely on admission to check for cardiac arrhythmias and excluded recent/current coronary ischemia. A chest x-ray may be useful in identifying undiagnosed congestive cardiac failure. The most appropriate imaging modality will depend upon what is available at the time, institutional factors, and patient factors – renal function, body habitus, and implanted devices, to name a few.

It is completely appropriate to proceed straight to surgical intervention without any imaging in some patient cohorts, namely, those with a good history, risk factors, and physical examination supportive of sudden embolic event. Any sugges-

	Description	Capp. refill	Muscle paralysis	Sensory loss	Arterial Doppler signals	Venous Doppler signals
I – Viable	Not immediately threatened	Intact	None	None	Audible	Audible
IIa – threatened	Salvageable if treated promptly	Slow	None	Partial	Inaudible	Audible
IIb – threatened	Salvageable if treated immediately	Slow/absent	Partial	Partial/complete	Inaudible	Audible
III – irreversible	Not salvageable	Absent. Fixed staining	Complete. Tense compartment	Complete	Inaudible	Inaudible

tion that there may be a proximal inflow stenosis or disease should ideally be investigated further with an imaging modality that is most appropriate and available at the time of presentation to the institution.

11.4.1   Arterial Duplex Ultrasound

Duplex ultrasound combines B-mode with color Doppler to assess both the arterial anatomy and blood flow characteristics. Ultrasound is noninvasive, inexpensive, and has good sensitivity and specificity in identifying lesions; however, it is highly operator dependent. Furthermore, it can be difficult to assess iliac vessels behind bowel gas.

11.4.2   Computed Tomographic Angiography

With recent technological improvements (multidetector, thinner slices), computed tomographic angiography (CTA) produces high spatial resolution images of the peripheral arterial tree. It can also assess lesions that have been previously stented. Arterial calcification, however, causes beam-hardening artifact, making interpretation of some lesions difficult, especially in small caliber vessels.

11.4.3   Magnetic Resonance Angiography

Magnetic resonance angiography (MRA) provides good-quality imaging of the arterial tree. MRA can assess the true lumen of a thrombosed aneurysmal vessel and the quality of potential venous conduit for a bypass. It is not impeded by vessel calcification, but steel stents or clips can cause a signal void and impede image quality.

11.4.4   Catheter Angiography (Digital Subtraction Angiography)

Catheter angiography (DSA) is the gold standard of peripheral arterial imaging. It has the benefit of being able to proceed to intervention if required; however, unlike the other modalities mentioned above, it is an invasive procedure.

11.5   Management

The management approach to the ischemic limb is dictated by a number of factors: physiological state of the patient, viability of the limb at the time of presentation, and the resources and surgical expertise available. Systemic anticoagulation (usually with unfractionated heparin) is the first and most important step for all patients presenting with acute limb ischemia, as it prevents propagation of thrombus.

Perhaps the most important decision that needs to be made is whether to attempt limb salvage, manage the patient nonoperatively, or proceed directly to a major limb amputation.

An ischemic limb that is viable and not imminently threatened (Rutherford Class I) can often initially be managed conservatively with systemic anticoagulation and imaging performed in a semiurgent manner. This allows time to assess for improvement in the limb with heparin as collaterals provide enough flow to maintain limb viability. A delayed intervention, endovascular or open, can then be considered in a planned fashion if the persisting symptoms warrant revascularization.

An imminently threatened limb (Rutherford Class II) usually has motor impairment and needs urgent treatment with expedited imaging, if clinically required, and revascularization. Tender muscle compartments are an ominous sign for underlying significant muscle ischemia, and revascularization should be attempted urgently. Following systemic anticoagulation, the patient must be transferred for operative intervention. Ideally, a noninvasive axial imaging study is obtained prior to surgery to aid operative planning, but surgical treatment should not be unduly and unreasonable delayed to allow imaging to be obtained. On-table angiography should be used in cases where time or resources will not allow for expedited imaging.

An irreversibly ischemic leg should not be revascularized as reperfusion syndrome can prove fatal. These cases should be considered for a primary limb amputation or palliative care in the medically comorbid patient with poor quality of life.

11.6 Operative Surgery

11.6.1 Brachial Embolectomy

In the vast majority of cases of acute upper extremity ischemia, embolectomy can be satisfactorily achieved through an ante-brachial approach. In situations where the acute occlusion or embolus is present in the distal axillary artery or upper brachial artery, a "high" brachial approach is indicated. Variations in brachial anatomy must be kept in mind with up to 20% of patients having a high brachial bifurcation in the upper arm.

11.6.1.1 Antecubital Approach

The procedure can usually be performed under local anesthetic with sedation. The entire arm (except the hand) is prepped and draped with the hand isolated in a clear plastic isolation bag so that the color of the hand can be monitored. A transverse incision is made 1–2 cm distal to the elbow crease where the brachial bifurcation is usually situated. The bicipital aponeurosis is opened longitudinally and the brachial artery is dissected out and isolated with vessel loops. The brachial bifurcation is identified, and the proximal radial and ulnar arteries are also looped as this allows selective thrombectomy of the forearm arteries. Systemic heparin is usually continued during the procedure – an additional bolus can be given before the vessels are clamped. A transverse arteriotomy just proximal to the brachial bifurcation is used. Visible clot is removed with a pair of forceps. A #3 Fogarty catheter is passed upstream proximally into the brachial artery, gently inflated, and withdrawn. This process is repeated once or twice until good pulsatile inflow is restored. The #3 or #2 Fogarty catheter (depending on the size of vessel) is then passed individually into the forearm arteries and thrombectomy is performed in a similar manner after which the vessels are flushed with heparinized saline. The arteriotomy is closed with an interrupted 5/0 or 6/0 polypropylene suture and the clamps released. The hand is then assessed for color, capillary return, and presence of wrist pulses. Restoring flow into one forearm artery is usually enough to maintain a viable hand. The absence of a palpable pulse, poor Doppler signals at the wrist, or sluggish capillary refill would suggest inadequate hand perfusion. Intraoperative angiography, if available in the operating room, is performed if there is still poor perfusion despite repeated thrombectomy.

11.6.1.2 "High Brachial"/Axillary Approach

In uncommon cases where the embolus is located either in the upper arm or the axillary artery, as confirmed on imaging, a longitudinal incision should be placed on the medial aspect of the upper arm. After dissection through the superficial tissues, the deep fascia of the arm is opened longitudinally and the brachial artery is carefully dissected out. At this level, branches of the brachial plexus often accompany it, with the median nerve most at risk during the dissection. The vessel is isolated with vessel loops and following vessel clamping an arteriotomy is made in a healthy soft part of the vessel. Embolectomy is most performed with #3 or #4 Fogarty catheters, depending on the size of the vessel.

Care must be taken when passing the Fogarty catheter upstream into the vessels, especially if the proximal axillary artery is involved. There is a small risk that thrombus or clot could be pushed into the vertebral artery either while advancing the Fogarty catheter, or during inflation and withdrawal. It is important when dealing with an ischemic arm where the brachial pulse is not palpable in the middle or upper arm that anatomic information is gained prior to the surgery with the use of noninvasive imaging (e.g., CTA or duplex ultrasound) so that the proximal extent of the thrombus is clearly identified. Prior to passing the catheter into the vessels, it is useful to estimate the length that the catheter should be advanced by placing the catheter externally on the patient along the course of the vessel. This also ensures that the catheter is not passed into the aortic arch and minimizes the risk of atheroembolism into the carotid circulation, particularly on the right side.

11.6.2   Femoral Embolectomy

The procedure is performed under local or general anesthetic, depending on the patient's body habitus, comorbidities, and the operator's level of experience. The patient is placed supine and the abdomen and ipsilateral leg prepped and draped in a standard fashion down to the ankle level. The ipsilateral foot is isolated in a clear plastic bag so that color and capillary refill can be assessed during the case. A vertical incision is made over the femoral pulse or mid-inguinal point if the femoral pulse cannot be felt. The incision is deepened, carefully ligating lymphatics and superficial epigastric veins as they are encountered. Following longitudinal division of the femoral sheath, the common femoral artery (CFA) is identified and the small side branches are isolated and encircled with vessel loops (Fig. 11.2). A segment of 5 cm of artery should be enough to perform a standard femoral embolectomy. The profunda femoris and superficial femoral artery (SFA) need to be dissected out and looped in order to allow the operator to selectively guide the thrombectomy catheters into each of these vessels. Profunda femoris most often branches from the posterior-lateral aspect of the femoral bifurcation and is crossed in the proximal part by the lateral femoral circumflex vein, which is usually divided to prevent iatrogenic injury.

If the patient is not already systemically heparinized, 50–100 IU/kg of intravenous unfractionated heparin is given and the vessel clamped or occluded with vessel loops. Provided the common femoral artery is not too heavily calcified or diseased, a transverse arteriotomy is created using a #11 blade scalpel and extended using Potts scissors. A diseased artery is often best opened longitudinally to allow for a femoral endarterectomy if needed. Once the vessel is opened, any thrombus can be extracted with forceps. Priority is first to ensure adequate inflow. Depending on the size of the vessels and the location of the clot, a #4 or #5 Fogarty catheter is passed proximally in the vessel into the external iliac artery with the vessel being controlled using vessel loops. The catheter is inflated gently until balloon and vessel wall contact is felt and withdrawn. This is repeated until pulsatile anterograde bleeding is seen. At least one "clean pass" of the catheter should be achieved before infusing the thrombectomized vessel with heparinized saline and reclamping. Similarly, this process is repeated with the profunda and SFA using #4 or #3 Fogarty catheters. The transverse arteriotomy is then closed with an interrupted 6/0 polypropylene suture and flow to the leg is released. In the case of a longitudinal arteriotomy, a patch should be used to close the vessel.

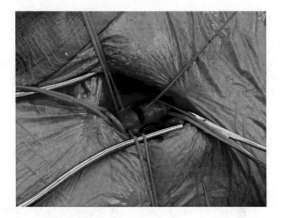

Fig. 11.2 Femoral embolectomy

11.6.2.1   Assessment of Foot Perfusion

If a foot pulse cannot be felt after a few minutes of reperfusion, a continuous wave handheld Doppler should be used to insonate the Doppler signals in the feet. A decision about whether to stop or proceed further with the operation is dependent on color and capillary refill of the foot, as well as Doppler signals. A biphasic Doppler signal in at least one foot/distal tibial vessel is usually adequate to maintain a viable leg/foot.

Following reperfusion, if the color of the foot fails to improve and the foot is still deemed to be critically ischemic, a decision needs to be made as to how to proceed. A palpable popliteal pulse indicates residual distal popliteal or tibial thrombus/embolus. In this case, a popliteal/tibial thrombectomy may be indicated.

If a popliteal pulse is absent despite femoral embolectomy or if the Fogarty catheter is not able to advance past a particular point in the thigh, residual or chronic occlusive disease must be suspected and at this stage, intraoperative angiography should be considered.

A small (18 or 20-gauge) IV cannula or Angiocath is inserted into the common femoral artery and attached to small extension tubing. Iodinated contrast (e.g., Omnipaque) is injected into the vessel under image intensifier guidance to perform a digital subtraction angiography. The distal leg run-off is assessed with a view to either further distal thrombectomy, or potentially a femoro-popliteal, or femoro-distal bypass graft.

11.6.3   Popliteal Embolectomy/Thrombectomy

The below knee popliteal artery is most easily approached through a longitudinal medial calf incision, approximately 1–2 cm posterior to the border of the tibial. On deepening the incision through subcutaneous tissue, care must be taken to not injure the great saphenous vein, which is important as a potential bypass conduit, or vein patch. The deep fascia is opened and the medial head of the gastrocnemius is retracted posteriorly. The below knee popliteal fossa is entered – the popliteal artery is most commonly situated in between paired popliteal veins or behind a single popliteal vein; the tibial nerve is situated more posteriorly. The popliteal artery is dissected out and encircled with a vessel loop. Ideally the dissection is continued distally with partial division of the soleus muscle to expose the origin of the anterior tibial artery (ATA) and the tibio-peroneal trunk (TPT). The patient is then systemically heparinized, if not already done, or an additional bolus of heparin is administered. If the operator is confident about the diagnosis of popliteal embolus and the vessel is of reasonable size (>6 mm), a transverse arteriotomy can be made with a view to primary closure. If not, a longitudinal arteriotomy in the distal popliteal artery, crossing the origin of the ATA and ending in the proximal TPT, allows selective thrombectomy of the ATA and TPT. The main advantage of the longitudinal arteriotomy is that it can be used as the site of a distal anastomosis should popliteal inflow restoration be unsuccessful and a distal bypass needed. In a similar fashion to the femoral thrombectomy outlined above, a #4 Fogarty is passed upstream into the above knee popliteal or superficial femoral artery, inflated, and retrieved. Similarly, the tibial vessels are thrombectomized using a #3 Fogarty catheter. Some thought could be given to administering a small bolus of a thrombolytic agent (e.g., Urokinase) into the tibial vessels following thrombectomy, provided there are no contraindications to thrombolysis. Occluded smaller side branches and important collateral pathways that are not targeted or treated with the Fogarty catheter may potentially be reopened with the infusion of a thrombolytic agent. If satisfactory inflow and outflow thrombectomy has been achieved, the arteriotomy is closed with an interrupted 6/0 polypropylene suture in the case of a transverse arteriotomy, or using a vein patch if a longitudinal arteriotomy was made. Once clamps are released, the foot perfusion is reassessed in a few minutes.

If the capillary refill or color fails to improve and/or Doppler signals are absent, an on-table angiography needs to be considered to ascertain the level of persisting occlusion with a view to re-embolectomy. Alternatively, a retrograde tibial embolectomy with retrograde passage of the Fogarty catheter through the pedal arteries can be considered but is usually an end-of-the-line measure to try to salvage a severely threatened limb.

11.6.4 Compartment Syndrome

Though more commonly seen in the setting of trauma, compartment syndrome can occur within hours to days of reperfusion of an ischemic limb. Failure to recognize and decompress the compartments can compromise the limb and put the patient's life at risk.

Compartment syndrome occurs when pressure within a fascial compartment increases to the point that it exceeds the perfusion pressure of the tissue and compromises circulation. The lower leg is particularly at risk given the tough facial sheaths, which enclose the four muscular compartments (anterior, lateral, superficial posterior, deep posterior). Also, previously ischemic tissue is less tolerant of increased tissue pressure.

Patients can describe severe pain not relieved by analgesia, as well as paresthesia, numbness, or muscle weakness in the affected limb. On examination, typical findings include pain with passive stretch of the muscle, tense muscle that has a "wood-like" feeling, and motor-sensory deficits ranging from paresthesia to paralysis. Compartment pressure measurements can be a helpful adjunct to the examination findings; however, a single normal result does not rule out the diagnosis. Pressures that are within 20–30 mmHg of the diastolic pressure are worrying and suggestive of compartment syndrome.

11.6.4.1 Lower Limb Fasciotomy

Lower limb fasciotomy for below knee muscle compartments is most often performed to allow for muscle edema post arterial reperfusion following prolonged ischemia. The authors' preferred technique to decompress all four muscle compartments in the lower leg involves a two-incision technique, with generous longitudinal incisions on the medial and lateral aspects of the leg.

The medial longitudinal skin incision extends from the upper calf inferiorly, approximately 1 cm posterior to the posterior edge of the tibia, down to the distal calf. Care must be taken to identify and preserve the saphenous nerve and vein where possible. The deep muscle fascia is released longitudinally and the superficial posterior compartment is opened. The soleus is freed from its tibial attachment. Decompression of the deep posterior compartment is best done from the distal part of the wound where the deep posterior compartment lies just below the subcutaneous tissue. Identifying and releasing the fascia overlying flexor digitorum longus frees the deep posterior compartment.

The lateral incision is made from the proximal shin between the tibia and fibula extending down to the distal leg, taking care to not injure the peroneal nerve as it spirals around the fibular head. Initially, a transverse incision is made in the deep fascia in the proximal aspect of the wound to help identify the exact location of the intercompartment septum that separates the anterior and lateral compartments. Once this is identified, these compartments are released by parallel longitudinal incisions in the deep fascia on either side of the septum.

Techniques such as "boot-lacing" with suture or silastic material can be used to keep the skin edges approximated, to allow for easier closure of the wounds in the next few days if clinically appropriate. Alternatively, a negative-pressure dressing can be applied with a view to primary closure or potentially delayed wound closure with a split-skin graft or closure by secondary intention (Fig. 11.3).

11.7 Summary

Treatment of acute limb ischemia remains a challenging clinical problem with several different variables influencing the decision-making process before, during, and following treatment of the acute problem. Upper limbs tend to have a good response following intervention with a very high limb salvage rate and most patients having no significant functional deficit. Lower limbs, however, tend to fare worse, with a not insignificant amputation rate. Perioperative mortality is largely due to the patients pre-existing comorbidities, predominantly cardiac. Preoperative cardiac status, duration of limb ischemia, malignancy-related limb ischemia, and the eventual need for major limb amputation are the major prognosticators for poor

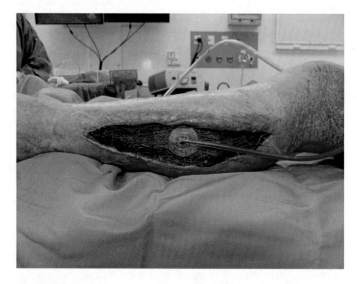

Fig. 11.3 Fasciotomy wound with negative pressure dressing

outcomes and higher mortality rate. Surgical techniques have largely remained the same over the last two decades with an increasing number of minimally invasive interventional procedures being utilized for acute limb ischemia. A multidisciplinary collaborative approach between interventional radiologists and surgeons is vital in improving limb salvage rates.

Bibliography

1. Cronenwett JL, Johnston KW, editors. Rutherford's vascular surgery, vol. 2. 8th ed. Philadelphia: Elsevier; 2014.
2. Hallett JW, Mills JL, Earnshaw JJ, Reekers TW, editors. Comprehensive vascular and endovascular surgery. 2nd ed. Philadelphia: Mosby; 2009.

3. Moore W, editor. Vascular and endovascular surgery: a comprehensive review. 8th ed. Philadelphia: Elsevier; 2013.
4. Norgren L, Hiatt WR, Dormandy JA, et al. Inter-society consensus for the management of peripheral arterial disease (TASC II). J Vasc Surg. 2007;33 Suppl 1:S1–75.

Chapter 12
Ruptured Abdominal Aortic Aneurysms and Major Vascular Injuries

Paolo Perini, Claudio Bianchini Massoni, and Antonio Freyrie

12.1 Ruptured AAA

Rupture of abdominal aortic aneurysm (AAA) represents one of the most common emergencies in surgery. If untreated, the natural history of this condition is always fatal. Pre-operative management, surgical or endovascular procedures and post-operative care are burdened by high morbidity and mortality, making this event one of the most challenging for surgical and medical staff.

P. Perini, MD (✉) • C. Bianchini Massoni, MD • A. Freyrie, MD
Department of Surgery, Unit of Vascular Surgery, University Hospital of Parma, Via Gramsci, 14, 43126 Parma, PR, Italy
e-mail: p.perini@live.com

© Springer International Publishing Switzerland 2017　　207
S. Di Saverio et al. (eds.), *Acute Care Surgery Handbook*,
DOI 10.1007/978-3-319-15341-4_12

12.1.1   Introduction

Ruptured abdominal aortic aneurysm (RAAA) is defined as bleeding outside the adventitia of a dilated aortic wall [1] (Fig. 12.1). The localisation of the rupture influences both symptoms and outcomes. Rupture in the peritoneal cavity (20 %) or in the retroperitoneal space (80 %) is the most frequent event [2]. In the latter case, the retroperitoneal tissue may temporarily reduce blood loss.

Arteriovenous fistula (mostly aorto-caval) and *aorto-enteric fistula* are rare events; in this case, the rupture occurs into the venous system or into the bowel lumen, respectively.

12.1.2   Epidemiology and Mortality

In a recent Norwegian study, the adjusted incidence rate of RAAA is 11.0 per 100.000 per year and is by far higher in males

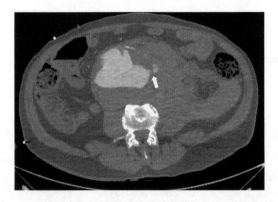

Fig. 12.1 Pre-operative computed tomography angiography (CTA) in a patient with RAAA. The *white arrow* depicts the site of aortic rupture in the anterior-left lateral wall. A blush of contrast media outside the aorta is evident, with voluminous intra-abdominal haematoma

(males: 17.6 per 100.00 per year *vs*. females: 4.7 per 100.00 per year) [3].

The risk of rupture mostly depends on the aneurysm diameter. According to recent data [4], cumulative yearly rupture rate is 3.5 % with diameter between 5.5 cm and 6 cm; 4.1 %, between 6.1 cm and 7 cm; and 6.3 %, >7 cm. Recent preliminary studies consider also additional parameters (geometrical AAA shape, female gender, arterial hypertension, smoking history, familiarity for AAA, intraluminal thrombus) to estimate individual AAA risk rupture [5, 6].

Patient died before reaching the hospital in about 45 % of cases and prior to undergo surgery in 25 % [7]. Among patients admitted to hospital for RAAA, intervention was not performed in 27 % of cases because of death, agonal status or patient's decision [3]. Considering operated patients, 30-day/in-hospital mortality after surgery is about 46–48.5 % [8, 9]. Overall mortality of this condition is about 75 % [9].

12.1.3   Clinical Presentation and Diagnosis

A RAAA is characterised by the classical triad: pain, shock and pulsatile mass. Anterior rupture into the peritoneal cavity induces sudden abdominal or back pain. Collapse and death occur often before reaching the hospital [2]. In case of posterior aneurysm rupture, back pain is the main symptom; this condition may or not be associated with abdominal pain and hypotension. Retroperitoneal tissues may contain the rupture, so that patients may reach cure [2]. Unusual clinical presentations are transient lower limb paralysis, right hypochondrial pain, hydronephrosis, testicular pain or ecchymosis [2]. Pulsatile mass is not always palpable (i.e. in case of obese patients or severe hypotension).

Rupture of abdominal aortic aneurysm into the venous system (inferior vena cava, left renal vein, iliac veins) occur in about 3–4 %

of RAAA with formation of *arteriovenous fistulae*. Adjunctive symptoms include abdominal bruit, dyspnoea, tachycardia, cyanosis, lower limb oedema, angina, palpitation, oliguria [2].

Rupture into the bowel creates an *aorto-enteric fistula* (<1%) inducing haematemesis, melena and/or haematochezia [2]. Primary aorto-enteric fistulae are rare. Secondary fistulae must be considered in case of previous surgical aortic repair. The third and fourth portions of the duodenum are the most frequently involved.

Despite this frequent overt clinical presentation, misdiagnosis can occur [10]. Most common differential diagnoses are renal colic, myocardial infarction, colonic inflammation, gastrointestinal perforation [10]. Supporting imaging includes duplex ultrasound to confirm suspected diagnosis [1]. Computed tomography angiography (CTA) has nearly 100% of accuracy [11] and provides important information for surgical intervention (lower renal artery, position of left renal vein, quality of the possible clamping zones) or endovascular procedure (length, diameter, calcification, tortuosity of iliac access and sealing zones).

12.1.4   Pre-operative Evaluation and Management

Smaller, peripheral hospitals are not equipped with a vascular surgery unit and, consequently, a rapid inter-hospital transfer is essential for a successful intervention. Geographical location of vascular surgery units should provide equity of access. Inter-hospital transfer is reported as an independent risk factor for mortality [12].

A standardised, multidisciplinary approach involving emergency specialists, vascular surgeons, anaesthesiologists and radiologists, and an efficient logistic (availability of duplex ultrasound and computed tomography, dedicated operating or hybrid room, intra-operative autotransfusion) are mandatory.

Rapid imaging, trained physicians, nurses and other personnel, rapid availability of blood products and standard protocols are crucial for an adequate management [12].

Data on benefits from upfront transfusions are contradictory. Less recent publications [13–15] reported that, in case of haemorrhagic shock, massive fluid replacement could exacerbate the blood loss, inducing iatrogenic coagulopathy. By contrast, intravenous fluid transfusion <500 ml during pre-hospital phase with a target systolic blood pressure between 50 and 100 mmHg (*permissive hypotension*) may encourage clot formation. A recent publication states that aggressive transfusion before proximal clamping is a risk factor for death, independently from systolic blood pressure [16]. Data from prospective studies are lacking, and pre-operative transfusion policy varies among different centres.

According to the Guidelines of the European Society for Vascular Surgery [1], patients with a known abdominal aortic aneurysm, symptoms and shock should be immediately transferred to the operating room (after emergency ultrasound if available) [1]. In haemodynamically stable patients, urgent computed tomography angiography (CTA) is recommended. CTA has high accuracy in the diagnosis of RAAA providing data on aorto-iliac morphology [11], useful for decision-making processes. CTA can be performed in the majority of cases, and should be avoided only in severely unstable patients [10].

12.1.5 Operative Strategies: Open Repair

The intra-operative autotransfusion plays a role in reducing fresh frozen plasma use. Indeed, proportional greater use of autotransfusion is associated with lower mortality [17].

Median transperitoneal access is widely adopted, but left retroperitoneal approach (tenth intercostal space) is also described [18]. A rapid proximal control is required to stop the haemorrhage. It is crucial to preserve the integrity of the inferior vena cava, renal veins and oesophagus: this could be achieved with a subdiaphragmatic aortic cross-clamping. Then, it is suggested to rapidly isolate a more caudal segment of the aorta so the clamp can be moved distally, in a healthy portion of the vessel (preferably in an infrarenal position) for reducing the time of visceral ischaemia. In case of juxta- and infrarenal AAA, the preferred site of cross-clamping is supra- and infrarenal, respectively. Proximal control can be obtained also with intraluminal insertion of balloon catheter through the wall of the aneurysm [19] or by brachial [20] or femoral access [21].

Arterial reconstruction with aortoaortic tube or aortobiiliac bifurcated graft is performed depending on extension of aneurysmal disease (Figs. 12.2 and 12.3).

In case of tense abdomen and consequent difficult closure, open abdomen is left. After open surgical repair, primary closure of the abdomen is delayed in about 10 % [22] to avoid abdominal compartment syndrome with visceral organ dysfunctions.

12.1.6   Operative Strategies: Endovascular Repair

The first case of endovascular abdominal aortic aneurysm repair (EVAR) for RAAA treatment was reported in 1994 [23]. The lower invasiveness of the procedure compared with surgical treatment, and the possibility to perform it under local anaesthesia are the two characteristics that make EVAR an appealing option for RAAA.

However, aorto-iliac morphology must be fit for endovascular procedures in terms of access and sealing zones (both proximal and distal). An accurate pre-operative CTA evaluation is essential to plan the endovascular strategy and choose the most appropriate device. The rate of RAAA considered eligible for EVAR largely depends on personal endovascular skills and hospital organisation.

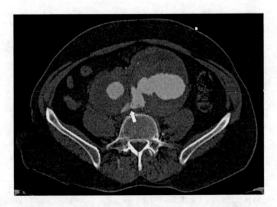

Fig. 12.2 Axial cut of a pre-operative CTA of a ruptured 11 cm aneurysm of the left common iliac artery, associated with a 5 cm aneurysm of the right common iliac artery. The *white arrow* indicates the rupture of the left common iliac artery aneurysm into the right iliac vein (arteriovenous fistula)

Aorto-uniiliac endograft deployment ensures a rapid control of bleeding. However, this procedure requires additional femorofemoral crossover bypass and contralateral iliac occluder placement. Bifurcated grafts are largely used in emergency, but an adequate stock of endografts is necessary which is unlikely to be available in all centres.

In case of haemodynamic instability, the occlusion of the supraceliac aorta with an inflatable balloon leads to haemorrhage control.

12.1.7 Post-operative Management and Complications

The post-operative development of intra-abdominal hypertension and abdominal compartment syndrome (ACS) is one of the most frequent complications after surgical or endovascular treatment of RAAA. ACS is defined as intra-abdominal pressure

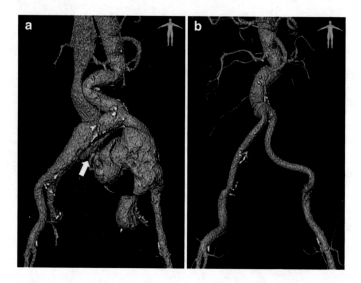

Fig. 12.3 Comparison between pre- and post-operative CTA through three-dimensional volume rendering reconstruction. (**a**) Pre-operative CTA showing the aneurysm rupture of the left common iliac artery into the venous system (*white arrow*). Visualisation of early passage of contrast media into the right iliac vein and the inferior vena cava. (**b**) Post-operative CTA after surgical aorto-bi-iliac grafting, with associated ligation of bilateral internal iliac arteries for hypogastric aneurysms

>20 mmHg associated with new organ dysfunction or failure [22]. ACS can also be present with an intra-abdominal pressure <20 mmHg in case of hypotension (mean arterial pressure <60 mmHg). Incidence of ACS is about 20 % after both surgical and endovascular treatment [24, 25]. Medical support consists of neuromuscolar blockade, positive end-expiratory pressure, albumin and diuretics [22]. Some Authors [26] described CT-guided puncture of the abdominal haematoma with drainage insertion and injection of tissue plasminogen activation to facilitate clot dissolution and abdominal decompression. Decompression laparotomy is still often required. Temporary

abdomen closure is needed to avoid bowel fistula formation and is obtained by meshes or patches and, sometimes, vacuum therapy [22].

Peri-operative myocardial ischaemia occurs in about 10–15 % of treated RAAA [27, 28] without statistical differences between open and endovascular treatments.

Pneumonia and respiratory complications are reported in about 15–25 % of cases, independently from strategy of RAAA treatment [27, 28].

Worsening of renal function after surgical procedure for RAAA is a common complication [29] caused by hypovolaemic shock, reperfusion and cross-clamping. During EVAR, iodinated contrast agent can cause nephrotoxicity. Severe acute renal failure occurred in 36 % of patients treated for RAAA with higher percentage after surgical repair (43 % after open repair vs. 26 % after EVAR) [30].

Bowel ischaemia is a high-mortality complication, that burden open surgery and endovascular treatment in 42 % and 23 % of cases, respectively [31, 32]. The pathogenesis of intestinal ischemia is multifactorial: hypotension, cross-clamping, embolisation, exclusion of hypogastric arteries or inferior mesenteric artery, reperfusion injury [32]. Sigmoidoscopy is recommended during the post-operative period for early diagnosis [32].

Multiple organ failure (MOF) occurs in about 5.8 % of cases [27], and it is an independent predictor for lower long-term survival [27].

12.1.8 Outcomes

Comparison between surgical and endovascular treatment of RAAA has been one of the most discussed topics in the last years. Data from several retrospective studies and randomised trials has been largely analysed [33–35] with risk of bias for clinical and anatomical characteristics and different enrolment criteria. A recent meta-analysis, analysing three randomised trials [36], showed no statistically significant difference in terms of 30- and 90-day mortality according to the surgical approach.

Even considering 1-year mortality, mortality was overlapping between surgical and endovascular intervention (38.6 % in EVAR group *vs.* 42.8 % in open repair group) [36].

12.2 Major Abdominal Vascular Injuries

Abdominal vascular injuries after a penetrating or blunt trauma are often lethal at the scene and never reach medical care [37]. Overall, these traumas are characterised by high mortality rates that can exceed 40 %, according to the most recent literature [38–41]. A rapid transfer to a trauma centre with adequate pre-hospital and emergency department treatment, a good medical judgement and an early surgical intervention are of vital importance to obtain a positive outcome.

12.2.1 Anatomy, Mechanism of Injury and Epidemiology

The abdomen is conventionally divided into three topographic zones, which not only define the anatomic area of the lesion, but also drive the therapeutic decisions [42]:

- *Zone 1*: it includes the midline retroperitoneum from the diaphragm to the sacral promontory. This zone is in turn subdivided according to the possible surgical approach as follows:

    - *Supramesocolic area*: suprarenal aorta with its major branches, suprarenal inferior vena cava (IVC), superior mesenteric vein.

- *Inframesocolic area*: infrarenal aorta and IVC, superior mesenteric artery distal to the middle colic artery, inferior mesenteric artery.

- *Zone 2*: it includes the right and left paracolic gutters and the renal vessels.
- *Zone 3*: it includes the pelvic retroperitoneum below the sacral promontory, with the iliac vessels and the presacral venous plexus.
- Portal vein, hepatic artery and retrohepatic IVC lesions are considered separately.

Abdominal traumas are distinguished in penetrating or blunt, according to the mechanism of injury. Penetrating trauma is accountable for most abdominal vascular lesions (90–95 % of patients [43, 44]) and is generally attributable to knife and gunshot injuries [45]. All abdominal vessels can be involved, and all types of vascular damage can occur (tearing, transection, intimal dissection, thrombosis, pseudoaneurysm, arteriovenous fistula). High-velocity bullets can also determine vascular lesions by means of the shock wave and transient cavitation, leading – usually – to acute thrombosis of nearby arteries [46]. Rare causes of penetrating aortic trauma include misplacement of spinal fixation screws, and laceration from spinal fractures [47, 48].

Blunt abdominal traumas are mostly associated with high-speed motor vehicle collisions (steering-wheel, seat-belt and lap-belt injuries), and vascular injuries may be secondary to:

1. Compression/direct anteroposterior crushing

2. Rapid deceleration (avulsion or intimal tear and subsequent thrombosis)

3. Direct laceration by a bone fragment dislocation

Blunt abdominal aortic injuries represent about 4–5 % of blunt aortic injuries [49].

In 2009, Azizzadeh et al. [50] proposed a classification to guide management of aortic injuries based on imaging appearances:

- *Grade I*: intimal tear
- *Grade II*: intramural haematoma
- *Grade III*: pseudoaneurysm (the most common to present clinically)
- *Grade IV*: rupture

Abdominal arterial and venous lesions occur with the same incidence [42]. Most frequently injured vessel are the IVC (25 % of injuries in a large series of abdominal vascular traumas [43]), followed by the aorta (21 %), the iliac arteries and veins, the superior mesenteric vein and the superior mesenteric artery. The majority of the patients have more than one vascular lesion.

12.2.2   Clinical Presentation and Diagnosis

The clinical presentation depends on many variables:

- The mechanism of injury (penetrating *vs.* blunt)
- The injured vessel
- The size and type of the lesion (i.e. the presence of a retro-peritoneal hematoma *vs.* a free rupture)
- The presence of associated injuries
- Time elapsed since the injury

Patients with penetrating wounds and associated major vascular lesions often arrive at the hospital in hypovolaemic shock, and the outcome is extremely poor (76.1 % mortality in case of aortic injuries [51]). Patients may also be haemodynamically stable because of vessel thrombosis or contained rupture; in these cases, the diagnosis is usually made intra-operatively.

In one-third of the patients with blunt vascular trauma, the diagnosis is delayed. In fact, only 2/3 of the cases are associated with significant bleeding or early ischemic changes.

Immediate laparotomy (without pre-operative imaging) is necessary only in case of severe instability after a penetrating trauma. In all other cases, it is mandatory to perform a pre-operative whole-body CTA [52]. In fact, this technique detects not only the type of the vascular damage, but also the presence and the gravity of associated injuries.

Digital subtraction angiography (DSA) has no more a role as a diagnostic tool during the acute stage. However, it remains a valuable tool in endovascular repair.

12.2.3   Pre-operative Evaluation and Management

Severely injured patients should be transferred directly to an appropriate trauma facility, and the time elapsed between injury and bleeding control should be minimised, according to the latest *'European guideline on management of major bleeding and coagulopathy following trauma'* [53]. The concept of 'damage control resuscitation' (DCR) aims to avoid the 'lethal triad' composed by hypothermia, acidosis and coagulopathy. The DCR aims to achieve a 'permissive hypotension' (systolic blood pressure of 80–90 mmHg), by using a restricted volume replacement strategy (and, in case, vasopressors) to achieve target blood pressure until bleeding can be controlled. Coagulation should be monitored repeatedly, and possibly corrected (also using anti-fibrinolytic agents). At the same time, laparotomic damage control surgery (DCS) should be started [54].

Haemodynamically stable patients should undergo whole-body CTA. Pre-operative imaging, in fact, guides the operative strategy (surgical *vs*. endovascular *vs*. conservative treatment).

12.2.4 Operative Strategies: Surgical Treatment

In case of unstable, severely injured patients, urgent abdominal DCS is performed. It consists of three components [53]:

1. Control of bleeding

2. Restitution of blood flow where necessary

3. Control of contamination

Haemorrhage should be arrested as rapidly as possible, with temporary control of bleeding by direct compression and aortic cross-clamping – if necessary – at the diaphragm. The abdomen is packed and temporary abdominal closure is performed. Traditional organ repairs should be delayed to a later phase ('second look laparotomy').

In the haemodynamically stable patient, primary definitive surgical management is recommended [53].

The abdomen should be entered through a long midline incision. All haematomas due to penetrating trauma should be explored. Exploration of retroperitoneal hematomas due to blunt trauma should be limited to expanding, pulsatile or leaking hematomas.

The exploration of each anatomic zone requires a different technical manoeuvre:

- Zone 1, supramesocolic: medial rotation of the viscera in the left upper abdomen; for the supramesocolic IVC, medial rotation of the right colon and hepatic flexure and Kocher manoeuvre
- Zone 1, inframesocolic: cephalic retraction of the transverse colon, displacement of the small bowel to the right

- Zone 2: left, mobilisation of the left colon; right, medial rotation of the right colon, duodenum and head of the pancreas
- Zone 3: dissection of the paracolic peritoneum and medial rotation of the colon, or direct dissection over the vessels

Supramesocolic aortic injuries are usually repaired with direct suture (with pledget interposition if necessary), while pararenal and infrarenal aortic lesions are usually fixed with interposition grafts, as it is customary in chronic diseases. Omental wrapping should be considered to reduce postoperative graft infection if a prosthetic reconstruction of a major vessel is required.

Simple ligation should be considered in case of venous injuries or visceral vessel lesions (especially for the celiac trunk [55] and for the inferior mesenteric artery).

The abdomen should be never closed primarily because of the high incidence of ACS.

12.2.5   Operative Strategies: Endovascular Treatment

There has been a recent shift to endovascular repair, with satisfactory outcomes. In fact, endovascular repair avoids the potential for surgical graft infection from concurrent bowel injury, and should be considered for each stable patient, especially in blunt traumas.

Endovascular management has a definitive role in selected cases: limited dissections, pseudoaneurysms, aorto-caval fistulae. The damage can be repaired by endografts following the same indications of EVAR (i.e. for ruptures or fistulae, see Fig. 12.4), bare metal stents (in case of dissection with ischaemia) or embolisation (with coils [56], plugs or glue, i.e. in case of pseudoaneurysms or bleeding from small vessels).

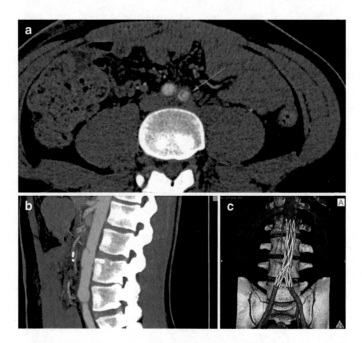

Fig. 12.4 A case of symptomatic aorto-iliac dissection after a blunt trauma (train accident). (**a**) Axial cut depicting the dissection of the left iliac artery (*arrow*). (**b**) Pre-operative maximum intensity projection that shows the dissection in the infrarenal aorta (*arrow*) and the left iliac artery. (**c**) Post-operative 3D volume rendering showing the implanted endograft and the resolution of the dissection

The placing of an intra-aortic occlusion balloon in the early stages of trauma management may be used as a 'bridge' to surgery and/or embolisation [57].

12.2.6   Operative Strategies: Conservative Treatment

Non-operative treatment may be considered in minimal aortic injuries (small intimal tear and intramural hematoma). A conservative management with blood pressure control, anti-platelet therapy and close follow-up demonstrated to be safe and feasible in Grade I and II aorto-iliac lesions [40, 58].

Observation may also be considered in non-expanding retroperitoneal haematomas in stable patients.

12.2.7 Post-operative Management, Complications and Outcomes

The post-operative management is comparable to that for RAAA. Complication rates are similar, especially the incidence of ACS or MOF. In addition, there is a higher risk of contamination, sepsis and graft infection, particularly in case of open wounds or associated bowel injury.

Despite advances in trauma management, the outcome is generally poor. Mortality after a blunt trauma is 27 %, 65–85 % after a penetrating aortic wound [40, 42, 59, 60]. The prognosis is worse in case of suprarenal lesions.

References

1. Moll FL, et al. Management of abdominal aortic aneurysms clinical practice guidelines of the European society for vascular surgery. Eur J Vasc Endovasc Surg. 2011;41 Suppl 1:S1–58.
2. Assar AN, Zarins CK. Ruptured abdominal aortic aneurysm: a surgical emergency with many clinical presentations. Postgrad Med J. 2009;85(1003):268–73.
3. Reite A, et al. Epidemiology of ruptured abdominal aortic aneurysms in a well-defined Norwegian population with trends in incidence, intervention rate, and mortality. J Vasc Surg. 2015;61(5):1168–74.
4. Parkinson F, et al. Rupture rates of untreated large abdominal aortic aneurysms in patients unfit for elective repair. J Vasc Surg. 2015;61(6):1606–12.
5. Erhart P, et al. Finite element analysis in asymptomatic, symptomatic, and ruptured abdominal aortic aneurysms: in search of new rupture risk predictors. Eur J Vasc Endovasc Surg. 2015;49(3):239–45.

6. Khosla S, et al. Meta-analysis of peak wall stress in ruptured, symptomatic and intact abdominal aortic aneurysms. Br J Surg. 2014;101(11):1350–7; discussion 1357.

7. Taylor Jr LM, Porter JM. Basic data related to clinical decision-making in abdominal aortic aneurysms. Ann Vasc Surg. 1987;1(4):502–4.

8. Hoornweg LL, et al. Meta analysis on mortality of ruptured abdominal aortic aneurysms. Eur J Vasc Endovasc Surg. 2008;35(5):558–70.

9. Lindholt JS, Sogaard R, Laustsen J. Prognosis of ruptured abdominal aortic aneurysms in Denmark from 1994–2008. Clin Epidemiol. 2012;4:111–3.

10. Azhar B, et al. Misdiagnosis of ruptured abdominal aortic aneurysm: systematic review and meta-analysis. J Endovasc Ther. 2014;21(4):568–75.

11. Biancari F, et al. Diagnostic accuracy of computed tomography in patients with suspected abdominal aortic aneurysm rupture. Eur J Vasc Endovasc Surg. 2013;45(3):227–30.

12. Mell MW, et al. Interfacility transfer and mortality for patients with ruptured abdominal aortic aneurysm. J Vasc Surg. 2014;60(3):553–7.

13. Dries DJ. Hypotensive resuscitation. Shock. 1996;6(5):311–6.

14. Capone AC, et al. Improved outcome with fluid restriction in treatment of uncontrolled hemorrhagic shock. J Am Coll Surg. 1995;180(1):49–56.

15. Owens TM, et al. Limiting initial resuscitation of uncontrolled hemorrhage reduces internal bleeding and subsequent volume requirements. J Trauma. 1995;39(2):200–7; discussion 208–9.

16. Dick F, et al. Delayed volume resuscitation during initial management of ruptured abdominal aortic aneurysm. J Vasc Surg. 2013;57(4):943–50.

17. Kauvar DS, Sarfati MR, Kraiss LW. Intraoperative blood product resuscitation and mortality in ruptured abdominal aortic aneurysm. J Vasc Surg. 2012;55(3):688–92.

18. Darling 3rd RC, et al. Advances in the surgical repair of ruptured abdominal aortic aneurysms. Cardiovasc Surg. 1996;4(6):720–3.

19. Lorenzi M, Mancini S, Mancini S. Graft reconstruction using an intraluminal balloon catheter in ruptured abdominal aortic aneurysms. Eur J Surg. 1998;164(2):147–8.

20. Matsuda H, et al. Transbrachial arterial insertion of aortic occlusion balloon catheter in patients with shock from ruptured abdominal aortic aneurysm. J Vasc Surg. 2003;38(6):1293–6.

21. Raux M, et al. Endovascular balloon occlusion is associated with reduced intraoperative mortality of unstable patients with ruptured abdominal aortic aneurysm but fails to improve other outcomes. J Vasc Surg. 2015;61(2):304–8.

22. Bjorck M. Management of the tense abdomen or difficult abdominal closure after operation for ruptured abdominal aortic aneurysms. Semin Vasc Surg. 2012;25(1):35–8.

23. Yusuf SW, et al. Emergency endovascular repair of leaking aortic aneurysm. Lancet. 1994;344(8937):1645.

24. Djavani K, Wanhainen A, Bjorck M. Intra-abdominal hypertension and abdominal compartment syndrome following surgery for ruptured abdominal aortic aneurysm. Eur J Vasc Endovasc Surg. 2006;31(6):581–4.

25. Mayer D, et al. Open abdomen treatment following endovascular repair of ruptured abdominal aortic aneurysms. J Vasc Surg. 2009;50(1):1–7.

26. Horer T, et al. Tissue plasminogen activator-assisted hematoma evacuation to relieve abdominal compartment syndrome after endovascular repair of ruptured abdominal aortic aneurysm. J Endovasc Ther. 2012;19(2):144–8.

27. Barakat HM, et al. Outcomes after open repair of ruptured abdominal aortic aneurysms in octogenarians: a 20-year, single-center experience. Ann Vasc Surg. 2014;28(1):80–6.

28. von Meijenfeldt GC, et al. Differences in mortality, risk factors, and complications after open and endovascular repair of ruptured abdominal aortic aneurysms. Eur J Vasc Endovasc Surg. 2014;47(5):479–86.

29. van Beek SC, et al. Acute kidney injury defined according to the 'Risk', 'Injury', 'Failure', 'Loss', and 'End-stage' (RIFLE) criteria after repair for a ruptured abdominal aortic aneurysm. J Vasc Surg. 2014;60(5):1159–67, 1167.e1.

30. Ambler GK, et al. Incidence and outcomes of severe renal impairment following ruptured abdominal aortic aneurysm repair. Eur J Vasc Endovasc Surg. 2015;50(4):443–9.

31. Champagne BJ, et al. Outcome of aggressive surveillance colonoscopy in ruptured abdominal aortic aneurysm. J Vasc Surg. 2004;39(4):792–6.

32. Champagne BJ, et al. Incidence of colonic ischemia after repair of ruptured abdominal aortic aneurysm with endograft. J Am Coll Surg. 2007;204(4):597–602.

33. Pini R, et al. The influence of study design on the evaluation of ruptured abdominal aortic aneurysm treatment. Ann Vasc Surg. 2014;28(6):1568–80.

34. Luebke T, Brunkwall J. Risk-adjusted meta-analysis of 30-day mortality of endovascular versus open repair for ruptured abdominal aortic aneurysms. Ann Vasc Surg. 2015;29(4):845–63.

35. Badger S, et al. Endovascular treatment for ruptured abdominal aortic aneurysm. Cochrane Database Syst Rev. 2014;(7):CD005261.

36. Sweeting MJ, et al. Ruptured aneurysm trials: the importance of longer-term outcomes and meta-analysis for 1-year mortality. Eur J Vasc Endovasc Surg. 2015;50(3):297–302.

37. Gunn ML. Imaging of aortic and branch vessel trauma. Radiol Clin North Am. 2012;50(1):85–103.

38. Asensio JA, et al. Abdominal vascular injuries: the trauma surgeon's challenge. Surg Today. 2001;31(11):949–57.

39. Asensio JA, et al. Multiinstitutional experience with the management of superior mesenteric artery injuries. J Am Coll Surg. 2001;193(4):354–65; discussion 365–6.

40. Shalhub S, et al. Blunt abdominal aortic injury. J Vasc Surg. 2012;55(5):1277–85.

41. Tashiro J, et al. Mechanism and mortality of pediatric aortic injuries. J Surg Res. 2015;198(2):456–61.

42. Cronenwett JL, Johnston KW. Rutherford's vascular surgery. Philadelphia: Saunders/Elsevier; 2014. p. 1. online resource.

43. Asensio JA, et al. Operative management and outcome of 302 abdominal vascular injuries. Am J Surg. 2000;180(6):528–33; discussion 533–4.

44. Feliciano DV, Moore EE, Biffl WL. Western trauma association critical decisions in trauma: management of abdominal vascular trauma. J Trauma Acute Care Surg. 2015;79(6):1079–88.

45. Dosios TJ, et al. Blunt and penetrating trauma of the thoracic aorta and aortic arch branches: an autopsy study. J Trauma. 2000;49(4):696–703.

46. Chapellier X, Sockeel P, Baranger B. Management of penetrating abdominal vessel injuries. J Visc Surg. 2010;147(2):e1–12.

47. Lopera JE, et al. Aortoiliac vascular injuries after misplacement of fixation screws. J Trauma. 2010;69(4):870–5.

48. Dudko S, et al. Laceration of abdominal aorta by a fragment of fractured L2 vertebral body after a low-energy injury: a case report and review of literature. Spine (Phila Pa 1976). 2012;37(22):E1406–9.

49. Gunn M, Campbell M, Hoffer EK. Traumatic abdominal aortic injury treated by endovascular stent placement. Emerg Radiol. 2007;13(6):329–31.

50. Azizzadeh A, et al. Blunt traumatic aortic injury: initial experience with endovascular repair. J Vasc Surg. 2009;49(6):1403–8.

51. Demetriades D, et al. Mortality and prognostic factors in penetrating injuries of the aorta. J Trauma. 1996;40(5):761–3.

52. Mellnick VM, et al. CT features of blunt abdominal aortic injury. Emerg Radiol. 2012;19(4):301–7.

53. Rossaint R, et al. The European guideline on management of major bleeding and coagulopathy following trauma: fourth edition. Crit Care. 2016;20(1):100.
54. Sorrentino TA, et al. Effect of damage control surgery on major abdominal vascular trauma. J Surg Res. 2012;177(2):320–5.
55. Perini P, et al. Percutaneous embolization of symptomatic dissecting aneurysms of the celiac artery. Acta Radiol. 2014;55(9):1076–81.
56. Salsamendi J, et al. Endovascular coil embolization in the treatment of a rare case of post-traumatic abdominal aortic pseudoaneurysms: brief report and review of literature. Ann Vasc Surg. 2016;30:310 e1–8.
57. Horer TM, et al. Aorta balloon occlusion in trauma: three cases demonstrating multidisciplinary approach already on patient's arrival to the emergency room. Cardiovasc Intervent Radiol. 2016;39(2):284–9.
58. Charlton-Ouw KM, et al. Observation may be safe in selected cases of blunt traumatic abdominal aortic injury. Ann Vasc Surg. 2016;30:34–9.
59. Inaba K, et al. Blunt abdominal aortic trauma in association with thoracolumbar spine fractures. Injury. 2001;32(3):201–7.
60. Demetriades D, et al. Selective nonoperative management of gunshot wounds of the anterior abdomen. Arch Surg. 1997;132(2):178–83.

Chapter 13
Obstetrics-Gynecology Emergencies

Bruno M. Pereira and Gustavo P. Fraga

13.1 Introduction

This chapter's main objective is to assist the acute care surgeon in clearing his thoughts when confronted with an acute abdomen on a female patient and, therefore, facilitate diagnostic and emergency care management. It is paramount that the acute care surgeon finds himself prepared for different kinds of emergency scenarios including those involving obstetrics and gynecology (OB/GYN) situations. In such setting, it is important to first recognize the chief complaints that motivated the patient to call for emergency assistance, as many other diagnoses different than OB/GYN causes could appear. Figure 13.1 shows the most common differential diagnosis for acute abdominal pain on a female patient.

B.M. Pereira, MD, MHSc, PhD • G.P. Fraga, MD, PhD (✉)
Division of Trauma Surgery, Department of Surgery, School of Medical Sciences, University of Campinas, Campinas, SP, Brazil
e-mail: fragap2008@gmail.com

© Springer International Publishing Switzerland 2017   229
S. Di Saverio et al. (eds.), *Acute Care Surgery Handbook*,
DOI 10.1007/978-3-319-15341-4_13

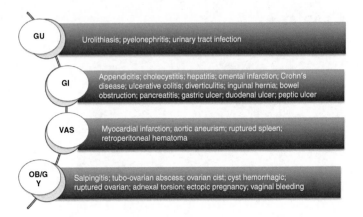

Fig. 13.1 Acute abdominal pain differential diagnosis for female individual in the emergency setting

Diagnosis of an OB/GYN emergency can take place in a hospital or other urgent care facility. The physician needs to take the patient's medical history and perform a general and pelvic physical examination. It is crucial that on any suspicious case of either an obstetric or gynecologic emergency a specialist must be consulted. Aside from that, any patient that presents herself with signs of hemorrhagic shock must be treated accordingly with life support measurements before searching for any diagnosis.

On the following sections, authors will focus at the main important OB/GYN chief complaints in the emergency room (ER) which basically belongs to two big groups: (1) vaginal bleeding and (2) lower abdominal or pelvic pain.

13.2   Vaginal Bleeding

Gynecologic bleeding usually presents into two main cohorts: those who have abnormal uterine hemorrhage (AUB) and those who have a cause based on ovulation, which is not necessarily characterized as an emergency situation. Obstetric causes of vaginal bleeding can include trauma during pregnancy, vulvar/vaginal trauma, ectopic and molar pregnancy, abruptio placentae, placenta previa, uterine rupture, and abortion.

13.2.1   Abnormal Uterine Bleeding (AUB)

In general AUB is not a life-threatening cause of bleeding, except for ruptured ectopic pregnancy. It may occur as menorrhagia – bleeding greater than 7 days presenting at regular intervals – or metrorrhagia – uterine bleeding presenting at irregular intervals. As AUB is treated based on the root cause, the emergency physician and acute care surgeon must have in mind an organized mechanism to quickly perform the diagnosis. Figure 13.2 exhibits a flowchart to assist nonspecialist physician in breaking down the diagnosis into its compartment causes. As each cause can be different from the others, a diagnostic direction is proposed.

Many patients suffering of AUB end up developing symptomatic anemia due to blood loss. It is relevant to emphasize that normal menstrual cycle has an interval of 28 days (±7 days). When menstrual cycle occurs either before 21 days or after 35 days it is consider abnormal. Nonetheless, the average length of menses is 4 days; thus, menses lasting than 7 days are also considered abnormally long [1–4].

Once finding the cause of patient's bleeding, laboratory evaluation should proceed including complete blood count, coagulation panel, liver function tests, thyroid-stimulating hormone, and pregnancy test. OB/GYN specialist must be consulted for specific examination of the vagina; if a foreign body is present, such as an intrauterine device, it should be removed and sent for culture. In regard to AUB treatment, acute care surgeon or emergency physician should follow the steps proposed on Fig. 13.2. Adolescent patients who present with AUB

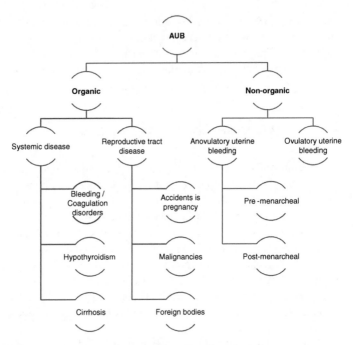

Fig. 13.2 Abnormal uterine bleeding causes

at the emergency room are at high risk for having a coagulation defect. Labs must be obtained including von Willebrand factor and evaluation for prothrombin deficiency. Beyond less common causes seen at the emergency room, pregnancy is a common cause of AUB. It can be presenting as a threatened, incomplete, or missed abortion or either on those who have an ectopic pregnancy. Many of these patients can be followed by the specialist with serial beta-hCG levels and transvaginal ultrasound. Nevertheless, the acute care surgeon may face a case of a young lady in hemorrhagic shock with positive history for pregnancy. In such cases, ACS has to be prepared for a definitive treatment through exploratory laparotomy. If there is concern that the patient may also have a gestational trophoblastic neoplastic process, counseling on the risk for hysterectomy is advised [2–5].

Over again, patients presenting with hemodynamic instability, medical supportive care must be taken in place including ventilatory support and blood product transfusion – sometimes requiring massive transfusion protocol. Emergency room health care providers may be aware that in severe AUB cases high-dose estrogen for stabilization of the endometrial lining may be needed as a life-saving measure although patient may only respond to the hormonal therapy within 6–12 h. It is worth to remember that this specific treatment may increase risk for deep vein thrombotic events which could be a great issue in severe cases of AUB coursing with hemorrhagic shock as the doctor may not be able to employ anticoagulant therapy. In this example, compressive leg stockings and intermittent self-compression devices may play a good prophylactic step [3, 4, 6].

When a pregnant patient presents to the ER with vaginal bleeding, the risk of abortion may be real. In Fig. 13.3, we propose a flowchart to facilitate decision making in emergency room.

In regard to ectopic pregnancy (EP), specifically, it worth to remember that young women with past history of salpingitis or any other inflammatory gynecologic or pelvic disease are on risk for EP. When fallopian tube presents with acute or chronic inflammation, its luminal diameter decreases and the oocyte may have difficulty navigating the tubal length into the intrauterine environ favoring fallopian tube embryo implantation rather than in the uterus. Patients who have ectopic pregnancy are found with abdominal pain, amenorrhea, and/or irregular vaginal bleeding most prevalently as well as ipsilateral adnexal tenderness and eventually adnexal mass. Not all patients present with rebound tenderness or peritoneal signs. Diagnosis of an ectopic pregnancy must be made based upon past/actual history, physical examination, lab exams – including CBC, quantitative

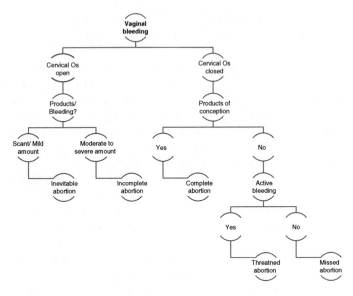

Fig. 13.3 Vaginal bleeding and pregnancy at the ER

beta-human chorionic gonadotropin (β-hCG) on admission and 48 h later (if the diagnosis remain unclear), blood type – and transvaginal ultrasound (TVUS). Association of TVUS and β-hCG has proven to allow earlier diagnosis of ectopic pregnancy and abnormal gestations. After initial assessment, an OB/GYN must be consulted for further investigation and direct treatment, unless ruptured ectopic pregnancy is diagnosed and surgical treatment is immediately required. In this last scenario, laparoscopic approach is possible on a hemodynamically stable patient and has shown to have fewer postoperative pelvic adhesions, less estimated blood loss, decreased hospital length of stay, and improved recovery time. Salpingectomy or salpingostomy may be performed as indicated [7].

13.2.2 *Vulvar and Vaginal Trauma*

Vulva and vaginal bleeding are usually secondary to local trauma such as fall on a bicycle, sports-related injuries, and automobile crashes [8]. Injuries not involved in blunt trauma can also be due to rupture of a varicosity in the late antepartum period, during labor or postpartum period when venous pelvic congestion is installed. Sex abuse should be strongly considered when pelvic examination includes hymeneal abnormal findings or labial tearing in a pediatric or adolescent patient [9].

If patient is admitted with involvement in recent trauma mechanism, pelvic fractures should be ruled out initially. In the setting of blunt or penetrating injury, especially with associated pelvic fractures, trauma to the bladder, bowel, and peritoneal cavity must also be considered. If gross or microscopic hematuria is found, a CT scan with a voiding cystourethrogram should be obtained before placement of a Foley catheter, as already defined by ATLS®. Figure 13.4 illustrates a case admitted on our institution with severe open book pelvic trauma associated with vulvar trauma. In this specific case, a young lady involved on a motor vehicle crash sustaining a pelvic fracture (Tile B), left femur and ankle fractures presented in hemorrhagic shock and was treated according to the ATLS® principles at the emergency room [10–12].

Before examination, intravenous, topical, or regional anesthesia may be required. Careful notation of the hematoma size and location should be made. Rectovaginal examination is important to assess extension into the retroperitoneal spaces. In the pediatric patient, the parent's assistance is recommended to help position the child for the examination. Visualization is best obtained with the child either in a frog-leg position or lying down in a knee-to-chest position. The vaginal vault should be well irrigated with warm saline and any foreign bodies removed.

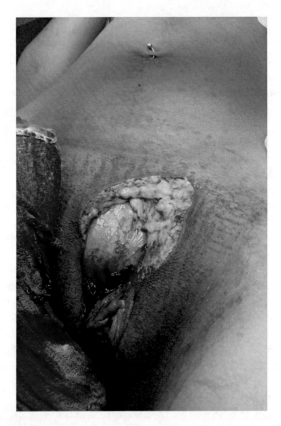

Fig. 13.4 Young lady admitted on our institution after blunt trauma (MVC), sustaining a Tile B pelvic fracture, vulvar trauma, bladder exposition, femur and ankle fractures

A CBC may be drawn in the setting of hemodynamic instability or rapidly expanding hematoma. For the vast majority of patients, little benefit is found in obtaining laboratory or radiographic data unless the injury is traumatic and there is concern for ureteral or sigmoid injury.

Management of vulvar and vaginal hematomas is usually conservative unless the hematoma exceeds 10 cm in diameter or if it is rapidly expanding. Most hematomas are venous in origin presenting as consistent dark bleeding; however, a rapidly expanding hematoma could indicate an arterial injury and attempts should be made to identify this vessel for control and ligation. Venous hematomas are typically self-limiting in nature and more difficult to control surgically than arterial hematomas [3, 8].

Of note, vaginal hematomas have the ability to expand into the retroperitoneal pelvic spaces allowing for significant blood loss. Most patients respond to ice packs and compression. In cases wherein the bleeding site cannot be identified, interventional radiology is useful and treatment can be performed through angioembolization. If necessary, a cystoscopy can be performed to evaluate function of the ureters. A Foley catheter should be placed because urinary retention can occur with significant hematoma expansion. Before placing a Foley's catheter, careful examination is recommended, and in any doubtful case a retrograde cystourethrogram should be obtained prior to inserting the catheter. In the setting of a chronic, expanding hematoma, debridement and placement of a drain is recommended. The patient should be aware that complete resolution may take several weeks. Once healed, there is usually minimal scarring or sequelae.

13.2.3 Trauma in Pregnancy

Trauma is highly prevalent and taken as the third cause of death worldwide. It complicates 6–7% of all pregnancies and is the leading nonobstetric cause of maternal morbidity and mortality. Trauma also is the leading cause of non-pregnancy-related death in women under 40 years of age in the United States, accounting for 46% of maternal deaths. Blunt abdominal trauma specifically is associated with 3–38 % of fetal mortality and may be the result of motor vehicle crash (MVC) – leading cause of maternal trauma cases, falls, pedestrian hit by car (PHBC), direct abdominal trauma and assault [13–15]. All these reported trauma mechanisms are related to maternal and fetal death when pregnant women present to the ER on hypovolemic shock due to traumatic bleeding. When high-energy mechanism is involved and blunt trauma and hemorrhagic shock is not the cause of mother and/or fetal death, abruption is the next leading cause of fetal mortality followed by uterine disruption. In regard to penetrating trauma, maternal mortality occurs in less than 5 % of the cases. Visceral trauma is also lower in pregnant woman when compared to nonpregnant population. Gunshot wounds (GSW) to the pregnant woman abdomen result in up to 70 % of fetal injury or death (which includes direct fetal trauma or preterm delivery).

Treatment guidelines for blunt or penetrating injuries are similar to those for nonpregnant patients [5, 14, 16, 17]. Management options include immediate surgical exploration, FAST (Focused Assessment Sonography for Trauma), laparoscopy, CT imaging, local wound exploration, and/or observation. Radiographic studies are helpful in localizing a missile or shrapnel that has not exited. Management often is individualized and should involve a multidisciplinary team, including ERP, trauma surgeons, and obstetricians.

The incidence of burns in pregnancy is relatively low and is difficult to determine. Maternal and fetal mortality are directly related to the type, location, and severity of the burn sustained, in addition to the presence of complications. Fetal outcome also is related to gestational age. The fetal loss rate is approximately 56 % when patients sustain burns over 15–25 % of the total body surface area (TBSA). Fetal mortality is as high as 63 % when 25–50 % of the TBSA is burned and approaches 100 % when burns exceed 50 % of TBSA. Burns are managed aggressively using treatment protocols for nonpregnant victims [15, 17–21].

In regard to falls, it accounts for 3–31 % of injuries. The morbidity associated with falls is modest and typically is associated with a less than 10 % incidence of maternal or fetal complications. The gravid female has an increase in spinal lordosis that allows the shifting of her center of gravity over her legs. This change in the center of gravity contributes to more falls as pregnancy progresses. As such, overly aggressive, high-impact activity should be avoided as pregnancy advances. The degree of injury is related to the distance and high of the fall and the specific body part involved. When patients fall, they fall primarily on their buttocks, side, or onto their abdomen. The nature of injuries includes bruises, cuts, ankle sprains, strains, and fractures. Associated complications include preterm labor, abruption, uterine rupture, low birth weight neonates, and stillbirths [16, 17, 22–25].

The prevalence of assault and domestic violence ranges from 10 to 30 % and is associated with a 5 % risk of fetal death. Abused pregnant women have a threefold higher risk of being victims of attempted and completed homicide than do nonabused controls. Most often the abuser is the patient's boyfriend or partner. Pregnancy and the postpartum period may escalate the incidence and severity of the abuse, and the uterus and fetus may sustain the brunt of the force. Common sites of abuse include the face, head, breasts, and abdomen. Patient under suspicious involvement on an assault or domestic violence event must be clinically evaluated on privacy and interrogated for any kind of abuse. Police intervention is necessary in positive cases [26–30].

13.2.4 Anatomical and Physiological Considerations of Pregnant Women in the Trauma Scenario

When managing the pregnant victim of trauma, appreciation of the anatomic and physiologic changes associated with pregnancy is critical. Before 13 weeks' gestation the uterus has not yet become an abdominal organ and is protected by the bony pelvis. Fetal loss in the first trimester is less likely the result of direct trauma (occurring less than 1 % of the time) but instead is likely to be caused by uterine hypoperfusion resulting from maternal hypotension or death. As the uterus enlarges, it displaces the bowel to cephalad position, thereby protecting these structures, but rendering the fetus more vulnerable to injury. Thinning of the uterine wall with fetal growth and the relative decrease in amniotic fluid volume also contribute to fetal vulnerability. In regard to amniotic fluid, specifically, attention to amniotic fluid embolism (AFE) is advised in trauma case scenarios. AFE is a rare but potentially fatal complication of pregnancy [14, 17].

Back to anatomic considerations, the bladder is displaced cephalad by the enlarging uterus, making it susceptible to injury; therefore, hematuria cases after traumatic injuries must be evaluated aggressively. Splenic injuries occur most commonly in the third trimester and may occur after even apparently mild trauma. Engorgement of the spleen renders it vulnerable to injury and excessive blood loss. Injuries to the liver or spleen may result in abdominal pain, shoulder pain, and elevated transaminases [13, 14]. It is important to highlight that nowadays most solid organs trauma, are eligible for non-operative management (NOM) [31–33] as well some inflammatory urgencies including in pregnant population with safety [34].

Pelvic fractures commonly are associated with blunt trauma and are the most common trauma resulting in direct fetal injury manifested by skull fractures and brain injury, particularly when the head is engaged into the bony pelvis. Fetal mortality can approach 25 % in these cases [17, 35]. Attention is advised to pelvic trauma-associated injuries to the bladder, urethra, and rectosigmoid colon [36, 37]. Pelvic radiographs required as part of the ATLS® protocol for assessing trauma in the ER must be interpreted with caution, because there is a normal widening of the sacroiliac joints and symphysis pubis with pregnancy.

Physiologic changes begin as early as the first trimester and can alter or mimic maternal response to trauma, thereby confounding ERP or trauma surgeon evaluation. The pregnant woman is physiologically prepared for the blood loss associated with delivery. Blood volume increases by approximately 50 %, and there is a 30 % increase in erythrocyte volume. With that said, a pregnant trauma patient can bleed up to 2000 mL of blood (or 30–40 % of her blood volume) before manifesting shifts in heart rate or blood pressure.

Cardiac output increases up to 50 % beginning in the first trimester and peaks somewhere between 20 and 30 weeks' gestation. Cardiac output remains at third trimester values for the first 48 h postpartum and then decreases gradually to nonpregnant values over the following 2 weeks. Uterine blood flow comprises about 20 % of cardiac output, increases up to 600 mL/min during pregnancy, and can serve as a significant source of hemorrhage in the face of trauma. Uterine blood flow has no autoregulation and, therefore, is dependent on maternal mean arterial blood pressure. As such, changes in blood pressure can impact uterine blood flow negatively, thereby compromising fetal perfusion and oxygenation. By 20 weeks' gestation the enlarging uterus is capable of aortocaval compression, which can compromise venous return to the heart and reduce cardiac output. When the pregnant woman is supine, aortocaval compression reduces cardiac output by approximately 30 % and can result in maternal pallor, sweating, nausea, vomiting, hypotension, tachycardia, and mental status changes. Blood pressure is lower in pregnancy secondary to decreased systemic vascular resistance. Lower vascular resistance is the result primarily of the vasodilatory effects of progesterone and the low resistance of the placental bed. Also, the increase of plasma volume over red blood cell volume results in hemodilution and, therefore, a physiologic anemia. Systolic and diastolic blood pressures decrease by 5–15 mmHg, reaching a nadir at 28 weeks' gestation and gradually returning to normal at term. Central venous pressure drops slowly from 9 mmHg to about 4 mmHg by term. Estrogen-mediated increases in myocardial alpha receptors result in heart rate increases of approximately 15 beats per minute [14]. ECG changes during pregnancy are common. Normal findings include sinus tachycardia, ectopic beats, left axis deviation, inverted or flattened T waves, and a Q wave in lead III. The increased metabolic demands of pregnancy increase oxygen consumption by 15–20 %. Minute ventilation increases by 50 %, largely as a result of increased tidal volume, because respiratory rate changes minimally. The diaphragm moves approximately 4 cm upward in pregnancy, and the thoracic anteroposterior diameter increases. Intra-abdominal pressure as well intra-thoracic pressure increases. These anatomic alterations, in addition to the enlarging uterus, cause decreased expiratory reserve and residual lung volumes, thereby decreasing functional residual capacity. The 20 % decrease in functional residual capacity coupled with increased oxygen consumption of pregnancy results in rapid maternal desaturation in the face of depressed respiration or apnea. The regular pregnant mother compensates in a state of mild respiratory alkalosis. Elevated progesterone levels act on the medullary respiratory center stimulating ventilatory drive causing a decrease in $PaCO_2$ values to levels approaching 25–30 mmHg.

There is a compensatory renal excretion of bicarbonate resulting in serum levels of 17–22 mEq/L, thereby maintaining an arterial pH of 7.40–7.45. The increased minute ventilation results in PaO_2 levels that is higher than nonpregnant values, ranging between 104 mmHg and 108 mmHg. Maternal oxygen saturation should be maintained at 95 % to maintain a PaO_2 greater than 70 mmHg, optimizing oxygen diffusion across the placenta. Fetal oxygenation is maintained when maternal PaO_2 remains above 60–70 mmHg, and it is compromised immediately at lower levels. The smooth muscle relaxation effects of progesterone contribute to decreased gastric tone and motility as well as reduced lower esophageal sphincter tone. These changes, in addition to the cephalad displacement of the stomach, result in an increased risk of aspiration when the trauma victim is unable to protect her airway. Normal chest radiographic findings in a pregnant patient include mild cardiomegaly, a widened mediastinum, an increased anteroposterior diameter, and prominence of the pulmonary vasculature [14, 16].

Normal pregnancy complaints include nausea, vomiting, and abdominal pain, symptoms that can confound the examination of a trauma patient. Venous pooling in the lower extremities can lead to more extensive blood loss with lower extremity injuries and can predispose the patient to deep venous thrombosis. The increased engorgement of pelvic vessels associated with pregnancy also places the patient at increased risk of retroperitoneal hemorrhage and hematomas following lower abdominal and pelvic trauma [13]. It is normal to have a leukocytosis during pregnancy with a count ranging from 5,000 to 25,000 per mm^3. Most pro-coagulant factors also are increased during pregnancy and may be beneficial for the patient in achieving hemostasis after injury. Fibrinogen levels normally approach 400 mg/dL. Therefore, findings of a normal or low fibrinogen level, in addition to elevated fibrin degradation products and low platelets, suggest disseminated intravascular coagulation. Increase in pro-coagulants, in addition to venous stasis and endothelial damage, place the pregnant patient at risk for thromboembolic complications including pulmonary embolism. Therefore, when possible, thromboembolic prophylaxis is recommended following trauma.

13.2.5 Abruption

Abruption occurs with 1–5 % of minor injuries and 20–50 % of major life-threatening injuries. It also occurs at a higher rate in women suffering trauma than in the general obstetric population [15–17]. Next to maternal death, abruption is the most frequent cause of fetal death from trauma (1 out of 400 cases of abruption) [38]. Abruption occurs when acceleration-deceleration injuries result in shearing forces that separate the relatively elastic myometrium from the inelastic placenta [39]. Other predisposing conditions include maternal hypertension, preeclampsia, multiple births, and previous abruption.

Placental injury results in the release of thromboplastin into the circulation, and uterine injury releases plasminogen activator, resulting in fibrinolysis. These processes can lead to disseminated intravascular coagulation. The patient may complain of abdominal pain, bleeding, and/or back pain. Examination may demonstrate vaginal bleeding and a tender, rigid uterus. The pregnant trauma patient should be admitted, and continuous fetal monitoring should be initiated if the fetus is viable. Electronic fetal monitoring is the most sensitive tool in identifying abruption. Cardiotocography has demonstrated a 100 % negative predictive value for adverse outcomes when monitoring was reassuring and there were no significant early clinical findings. Initial external fetal monitoring for a minimum of 4 h is recommended for all patients of 20 weeks' gestation who have experienced any multisystem or minor abdominal trauma. Monitoring should be continued if there is evidence of persistent contractions, uterine tenderness, vaginal bleeding, significant maternal injury, rupture of membranes, or a nonreassuring fetal heart rate pattern [39]. Monitoring may be discontinued and the patient discharged by obstetrician if laboratory evaluation is normal, the fetal tracing is reassuring, contraction frequency is less than 1 per 10 min, and there is no evidence of vaginal bleeding or nonreassuring maternal status.

13.2.6   Fetal-Maternal Hemorrhage

Fetal-maternal hemorrhage occurs in 10–30 % of pregnant trauma patients. It occurs more commonly in women who suffer abdominal trauma with an anterior placenta. Injury severity is not related to the incidence of fetal-maternal hemorrhage. Fetal risks of fetal-maternal hemorrhage include anemia, arrhythmias, and exsanguination with resultant fetal distress and death. Maternal risks include Rh sensitization. Less than 1 mL of Rh-positive fetal blood can result in sensitization in an Rh-negative woman. The Kleihauer-Betke blood test assesses for hemorrhage of fetal cells into maternal circulation. It allows quantification of the amount of fetal red blood cells introduced into the maternal bloodstream. All Rh-negative pregnant trauma victims should receive 300 mg of Rh-immune globulin within the first 72 h of fetomaternal hemorrhage and another 300 mg for each additional 30 mL of estimated fetal blood identified in the maternal circulation. Kleihauer-Betke testing is not indicated in Rh-positive women [35, 40].

13.2.7 Uterine Rupture

A rare complication of abdominal trauma in a pregnant woman is uterine rupture although it can also happen spontaneously during labor (1 in 1400 deliveries). Uterine rupture accounts for approximately 0.6 % of all injuries during pregnancy and can result in a very high maternal mortality rate and nearly universal fetal death rate. Uterine rupture occurs most commonly with rapid deceleration or direct compression injuries and is found most often in women who have had prior cesarean deliveries. The risk for uterine rupture tends to increase with advancing gestational age and with increasing severity of direct abdominal trauma. Prior C-section is the most important risk factor. The uterine wall separates, thereby rupturing the membranes and allowing extrusion of the umbilical cord and fetal parts into the abdomen. This rupture often is accompanied by extensive intra-abdominal hemorrhage. Rupture of an unscarred uterus tends to occur posteriorly and commonly is associated with a bladder injury, presenting occasionally with blood or meconium in the urine [3, 13, 17, 38].

Symptoms of uterine rupture include rigid abdomen with severe abdominal diffuse pain and cessation of uterine contractions. Examination is remarkable for vaginal bleeding, a rigid abdomen, rebound tenderness, and an asymmetric uterus or fetal parts palpable through the abdomen. There may be no fetal heart rate, decreased fetal heart rate beat-to-beat variability, decelerations, or fetal tachycardia as a result of anemia or hypoxemia. The diagnosis is suggested on abdominal radiograph or ultrasound and may require emergent surgical management [3, 13, 17, 38].

13.2.8 Special Consideration: Emergency Cesarean Delivery

Emergency cesarean deliveries occasionally are performed for maternal or fetal indications. Emergency cesarean is indicated when the uterus interferes in trauma-related surgical interventions, cardiopulmonary resuscitation has been unsuccessful after 4 min, there is fetal compromise in a viable fetus with a stable mother, or there is obvious impending or recent maternal death. Fetal and maternal survival rates after emergency cesarean delivery at greater than 25 weeks' gestation have been documented to be as high as 45 % and 72 %, respectively. There was no fetal survival when no fetal heartbeat was heard before emergent delivery, whereas there was 75 % survival when fetal heart tones were present and gestational age was 26 weeks or more. Optimum infant survival has been described when cesarean delivery was performed within 5 min of maternal death [41–43]. It is recommended that cesarean delivery be performed if the patient has not responded after 4 min of resuscitation. Four minutes of resuscitation and 1 min to deliver the neonate is the basis for the "5-min rule". One may want to consider proceeding with delivery even if resuscitation efforts have extended beyond 4 min, because neonatal survival has been reported. In addition to optimizing fetal outcome, cesarean delivery removes aortocaval compression, resulting in a 60–80 % increase in cardiac output and optimizing chances for maternal survival [41, 42].

13.3   Lower Abdominal or Pelvic Pain

On the gynecologic patient, lower abdominal pain or pelvic pain is usually due to ischemic, inflammatory, or bleeding processes. Bellow you will find the most common examples of each in the emergency department.

13.3.1   Adnexal Torsion

Patients who present with adnexal torsion (AT) often complain about lower abdominal acute intermittent pain. It is mandatory to exclude other differential diagnosis such as acute appendicitis, adnexal abscess, pelvic inflammatory disease (PID), ruptured corpus luteum, or ectopic pregnancy. AT is associated with enlarged ovarian mass and ipsilateral lower abdominal or pelvic acute intermittent pain exacerbated by positional shifts. The episodes may have intermittently persisted for the past few days to weeks worsening in the last hours with no relief with regular painkillers. Gastrointestinal unspecific symptoms such as nausea and vomiting are also common which can lead some providers to miss or confuse the current clinical hypothesis with any differential diagnosis mentioned above. It is worth to remember though that AT is a consequence of ovarian tumors (such as dermoid tumors) in 50–60 % of the cases. If the torsion persists or progresses, the ovarian tissue begins to undergo necrosis, when physician usually observes worsening symptoms.

Pelvic ultrasound with color Doppler is highly predictive of AT; however, a normal Doppler flow should not exclude the diagnosis when there are clinical findings of acute abdomen. Abdominal and pelvic CT scan must be performed in doubtful cases.

Surgery is the treatment of choice for AT. Laparoscopy approach to patients who have AT is showing to be a good surgical strategy. Instead of performing a salpingo-oophorec-tomy, a laparoscopic evaluation with a gentle untwisting of the ovary and an oophoropexy can be safely performed with a success rate of approximately 88 % [44–55]. In the setting of severe vascular compromise, unilateral salpingo-oophorectomy is indicated. Care should be taken when surgically removing the adnexal mass before excision. The ureter runs inferiorly and laterally to the infundibulopelvic ligament and can be tented upward from the torsion process. In a pregnant patient, specifically, there have been successful cases of laparoscopic adnexal torsion reduction and oophoropexy. The incidence of adnexal torsion in pregnancy is 1 in 5000 pregnancies. Many authors recommend entering in an open manner (i.e., Hasson technique) as opposed to Veress needle or other indirect approach; however, there has been documentation of complications in all three approaches. Precautions should be taken as the uterus may be in the abdominal cavity and surgical pneumoperitoneum poses the risk for decreased uterine blood flow secondary to increased intra-abdominal pressure [49]. Fetal cardiac activity should be documented through cardiotocography, for instance, before and after the procedure and the patient should be positioned in the dorsal supine position with left lateral tilt during the operation. The pregnant patient should be counseled on risks, including premature, preterm rupture of membranes, and preterm delivery [54].

13.3.2 Pelvic Inflammatory Disease

Pelvic inflammatory disease (PID) is caused by polymicrobial infection of the upper genital tract, originating from urethral focus, vaginal or cervical. The virulence of the bacteria and patient's immune response define the progression: endometritis, salpingitis, pelviperitonite, oophoritis, perihepatitis (Fitz-Hugh-Curtis syndrome – Fig. 13.5), tubo-ovarian abscess [51]. The pathogens are usually sexually transmitted (chlamydia, gonococcus, mycoplasma, trichomonas casually and viruses) or endogenous. The two most common organisms responsible for tubo-ovarian abscess are *Neisseria gonorrhoeae* and *Chlamydia trachomatis*. This is important to guide antibiotic coverage.

PID is diagnosed clinically based on having three physical findings (major criteria) plus one additional finding (minor criteria) from a laboratory or radiographic result (Fig. 13.6). Patients who have infections of the upper genital tract may present in a similar fashion as those who have an ectopic pregnancy, hemorrhagic corpus luteal cyst, appendicitis, or endometriosis/endometrioma. PID may be treated on an outpatient basis; however, there are some indications for hospitalization of patients

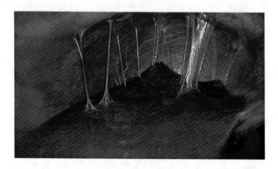

Fig. 13.5 Fitz-Hugh-Curtis syndrome, laparoscopic view from one of author's cases

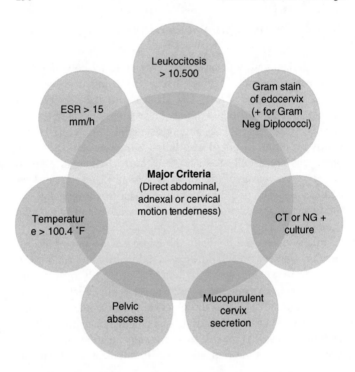

Fig. 13.6 PID diagnosis criteria: All major criteria required. One or more additional findings should be present (*ESR* erythrocyte sedimentation rate, *CT Chlamydia trachomatis, NG Neisseria gonorrhoeae*)

who have an acute PID picture. When evaluating a patient who has an adnexal mass and an acute abdomen in a setting of PID, a tubo-ovarian abscess should be considered. When the clinical picture is suggestive and there is no other possible diagnosis, starting treatment to decrease the prevalence of reproductive sequelae is advised. Diagnosis is determined by increased erythrocyte sedimentation rate and C-reactive protein; CBC; presence of leukocytes abundant in fresh examination of cervical discharge; and detection of gonococcal or chlamydial in endocervix. Diagnosis can also be complemented by pelvic ultrasound transabdominal/transvaginal, and/or CT/MRI. Laparoscopy allows more accurate diagnosis, though not proving endometritis [44–55].

The general treatment principles are: (1) rest and adequate analgesia; (2) deactivating intrauterine device in situ for fastest healing; (3) administering antibiotics including gonococcus, chlamydia, mycoplasma, aerobic bacteria (gram-positive and negative), anaerobic and facultative because the isolation of these pathogens is difficult and incomplete; (4) minimum antibiotic duration of 14 days; (5) in case of tubo-ovarian or pelvic abscess, drain if necessary; (6) monitoring the clinical and bacteriological findings for four to six weeks after the end of treatment. When treatment is out of hospital, the patient must be reassessed after 72 h. Hospitalize and prefer parenteral treatment when: (1) diagnostic is uncertain; (2) absence of clinical response, low adherence or intolerance to oral treatment; (3) severe cases (nausea and vomiting or high fever); (4) tubo-ovarian abscess or pelvic abscess; and (5) pregnancy. Clinical improvement into the first 3 days of treatment by parenteral lines (decrease of temperature, decrease of abdominal pain, and pelvic caused) physician is authorized to move for oral treatment. Specialist must be consulted as early as possible. Laparoscopy may be indicated in refractory cases [47, 48, 50, 52].

References

1. Caserta D, Toro G, Porretta M, Mancini E, Moscarini M. Hysteroscopic vs histologic diagnosis. Study of 222 cases of abnormal uterine hemorrhage. Minerva Ginecol. 1999;51(5):169–72.
2. Chen YT, Xu LF, Sun HL, Li HQ, Hu RM, Tan QY. Clinical efficacy and safety of uterine artery chemoembolization in abnormal placental implantation complicated with postpartum hemorrhage. Zhonghua Fu Chan Ke Za Zhi. 2010;45(4):273–7.

3. Mirza FG, Gaddipati S. Obstetric emergencies. Semin Perinatol. 2009;33(2):97–103.

4. Roth CK, Parfitt SE, Hering SL, Dent SA. Developing protocols for obstetric emergencies. Nurs Womens Health. 2014;18(5):378–90.

5. Green M, Rider C, Ratcliff D, Woodring BC. Developing a aystematic approach to obstetric emergencies. J Obstet Gynecol Neonatal Nurs JOGNN/NAACOG. 2015;44(5):677–82.

6. Sokol E, Peddinti R. Causes and diagnosis of abnormal vaginal bleeding. Pediatr Ann. 2015;44(7):e164–7.

7. Taran FA, Kagan KO, Hubner M, Hoopmann M, Wallwiener D, Brucker S. The diagnosis and treatment of ectopic pregnancy. Dtsch Arztebl Int. 2015;112(41):693–704.

8. Hoefgen HR, Merritt DF. Rope swing injuries resulting in vulvar trauma. J Pediatr Adolesc Gynecol. 2015;28(1):e13–5.

9. Walsh K, Latzman NE, Latzman RD. Pathway from child sexual and physical abuse to risky sex among emerging adults: the role of trauma-related intrusions and alcohol problems. J Adolesc Health Off publ Soc Adolesc Med. 2014;54(4):442–8.

10. Subcommittee A, American College of Surgeons' Committee on T, International Awg. Advanced trauma life support (ATLS(R)): the ninth edition. J Trauma Acute Care Surg. 2013;74(5):1363–6.

11. Mourad L. Tile classification of pelvic disruption. Orthop Nurs. 1997;16(3):34.

12. Osterhoff G, Scheyerer MJ, Fritz Y, Bouaicha S, Wanner GA, Simmen HP, et al. Comparing the predictive value of the pelvic ring injury classification systems by Tile and by Young and Burgess. Injury. 2014;45(4):742–7.

13. Daponte A, Khan N, Smith MD, Degiannis E. Trauma in pregnancy. S Afr J Surg Suid-Afrikaanse tydskrif vir chirurgie. 2003;41(2):51–4; discussion 5.

14. Shah AJ, Kilcline BA. Trauma in pregnancy. Emerg Med Clin North Am. 2003;21(3):615–29.

15. Battaloglu E, McDonnell D, Chu J, Lecky F, Porter SK. Epidemiology and outcomes of pregnancy and obstetric complications in trauma in the United Kingdom. Injury. 2016;47(1):184–7.

16. Cheng HT, Wang YC, Lo HC, Su LT, Lin CH, Sung FC, et al. Trauma during pregnancy: a population-based analysis of maternal outcome. World J Surg. 2012;36(12):2767–75.

17. El-Kady D, Gilbert WM, Anderson J, Danielsen B, Towner D, Smith LH. Trauma during pregnancy: an analysis of maternal and fetal outcomes in a large population. Am J Obstet Gynecol. 2004; 190(6):1661–8.

18. Khales A, Achbouk A, Siah S, Ihrai H. Burns and pregnancy: report on two cases and review of the literature. Ann Burns Fire Disasters. 2010;23(2):72–4.

19. Maghsoudi H, Samnia R, Garadaghi A, Kianvar H. Burns in pregnancy. Burns J Int Soc Burn Inj. 2006;32(2):246–50.

20. Parikh P, Sunesara I, Lutz E, Kolb J, Sawardecker S, Martin Jr JN. Burns during pregnancy: implications for maternal-perinatal providers and guidelines for practice. Obstet Gynecol Surv. 2015;70(10):633–43.

21. Subrahmanyam M. Burns during pregnancy - effect on maternal and foetal outcomes. Ann Burns Fire Disasters. 2006;19(4):177–9.

22. Brewin D, Naninni A. Women's perspectives on falls and fall prevention during pregnancy. MCN Am J Matern Child Nurs. 2014;39(5):300–5.

23. Inanir A, Cakmak B, Hisim Y, Demirturk F. Evaluation of postural equilibrium and fall risk during pregnancy. Gait Posture. 2014;39(4):1122–5.

24. Ozturk G, Geler Kulcu D, Aydog E, Kaspar C, Ugurel B. Effects of lower back pain on postural equilibrium and fall risk during the third trimester of pregnancy. J Matern Fetal Neonatal Med Off J Eur Assoc Perinat Med Fed Asia Oceania Perinat Soc Int Soc Perinat Obstet. 2015;26:1–5.

25. Sisay Woldeyes W, Amenu D, Segni H. Uterine rupture in pregnancy following fall from a motorcycle: a horrid accident in pregnancy-a case report and review of the literature. Case Rep Obstet Gynecol. 2015;2015:715180.

26. Arslantas H, Adana F, Ergin F, Gey N, Bicer N, Kiransal N. Domestic violence during pregnancy in an eastern city of Turkey: a field study. J Interpers Violence. 2012;27(7):1293–313.

27. Finnbogadottir H, Dykes AK, Wann-Hansson C. Prevalence of domestic violence during pregnancy and related risk factors: a cross-sectional study in southern Sweden. BMC Womens Health. 2014;14:63.

28. Gharacheh M, Azadi S, Mohammadi N, Montazeri S, Khalajinia Z. Domestic violence during pregnancy and women's health-related quality of life. Glob J Health Sci. 2015;8(2):46251.

29. Mahapatro M, Gupta RN, Gupta V, Kundu AS. Domestic violence during pregnancy in India. J Interpers Violence. 2011;26(15):2973–90.

30. Wokoma TT, Jampala M, Bexhell H, Guthrie K, Lindow S. A comparative study of the prevalence of domestic violence in women requesting a termination of pregnancy and those attending the antenatal clinic. BJOG Int J Obstet Gynaecol. 2014;121(5):627–33.

31. Fernandes TM, Dorigatti AE, Pereira BM, Cruvinel Neto J, Zago TM, Fraga GP. Nonoperative management of splenic injury grade IV is safe using rigid protocol. Rev Col Bras Cir. 2013;40(4):323–9.

32. Pereira BM. Non-operative management of hepatic trauma and the interventional radiology: an update review. Indian J Surg. 2013;75(5):339–45.

33. Zago TM, Pereira BM, Nascimento B, Alves MS, Calderan TR, Fraga GP. Hepatic trauma: a 21-year experience. Rev Col Bras Cir. 2013;40(4):318–22.

34. Jorge AM, Keswani RN, Veerappan A, Soper NJ, Gawron AJ. Non-operative management of symptomatic cholelithiasis in pregnancy is associated with frequent hospitalizations. J Gastrointest Surg Off J Soc Surg Aliment Tract. 2015;19(4):598–603.

35. Weiss HB, Songer TJ, Fabio A. Fetal deaths related to maternal injury. JAMA. 2001;286(15):1863–8.

36. Pereira BM, de Campos CC, Calderan TR, Reis LO, Fraga GP. Bladder injuries after external trauma: 20 years experience report in a population-based cross-sectional view. World J Urol. 2013;31(4):913–7.

37. Pereira BM, Reis LO, Calderan TR, de Campos CC, Fraga GP. Penetrating bladder trauma: a high risk factor for associated rectal injury. Adv Urol. 2014;2014:386280.

38. Kuczkowski KM. Trauma in the pregnant patient. Curr Opin Anaesthesiol. 2004;17(2):145–50.

39. Atkinson AL, Santolaya-Forgas J, Blitzer DN, Santolaya JL, Matta P, Canterino J, et al. Risk factors for perinatal mortality in patients admitted to the hospital with the diagnosis of placental abruption. J Matern Fetal Neonatal Med Off J Eur Assoc Perinat Med Fed Asia and Oceania Perinat Soc Int Soc Perinat Obstet. 2015;28(5):594–7.

40. Atkinson AL, Santolaya-Forgas J, Matta P, Canterino J, Oyelese Y. The sensitivity of the Kleihauer-Betke test for placental abruption. J Obstet Gynaecol J Inst Obstet Gynaecol. 2015;35(2):139–41.

41. Aronsohn J, Danzer B, Overdyk F, Roseman A. Perimortem cesarean delivery in a pregnant patient with goiter, preeclampsia, and morbid obesity. A A Case Rep. 2015;4(4):41–3.

42. Katz VL. Perimortem cesarean delivery: its role in maternal mortality. Semin Perinatol. 2012;36(1):68–72.

43. Yildirim C, Goksu S, Kocoglu H, Gocmen A, Akdogan M, Gunay N. Perimortem cesarean delivery following severe maternal penetrating injury. Yonsei Med J. 2004;45(3):561–3.

44. Birgisson NE, Zhao Q, Secura GM, Madden T, Peipert JF. Positive testing for Neisseria gonorrhoeae and Chlamydia trachomatis and the risk

of pelvic inflammatory disease in IUD users. J Womens Health. 2015;24(5):354–9.

45. Brunham RC, Gottlieb SL, Paavonen J. Pelvic inflammatory disease. N Engl J Med. 2015;372(21):2039–48.

46. Cho HW, Koo YJ, Min KJ, Hong JH, Lee JK. Pelvic inflammatory disease in virgin women with tubo-ovarian abscess: a single-center experience and literature review. J Pediatr Adolesc Gynecol. 2015. [Epub ahead of print].

47. Crum-Cianflone NF. Pelvic inflammatory disease. N Engl J Med. 2015;373(7):686.

48. Duarte R, Fuhrich D, Ross JD. A review of antibiotic therapy for pelvic inflammatory disease. Int J Antimicrob Agents. 2015;46(3):272–7.

49. Fujishita A, Araki H, Yoshida S, Hamaguchi D, Nakayama D, Tsuda N, et al. Outcome of conservative laparoscopic surgery for adnexal torsion through one-stage or two-stage operation. J Obstet Gynaecol Res. 2015;41(3):411–7.

50. Kim HY, Yang JI, Moon C. Comparison of severe pelvic inflammatory disease, pyosalpinx and tubo-ovarian abscess. J Obstet Gynaecol Res. 2015;41(5):742–6.

51. Kim JS, Kim HC, Kim SW, Yang DM, Rhee SJ, Shin JS. Does the degree of perihepatitis have any relevance to the severity of the manifestations of pelvic inflammatory disease on multidetector computed tomography? J Comput Assist Tomogr. 2015;39(6):901–6.

52. Oliphant J, Azariah S. Pelvic inflammatory disease associated with Chlamydia trachomatis but not Mycoplasma genitalium in New Zealand. Sex Health. 2016;13(1):43–8.

53. Patil AR, Nandikoor S, Rao A, MJ G, Kheda A, Hari M, et al. Multimodality imaging in adnexal torsion. J Med Imaging Radiat Oncol. 2015;59(1):7–19.

54. Spinelli C, Piscioneri J, Strambi S. Adnexal torsion in adolescents: update and review of the literature. Curr Opin Obstet Gynecol. 2015;27(5):320–5.

55. Yaakov O, Zohav E, Kapustian V, Gdalevich M, Volodarsky M, Anteby EY, et al. Are ultrasonographic findings suggestive of ovarian stromal edema associated with ischemic adnexal torsion? Gynecol Obstet Invest. 2016;81(3):262–6.

Chapter 14
Genitourinary Emergencies

**Rodrigo Donalisio da Silva, Rodrigo Pessoa,
Nicholas Westfall, and Fernando J. Kim**

14.1 Bladder Trauma

14.1.1 Clinical Presentation

The most common cause of traumatic bladder injury (excluding iatrogenic causes) is motor vehicle collisions, followed by falls, industrial trauma, and blows to the lower abdomen [1]. Pelvic fracture is found in 60–90 % of patients with blunt bladder trauma, and 44 % of the patients with bladder injuries have at least one intra-abdominal organ-associated injury [2]. The majority of bladder ruptures are extraperitoneal. A combination of bladder and urethral trauma can be found in 4.1–15 % of the cases [2, 3].

Extraperitoneal ruptures are almost always associated with pelvic fracture [4]. The bladder can be injured on the same side

R.D. da Silva • R. Pessoa • N. Westfall • F.J. Kim (✉)
Denver Health Hospital and Authority, Denver, CO, USA
e-mail: Fernando.Kim@DHHA.org

© Springer International Publishing Switzerland 2017
S. Di Saverio et al. (eds.), *Acute Care Surgery Handbook*,
DOI 10.1007/978-3-319-15341-4_14

as the fracture due to distortion of the pelvic ring, which causes traction of the ligaments attached to the pelvic wall. When the bladder injury is found on the opposite side of the pelvic fracture, it is referred to as a contrecoup injury. The bladder wall can be perforated by bones fragments [3].

Bladder trauma is predicted by disruption of the pelvic circle with displacement greater than 1 cm, diastasis of the symphysis greater than 1 cm, and fractures of the rami pubis [5].

The bladder dome is the weakest point of the bladder. A sudden rise in intravesical pressure can cause bladder rupture at the bladder dome, leading to intraperitoneal bladder rupture and urinary leakage inside the peritoneal cavity. A full bladder at the time of the trauma is a risk factor for intraperitoneal bladder rupture [3].

The presence of visible hematuria may be indicative of bladder trauma and should be investigated [3]. The combination of visible hematuria with pelvic fracture is strongly associated with bladder injury. When this combination is present, patients should undergo radiological evaluation [6–8].

Patients with traumatic bladder injury may exhibit other signs and symptoms such as inability to void, abdominal tenderness, suprapubic bruising, urinary ascites, elevated creatinine levels, entrance/exit wounds at lower abdomen, perineum, or buttocks [3, 4, 9].

Bladder traumas can be graded according to AAST classification but usually surgeons classify the bladder injuries according to the mechanism of trauma (blunt vs. penetrating) and anatomical location (intraperitoneal, extraperitoneal, or combined intra-extraperitoneal).

14.1.2   Radiological Evaluation

The radiological diagnosis of bladder rupture can be made with different radiological examinations. The sensitivity and specificity of radiological examinations are different, but the radiological modality needs to be individualized for each patient depending on clinical presentation, trauma mechanism, potential associated injuries, and hemodynamic stability.

Classically, voising cystourethrogram (VCUG) is the diagnostic modality for suspected bladder rupture [7, 8, 10]. Cystography can be performed by filling the bladder with at least 350 ml of contrast material. Sensitivity (90–95%) and specificity (100%) of plain or CT cystography are similar [4]. Surgeons must be aware that clamping the Foley catheter during the excretory phase of CT or IVP is not recommended to diagnose bladder injury because this procedure lacks sensitivity to exclude bladder injuries [3, 10].

The presence of contrast material within bowel loops and/or outlining abdominal viscera is diagnostic for intraperitoneal bladder rupture. Extraperitoneal bladder ruptures are associated with extravasation of the contrast material in the perivesical soft tissue [3, 8].

Using ultrasound to diagnose the presence of fluid in the perivesical space and/or intraperitoneal space is possible; however, the use of ultrasound alone cannot be used to diagnose bladder rupture because fluid collection could be blood [3] (Figs. 14.1 and 14.2).

Cystoscopy is a minimally invasive procedure that can help identify the location and size of the bladder rupture as well as provide additional information regarding the lesion and the position of the ureters and bladder neck. Also, cystoscopy can be used to diagnose foreign bodies inside the bladder [11].

14.1.3 Management

14.1.3.1 Nonoperative

The nonoperative management of extraperitoneal bladder rupture is the standard treatment for patients that present with uncomplicated extraperitoneal bladder injuries [3, 7, 8]. Almost

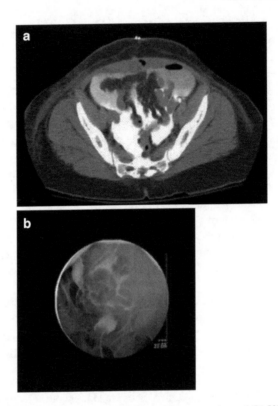

Fig. 14.1 Intraperitoneal bladder injury: (**a**) tomography and (**b**) VCUG

all blunt extraperitoneal bladder ruptures can be treated nonoperatively. Nonoperative management consists of continuous bladder drainage with a catheter, antibiotic prophylaxis, and clinical observation [3].

Orthopedic surgeons often choose to stabilize pelvic fractures with open reduction and internal fixation. Extraperitoneal bladder injuries should be repaired while pelvic fractures are surgically treated to reduce the risk of infection [3, 4]. If lapa-

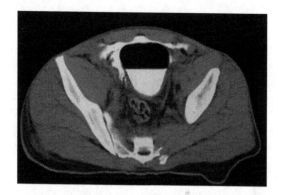

Fig. 14.2 Extraperitoneal bladder rupture

rotomy is performed to treat another abdominal injury in patients with extraperitoneal bladder rupture, latter complications can be avoided if the bladder injury is sutured during the same operation [7].

14.1.3.2 Operative Treatment of Bladder Ruptures

Bladder injuries are operatively managed in patients with intraperitoneal bladder ruptures, penetrating injuries, or for patients with extraperitoneal bladder ruptures with concomitant bladder neck involvement, bones fragments inside the bladder wall, concomitant rectal injury, or entrapment of the bladder wall [3, 9].

Bladder penetrating injuries should be treated with exploration, debridement of devitalized tissue, and primary wall suture [12]. Penetrating injuries caused by gunshot wounds require special attention. If a gunshot wound to the bladder is identified, the surgeon must assess the presence of enter and exit wounds. A midline cystotomy should be performed to inspect the bladder, treat the lesions, and evaluate the ureters bilaterally. A careful inspection for foreign bodies, fecal material, and bone fragments needs to be done before closing the bladder [9, 12].

Overall, approximately 40 % of penetrating bladder injuries is associated with rectal injuries. The diagnosis of concomitant rectal injury is challenging and only 25 % of rectal injuries can be identified during ordinary physical examination. If a rectal injury is suspected, proctoscopy or even proctosigmoidoscopy should be performed [13]. When the colon or the rectum adjacent to the bladder lesion is damaged, a fecal diversion may be necessary in up to 67 % of patients [13].

Laparoscopic management of blunt intraperitoneal ruptures can be safely performed in well-selected patients with no other intra-abdominal injuries or intracranial pressure issues. A single layer of suture can be performed, offering the patients the benefits of minimally invasive procedures such as faster recovery and better cosmetic results [14].

Urinary catheter insertion is necessary to prevent elevated intravesical pressure by reducing the leakages and allowing bladder healing [15]. Bladder injuries treated conservatively should be followed-up with a cystography, usually within 7–14 days. If no contrast extravasation is identified, the catheter can be safely removed [15]. If a leakage is found during the control cystography, radiological reevaluation can be performed 7 days later or, depending on the extent of the extravasation, size of the laceration, and presence of complications, surgeons can perform a surgical repair.

Simple injuries that required surgical repair do not need to undergo cystography before catheter removal. The catheter can be safely removed after 7–10 days [7, 15]. On the other hand, cystography is highly recommended before removing the catheter in cases of complex bladder injuries, lesions at the bladder neck, concomitant ureteral reimplantation, or high risk factors for wound healing (steroids, previous radiation, malnutrition, infection) [15].

14.2 Difficult Urinary Catheterization

Indwelling urethral catheters are often used for bladder drainage in the hospital setting. The indications for urethral catheter placement are broad and include patients with acute urinary retention, unstable patients in the emergency department or intensive care unit, patients undergoing major surgeries, and patients who present with hematuria. Placement of urethral catheters is usually performed by health care partners but adequate training is required [16].

Some patients may present with difficult urinary catheterization (DUC). In men, the most frequent causes of DUC are urethral strictures, benign prostatic hyperplasia, phimosis, meatal stenosis, penile edema, and bladder neck sclerosis following urologic procedures. Women can present with difficult urinary catheterization too, mostly caused by morbid obesity, atrophic vaginitis, intravaginal retraction of the urethral meatus, and previous pelvic procedures [17].

Several potential complications of difficult urinary catheterization (DUC) can cause acute and chronic complications including rectal perforation, meatal and urethral erosions, infection, false passages, and chronic urethral strictures. In order to avoid complications, the absolute need for placement of an indwelling urethral catheter must be assessed because unnecessary catheterization rates can be as high as 50 % [16]. Proper sterile technique with lubrication of the urethra using lidocaine gel is a key step to achieve successful catheterization and decrease the chances of urinary tract infection. Contrary to common perception, larger diameter catheters (18–22 French) are preferable to smaller catheters due to the firmness and better success rates. Finally, when facing a difficult catheterization, application of excessive pressure or force is not recommended as it may cause or increase the magnitude of iatrogenic injury to the urethra. It is crucial that urethral trauma be considered a

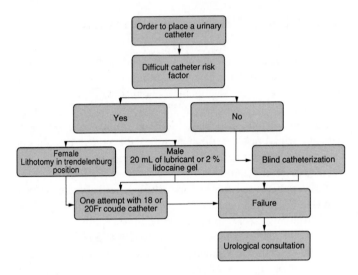

Fig. 14.3 Urology consultation flow chart

contraindication for urethral catheterization by the novice. Urology consultation is mandatory in such cases [18] (Fig. 14.3).

14.2.1 Difficult Female Catheterization

Morbidly obese females may require lithotomy with slight Trendelenburg position for better exposure. If the urethra is not yet visible, a vaginal speculum can be used to press the posterior vaginal wall downwards while an assistant retracts the labia majora to expose the meatus. Similarly, in older postmenopausal women, the meatus may be retracted posteriorly toward the vagina. In these cases, insertion of the first and second fingers into the vaginal introitus may guide the insertion of the Foley catheter by locating the urethral meatus above the introitus and about 2–3 cm below the clitoris. Female meatus stricture can be secondary to previous instrumentation, injury, and female circumcision. In these complex cases, urethral dilation with endoscopic approach is often necessary and is usually performed by the urology team [18].

14.2.2   Difficult Male Catheterization

Male patients admitted for heart failure, sepsis, hepatic failure, and trauma can present foreskin edema, making it difficult to visualize the urethral meatus. In this case, hand compression of the distal half of the penis with gauze or application of loose fitting elastic dressings for 10–20 min can reduce the swelling and a Foley catheter can be placed using standard sterile technique. Phimosis can also make it difficult or impossible to visualize the meatus. Pulling the foreskin outward can open a passage that allows visualization. In severe cases of phimosis, blind or endocopic approach may be necessary to introduce the catheter by aiming toward the 6 o'clock. Rarely, a dorsal slit is indicated [18].

To avoid complications caused by inflating the balloon inside the urethra or the prostate, the Foley retention balloon should only be inflated after the Foley catheter is introduced into the bladder up to the Y-hub bifurcation of the catheter and drainage of urine is visualized. Bedside bladder ultrasound is recommended when in doubt of catheter's placement [18].

To lubricate and locally anesthetize, 2 % lidocaine gel is used. Better results are obtained using 20 mL of the gel at least 10 min prior to the procedure. If lidocaine gel is not available, plain lubricating gel can be used [17, 18].

14.2.3   Catheter Selection

Multiple urethral catheters are commercially available. The most used in common practice are latex or silicone catheters, three-way Foley for continuous irrigation of the bladder, and

Coudé (curved tip) catheter. Catheter size is measured using the French scale, where 1 French equals 1/3 mm in diameter [17].

If no complications are known or anticipated, 16 or 18 French catheters are generally used for catheterization. Coudé catheters are used when patients are known to have a large prostate or history of difficult catheterization with clearance at 12 o'clock (high bladder neck). The tip should be directed anteriorly and upward in order to facilitate bypassing obstruction or false passages. Council tip catheters are designed to be placed over a stiff guidewire, preplaced under cystoscopic guidance by the urologist [18, 19].

14.2.4 Flexible Cystoscopy and Dilatation

Flexible cystoscopy under local anesthesia can assist the placement of Council tip catheters or suprapubic catheters under direct visualization. During the cystoscopy, a stiff guidewire is placed through the stenosis or false passage. The scope is then removed and a Council tip catheter is placed using the wire as a guide. If needed, "S" curved urethral dilators can be used to dilate the urethral stricture before urethral catheter placement [17] (Fig. 14.4).

Urethral dilation has traditionally been done blind with metal Van Buren sounds. The use of such sounds is encouraged only for very distal strictures or meatal stenosis. Similarly, filiforms and followers can also be used but false passages may occur. Currently, the use of sequential urethral dilators over the guidewire and under fluoroscopic guidance is often practiced [17].

14.2.5 Suprapubic Catheter

A suprapubic catheter (SP) can be inserted percutaneously in cases of catheterization failure or when total urethral disruption

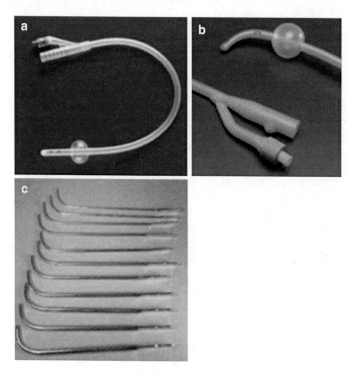

Fig. 14.4 (a) Silicon catheter, (b) Coude catheter, (c) S-curved dilators

is likely. SP tubes are placed using local anesthesia with or without the use of ultrasound placed 2 inches above the pubic bone in the midline [20].

Contraindications for percutaneous suprapubic tube placement include bladder cancer, unavoidable bowel injury due to previous surgery, uncorrected coagulopathies, and active anticoagulation, and abdominal wall abscess or cellulitis [18].

14.3 Ureteral Trauma

14.3.1 Clinical Presentation

Ureteral trauma has a low incidence and accounts for approximately 1–2.5 % of urinary tract trauma [21]. Most ureteral injuries are caused by penetrating trauma; gunshot wounds are especially common penetrating injuries [22]. Blunt trauma can damage the ureter in about 30 % of patients [21]. Missing of ureteral injuries is reported to be 11 % [23].

Clinical diagnosis of ureteral injuries is difficult. Ureteral injuries are usually associated with severe injuries to the abdomen, pelvic bone, and spine [21]. Around 50–70 % of patients with ureteral injuries will present gross hematuria; however, ureteral injury is also associated with other urological traumas such as kidney, bladder, and urethra, making hematuria an unreliable factor in the diagnosis of ureteral trauma [22, 24].

14.3.2 Radiological Evaluation

The radiological evaluation of ureteral trauma is a contrast-enhanced abdominal/pelvic CT with delayed imaging (CT-IVP) for stable trauma patients with suspected ureteral injuries [7, 8, 25]. The extravasation of contrast material of the ureter is the hallmark sign of ureteral injury. Other signs that can be suggestive of ureteral injury in suspected cases include the presence of hydronephrosis, urinoma, or free liquid in the abdomen. In cases that the CT-IVP was not able to confirm the diagnoses, retrograde pyelogram is the gold standard to confirm ureteral injury [24]. Plain pyelography or one-shot IVP should not be used because they can have up to 60 % false negative results in ureteral injuries [22, 24]. Patients that required laparotomy without imaging should have their ureters directly inspected, looking for lesions [8].

14.3.3 Management of Ureteral Trauma

14.3.3.1 Minimally Invasive Treatment

Management of ureteral injuries is influenced by several factors including the patient's clinical condition, mechanism of trauma, partial or complete ureteral injury, and time to diagnose ureteral injuries.

Nonoperative management of ureteral injuries caused by external trauma (excluding iatrogenic lesions) has a limited role in primary treatment. In most cases, patients will benefit from early definitive treatment of ureteral injuries, avoiding extensive fibrosis induced by urine extravasation. In this case, minimally invasive procedures can be performed to prevent complications caused by urine extravasation and restore renal function. Urine drainage can be performed using a ureteral stent and/or nephrostomy tube. In unstable patients, temporary urine drainage can be managed with the placement of a nephrostomy tube guided by ultrasound. This procedure can be performed in the ICU without needing to transfer patients to the operating room and help avoid the risks associated with the transfer of unstable patients. Finding coagulopathy is often considered a relative contraindication to percutaneous renal drainage; renal bleeding is always a risk of such procedures.

In very select cases of patients with ureteral injuries recognized early and with limited urine extravasation, a retrograde ureteropyelography can be performed to determine if the ureteral injury is complete or partial, as well the extent of the lesion. If the ureteral injury is partial, a ureteral stent can be inserted. Passing a guidewire under direct vision through an ureteroscopy is a good alternative to avoid placing the stent in the retroperitoneum [26]. The placement of ureteral stent in these patients allows a ureteral realignment and, in many cases, could spare the need of the nephrostomy tube [26].

In multitrauma patients, sometimes not all lesions can be treated in the same surgery, requiring an abbreviated laparotomy with damage control strategies.

14.3.3.2   Operative Treatment of Ureteral Injuries

Ureteral injuries will require surgical procedures in the majority of patients. Reviews of ureteral injury outcomes indicate that most types of ureteral trauma fare better with early operative repair as opposed to delayed repair or attempts at nonoperative management. There is an exception when considering limited iatrogenic injuries from endoscopy. This is the case for stab and gunshot wounds as well as avulsion injuries from blunt trauma.

Surgeons should directly inspect the ureter during urgent laparotomy in stable patients with suspect ureteral injuries and no preoperative images [8]. Unstable patients with identified ureteral injuries should be managed with temporary urinary drainage. Depending on the case, options can include placing a ureteral stent, ureteral ligation and nephrostomy tube, or nephrostomy tube alone.

Ureteral contusions recognized intraoperatively, due to either penetrating or blunt trauma, may be managed nonoperatively and simply observed; however, some reports suggest that the risk of late perforation and urinary extravasation may be reduced by intraoperative insertion of a ureteral stent. Depending of the ureteral viability and clinical scenario, primary repair may be necessary [8].

In stable patients, surgeons should repair traumatic ureteral injury at the time of the laparotomy [8, 25]. When possible, primary repair of the ureteral lesions proximal to the iliac vessels is the best repair option. Ureteral dissection needs to be meticulous and careful in order to avoid excessive dissection. Also, the ureter must remain with the peri-ureteric tissue because it is important for ureteric blood supply. All necrotic tissue or lesions caused by gunshot wounds should undergo debridement. Debridement of damaged tissue is the key to avoid dehiscence and fistula. Before performing ureteric anastomosis, the ureter ends need to be spatulated to enlarge ureter diameter and decrease the risks of stenosis. The anastomosis should be performed using absorbable sutures and watertight mucosa-mucosa sutures, with the placement of internal stenting. The placement of an external drain should be performed to be a sentinel for fistulas and to guide the urine drainage to the skin if fistula occurs. The ureter should be isolated in the retroperitoneum, closing the retroperitoneum when possible or with the placement of an omental wrap.

Midureter lesions that cannot be treated with primary uretero-uretero anastomosis can be treated with trans-ureteral anastomosis, crossing the proximal ureter across the midline and anastomosed to the contralateral ureter. This technique is associated stenosis of the anastomosis in 4% of patients and surgical revision in 10% of patients [27].

The management of the distal ureter is better treated with ureteroneocystostomy [7, 8]. Trauma to the distal ureter usually compromises the blood supply to the distal ureter, increasing the risk of postoperative complication. Distal ureteric injuries that compromise larger portions of the ureter may require bladder mobilization of contralateral bladder ligaments and bladder fixation in the psoas muscle tendon (psoas hitch). This procedure has success rates of 97% [27]. Extensive mid-lower ureteral injuries may require reconstruction by a tabularized bladder flap (Boari-flap) (figure), which has success rates of 81–88% [28]. When performing surgical reconstruction of the ureter, operative time and surgeon experience should be weighted to determine if the reconstructive procedure should be performed in the acute setting.

Autotrasplantation of the kidney is the last option for patients who have undergone multiple attempts of ureteral reconstruction or have extensive ureteral loss. The kidney is relocated in the pelvis, performing the anastomosis of the renal vessels to the iliac vessels and the ureteral reimplantaion is performed in the bladder (image) [29]. Ureteral substitution with intestinal flaps and autotransplantation are complex procedures and should not be attempted in the acute setting. These procedures should be performed in reconstruction centers by surgeons with significant experience using these techniques.

14.3.4 High Yield Anatomy and Surgical Tips and Tricks

The ureters are retroperitoneal organs with close anatomical relation with several other organs such as the colon, vena cava, aorta, iliac vessels, bladder, uterus, and psoas muscle. The blood supply changes according to the location (upper, mid, and lower ureter) and surgeons must be familiar with the ureteral anatomy to prevent ureteral injuries when performing surgical procedures in close related organs. This is especially important when bleeding and/or hematoma is present because properly identifying the ureter becomes difficult. Also, when dissection of the ureter is necessary, knowledge of ureteral blood supply is important to avoid ischemic injuries to the ureter.

The proximal and midureter have their blood supply coming directly from the aorta or common iliac vessels. This blood supply to the ureters is located primarily in the medial aspect of the ureter. In the ureter below the common iliac vessels, the blood supply is derived from the vesical arteries and the arterial branches, which are located on the lateral aspect of the ureter. An anastomotic chain between branches usually occurs in a single, long longitudinal vessel that runs between the ureteral adventitia and muscularis.

References

1. Hayes EE, Sandler CM, Corriere JN, McAninch JW. Management of the ruptured bladder secondary to blunt abdominal-trauma. J Urol. 1983;129(5):946–8.
2. Deibert CM, Spencer BA. The association between operative repair of bladder injury and improved survival: results from the National Trauma Data Bank. J Urol. 2011;186(1):151–5.
3. Gomez RG, Ceballos L, Coburn M, Corriere JN, Dixon CM, Lobel B, et al. Consensus statement on bladder injuries. BJU Int. 2004;94(1):27–32.
4. Wirth GJ, Peter R, Poletti PA, Iselin CE. Advances in the management of blunt traumatic bladder rupture: experience with 36 cases. BJU Int. 2010;106(9):1344–9.
5. Avey G, Blackmore CC, Wessells H, Wright JL, Talner LB. Radiographic and clinical predictors of bladder rupture in blunt trauma patients with pelvic fracture. Acad Radiol. 2006;13(5):573–9.
6. Morey AF, Iverson AJ, Swan A, Harmon WJ, Spore SS, Bhayani S, et al. Bladder rupture after blunt trauma: guidelines for diagnostic imaging. J Trauma. 2001;51(4):683–6.
7. Lynch TH, Martínez-Piñeiro L, Plas E, Serafetinides E, Türkeri L, Santucci RA, et al. EAU guidelines on urological trauma. Eur Urol. 2005;47(1):1–15.
8. Morey AF, Brandes S, Dugi DD, Armstrong JH, Breyer BN, Broghammer JA, et al. Urotrauma: AUA guideline. J Urol. 2014;192(2):327–35.
9. Tonkin JB, Tisdale BE, Jordan GH. Assessment and initial management of urologic trauma. Med Clin North Am. 2011;95(1):245–51.
10. Ramchandani P, Buckler PM. Imaging of genitourinary trauma. AJR Am J Roentgenol. 2009;192(6):1514–23.
11. Rafique M. Intravesical foreign bodies: review and current management strategies. Urol J. 2008;5(4):223–31.
12. Cinman NM, McAninch JW, Porten SP, Myers JB, Blaschko SD, Bagga HS, et al. Gunshot wounds to the lower urinary tract: a single-institution experience. J Trauma Acute Care Surg. 2013;74(3):725–30; discussion 30–1.
13. Pereira BM, Reis LO, Calderan TR, de Campos CC, Fraga GP. Penetrating bladder trauma: a high risk factor for associated rectal injury. Adv Urol. 2014;2014:386280.
14. Kim FJ, Chammas MF, Gewehr EV, Campagna A, Moore EE. Laparoscopic management of intraperitoneal bladder rupture

secondary to blunt abdominal trauma using intracorporeal single layer suturing technique. J Trauma. 2008;65(1):234–6.

15. Inaba K, Okoye OT, Browder T, Best C, Branco BC, Teixeira PG, et al. Prospective evaluation of the utility of routine postoperative cystogram after traumatic bladder injury. J Trauma Acute Care Surg. 2013;75(6):1019–23.

16. Jain P, Parada JP, David A, Smith LG. Overuse of the indwelling urinary-tract catheter in hospitalized medical patients. Arch Intern Med. 1995;155(13):1425–9.

17. Ghaffary C, Yohannes A, Villanueva C, Leslie SW. A practical approach to difficult urinary catheterizations. Curr Urol Rep. 2013;14(6):565–79.

18. Villanueva C, Hemstreet GP. Difficult catheterization: tricks of the trade. AUA Update Series. 2011;30:41–8.

19. Patel AR, Jones JS, Babineau D. Lidocaine 2% gel versus plain lubricating gel for pain reduction during flexible cystoscopy: a meta-analysis of prospective, randomized, controlled trials. J Urol. 2008;179(3):986–90.

20. Villanueva C, Hemstreet 3rd GP. Difficult male urethral catheterization: a review of different approaches. Int Braz J Urol Off J Braz Soc Urol. 2008;34(4):401–11; discussion 12.

21. Siram SM, Gerald SZ, Greene WR, Hughes K, Oyetunji TA, Chrouser K, et al. Ureteral trauma: patterns and mechanisms of injury of an uncommon condition. Am J Surg. 2010;199(4):566–70.

22. Elliott SP, McAninch JW. Ureteral injuries: external and iatrogenic. Urol Clin North Am. 2006;33(1):55–66, vi.

23. Shariat SF, Jenkins A, Roehrborn CG, Karam JA, Stage KH, Karakiewicz PI. Features and outcomes of patients with grade IV renal injury. BJU Int. 2008;102(6):728–33; discussion 33.

24. Brandes S, Coburn M, Armenakas N, McAninch J. Diagnosis and management of ureteric injury: an evidence-based analysis. BJU Int. 2004;94(3):277–89.

25. Serafetinides E, Kitrey ND, Djakovic N, Kuehhas FE, Lumen N, Sharma DM, et al. Review of the current management of upper urinary tract injuries by the EAU Trauma Guidelines Panel. Eur Urol. 2015;67(5):930–6.

26. Brandt AS, von Rundstedt FC, Lazica DA, Roth S. Ureteral realignment with the rendezvous procedure in complex ureteral injuries - aspects of technique and our experience. Aktuelle Urol. 2010;41(4):257–62.

27. Burks FN, Santucci RA. Management of iatrogenic ureteral injury. Ther Adv Urol. 2014;6(3):115–24.

28. Wenske S, Olsson CA, Benson MC. Outcomes of distal ureteral reconstruction through reimplantation with psoas hitch, Boari flap, or

ureteroneocystostomy for benign or malignant ureteral obstruction or injury. Urology. 2013;82(1):231–6.

29. Hau HM, Bartels M, Tautenhahn HM, Morgul MH, Fellmer P, Ho-Thi P, et al. Renal autotransplantation–a possibility in the treatment of complex renal vascular diseases and ureteric injuries. Ann Transplant. 2012;17(4):21–7.

Chapter 15
Critical Care in Acute Care Surgery

Kathryn L. Butler and George Velmahos

15.1   Introduction

Trauma, acute care surgery, and critical care have been inter-linked for over a century. The field of critical care arose during the Crimean War of the 1850s, when Florence Nightingale dedi-cated a separate treatment area to the most severely wounded soldiers [1]. Although anesthesiologists, pulmonologists, and emergency medicine physicians also staff intensive care units (ICUs), mastery of critical care principles remains fundamental

K.L. Butler, MD (✉)
Massachusetts General Hospital, Harvard Medical School,
Boston, MA, USA
e-mail: KLBUTLER@PARTNERS.ORG

G. Velmahos, MD, PhD, MSEd
Division of Trauma, Emergency Surgery, and Surgical Critical Care,
Massachusetts General Hospital, Harvard Medical School,
Boston, MA, USA
e-mail: GVELMAHOS@mgh.harvard.edu

© Springer International Publishing Switzerland 2017
S. Di Saverio et al. (eds.), *Acute Care Surgery Handbook*,
DOI 10.1007/978-3-319-15341-4_15

to an acute care surgeon's practice. As a single chapter cannot accommodate the breadth of the critical care literature, we focus here on content most relevant to the acute care surgeon: resuscitation and respiratory support.

15.2 Shock and Resuscitation

Among the most pivotal critical care skills for acute care surgeons are diagnosis and characterization of shock, and goal-directed resuscitation. Shock occurs when an injury or illness impairs end-organ perfusion. The natural course of shock is progressive end-organ ischemia, multiorgan failure, and death, and therefore timely diagnosis and treatment are paramount to patient survival.

Clinicians should suspect shock in any patient with signs of diminished tissue perfusion (see Table 15.1). Identification of shock mandates prompt acquisition of data to determine the etiology and class, both of which guide therapy.

Table 15.1 Clinical signs of shock

Sign	Pathophysiology
Hypotension	Low vasomotor tone or decreased cardiac output reduce mean arterial pressure
Oliguria/anuria	Decreased renal arterial blood flow
Depressed mental status	Decreased cerebral arterial blood flow
Metabolic/lactic acidosis	Tissue ischemia leading to increased anaerobic metabolism
Elevated liver function tests	Decreased portal and hepatic arterial blood flow
Coagulopathy	Disseminated vascular coagulation secondary to release of tissue factor in the setting of cytokine release or end-organ damage

15.2.1   Differentiation of Shock States

The equation for mean arterial pressure (MAP) vastly simplifies an understanding of shock. Considering MAP as the product of cardiac output (CO) and systemic vascular resistance (SVR), shock represents a perturbation of preload, contractility, systemic vascular resistance, or a combination of the three (Table 15.2). The challenge in differentiating between shock states lies in identifying which of these parameters requires restoration.

The first step is to assess for preload deficits through a determination of volume responsiveness. The concept of volume responsiveness arises from the Frank-Starling curve (Fig. 15.1). Along the steep slope of the Frank-Starling curve, increases in left ventricular (LV) end-diastolic volume (preload) translate into improved stroke volume (SV) and, therefore, cardiac output. Beyond the inflection point of the Frank-Starling curve, however, the myocardial fibers of the LV are maximally stretched, such that further volume loading does not increase stroke volume. In such patients, intravenous fluid boluses do not improve cardiac output.

In general, patients in shock whose blood pressure rises with volume are volume responsive and have either distributive or hypovolemic shock. In contrast, if fluids have minimal impact on cardiac output, clinicians should suspect cardiogenic or obstructive shock (Fig. 15.1). Note that although patients with

Table 15.2 Shock states as functions of mean arterial pressure (MAP=CO*SVR)

	Contractility		Preload	SVR
Hypovolemic	Early↑	Late↓	↓	↑
Distributive	No change,↑ or↓		↓	↓
Cardiogenic	↓		↑	↑
Obstructive	Early↑	Late↓	↓	↑

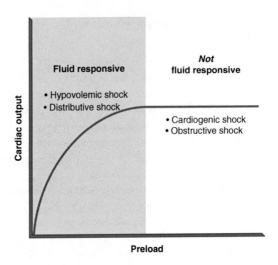

Fig. 15.1 The Frank-Starling curve

obstructive shock have deficient preload, they rarely improve with boluses because the inciting pathology (pneumothorax, pericardial tamponade, etc.) obstructs LV filling.

Administration of intravenous crystalloid is the simplest option to investigate volume responsiveness. However, injudicious fluid resuscitation delivers well-documented detrimental effects, including acute lung injury and compartment syndrome [2–9]. Clinicians should therefore consider an array of additional methods to measure volume responsiveness:

1. *Passive leg raise (PLR).* Noninvasive and reversible, this method requires lifting the legs of a supine patient 45°, which increases venous return from the lower extremities for an approximate total volume of 200 cc. A 10 % increase in pulse pressure with PLR has 79 % sensitivity and 85 % specificity for volume responsiveness [10]. Drawbacks of the PLR include unreliability in severely hypovolemic patients (in

whom total blood volume may be too low to detect a change), as well as in patients with abdominal hypertension.

2. *Pulse pressure variation (PPV)*. Changes in the arterial waveform throughout the cardiac cycle predict volume responsiveness in mechanically ventilated patients. During inspiration, increased intrathoracic pressure decreases venous return, shifting the interventricular septum to the right and improving LV compliance. Return of blood from the pulmonary veins to the left atrium increases, with the net effect of increased preload and, therefore, higher systolic blood pressure at end inspiration. During expiration, the decreased right ventricular (RV) volume seen on end inspiration translates into decreased LV preload, with a resultant drop in systolic blood pressure. Hypovolemia augments this pattern of pulse pressure variation. In mechanically ventilated patients, a PPV of ≥13 % during the respiratory cycle confers 94 % sensitivity and 96 % specificity for volume responsiveness [11, 12].

3. *Stroke volume variation (SVV)*. Recent technology termed pulse contour analysis (PCA) monopolizes upon stroke volume variation during mechanical ventilation to predict volume responsiveness. Although the specific algorithms vary, all PCA devices analyze the area beneath the arterial pressure waveform and correlate these measurements with stroke volume. The PiCCO system (Pulsion Medical Systems, Germany) accomplishes this through thermodilution techniques similar to the Swan-Ganz catheter. The Flo-Trac or Vigileo devices (Edward Lifesciences, USA), meanwhile, sample the waveform at regular intervals and apply statistical models to calculate SVV. The threshold above which SVV predicts volume responsiveness depends upon the device and is more accurate for tidal volumes >8 cc/kg, an important caveat given the low-tidal volume ventilation strategy now commonplace in surgical ICUs [13–15].

4. *IVC diameter.* Point-of-care ultrasound (POCUS) has gar-
nered enthusiasm over the past decade for its versatility,
reproducibility, noninvasiveness, and accuracy in skilled
hands. A common metric for fluid responsiveness using ultrasound is variation of inferior vena caval (IVC) diameter with
respiration. During positive pressure inspiration, the diameter of the IVC increases. Practitioners can quantify this
change with M-mode, and values >18 % correlate with volume responsiveness [16]. In contrast, static recordings of
IVC diameter warrant cautious interpretation, as high-tidal
volumes, right ventricular failure, and intra-abdominal hypertension confound measurements [16–18].

Although traditionally surrogates for volume status, central
venous pressure (CVP), and pulmonary capillary wedge pressure (PCWP) poorly predict fluid responsiveness and should not
guide shock workup and therapy [19]. The high and low
extremes of these measurements may correlate with hypovolemia and volume overload, respectively, but the vast middle
ground of values are inconclusive.

Once tests have confirmed a patient as volume responsive or
nonresponsive, further characterization of shock entails careful
attention to a patient's history, physical examination, and diagnostic study results. The algorithm in Fig. 15.2 outlines a basic
approach. Point-of-care ultrasound (POCUS) plays an increasingly important role in the diagnosis of shock [20], and as such,
Table 15.3 summarizes the key findings. POCUS is an evolving
practice, and an in-depth discussion of the technique is beyond
the scope of this chapter.

15.2.2   Management of Shock

The following sections detail the management of specific shock
variants. Acute care surgeons frequently encounter both septic
(distributive) shock and obstructive shock from abdominal com-

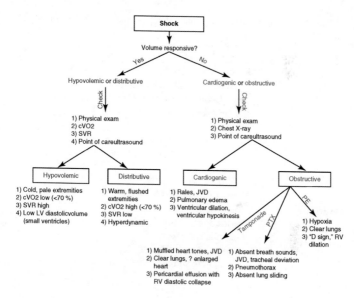

Fig. 15.2 Algorithm for characterization of shock. *cVO2* central venous oxygen saturation, *SVR* systemic vascular resistance, *LV* left ventricle, *JVD* jugular venous distension, *PTX* pneumothorax, *PE* pulmonary embolus, *RV* right ventricle

partment syndrome. This handbook dedicates separate chapters to these topics, and so the ensuing discussion will not duplicate such in-depth coverage.

For all diagnoses discussed below, monitoring of serum lactate, base deficit, and laboratory parameters of end-organ function (creatinine, liver function tests, coagulation factors) can guide therapy.

15.2.2.1 Hemorrhagic Shock

Massive hemorrhage subjects patients to hypothermia, acidosis, and coagulopathy, a "lethal triad" that further potentiates bleed-

Table 15.3 Point-of-care ultrasound (POCUS) findings in specific shock states

	POCUS findings

Hypovolemic	"Kissing ventricles:"
	  Collapse of ventricular walls during systole
	  Small ventricular diameter during diastole

Distributive	"Hyperdynamic:"
	  Increased heart rate
	  Increased contractility (early)
	  May have collapse of ventricular walls during systole, but end-diastolic ventricular diameter approximates normal

Cardiogenic	Dilated, hypokinetic LV

Obstructive	*Tamponade:*
	  Pericardial effusion
	  Diastolic collapse of RV
	Tension pneumothorax:
	  Absent lung sliding
	  Absent B-lines
	Pulmonary embolus:
	  "D-sign:" flattening of intra-ventricular septum due to RV hypertension, with "D"-shaped appearance of RV on parasternal short axis view
	  Dilated RV

LV, left ventricle; *RV*, right ventricle

ing. Survival depends upon rapid resuscitation with blood products through large-bore access, and correction of these abnormalities [21]. Patients in hemorrhagic shock must be warmed to normothermia, and coagulopathy and acidosis reversed through attentive resuscitation. A growing body of data supports the transfusion of fresh frozen plasma, packed red blood cells, and platelets in a 1:1:1 ratio to approximate whole blood and limit dilutional coagulopathy [22]. Patients with a large transfusion requirement must be closely monitored for electrolyte derangements, particularly hypocalcemia and hyperkalemia, and should undergo serial examinations for the development of compartment syndrome.

Recent research suggests promise in the use of thromboelastography (TEG) after trauma, transplant surgery, and cardiac surgery [23–25]. Unlike conventional coagulation tests, TEG elucidates the precise mechanism of coagulopathy (e.g., factor deficiency, fibrinogen deficiency, low or dysfunctional platelets, or fibrinolysis). Unfortunately, studies in nontrauma emergency surgery patients are lacking. The same paucity of data applies to tranexamic acid (TXA), an antifibrolytic agent that reduces mortality due to hemorrhage in trauma patients, but has not been studied in acute care surgery [26]. In theory, such agents could assist in the treatment of hemorrhagic shock in emergency surgery patients; however, further research is required to provide recommendations. In contrast, Factor VIIa, an adjunct in hemorrhagic shock that has generated controversy for years, incurs an unacceptable risk of thromboemoblic events and cannot be routinely recommended [27–29].

15.2.2.2 Obstructive Shock

Management of obstructive shock depends upon identification and reversal of the inciting process.

1. *Tension pneumothorax.* Treatment is needle decompression, followed by tube thoracostomy.

2. *Pericardial tamponade.* Pericardiocentisis with placement of a pigtail catheter relieves tamponade from simple effusion. For cardiac injury, pericardial window (in the stable patient) or median sternotomy (in the unstable patient) is indicated.

3. *Pulmonary embolus (PE).* Patients with pulmonary embolism sufficiently large to produce shock may benefit from catheter-directed thrombolysis, or in select scenarios, pulmonary thromboembolectomy. In stable patients, systemic anticoagulation is often sufficient.

15.2.2.3 Cardiogenic Shock

Management of cardiogenic shock focuses on restoration of cardiac output through pharmacologically enhanced contractility. Emergency surgeons encounter ventricular failure most frequently in the setting of concurrent sepsis, i.e., sepsis-induced cardiomyopathy. Such patients suffer from poor vasomotor tone in addition to depressed contractility, and so their management varies slightly from that of the nonseptic patient in heart failure.

In all cases of cardiogenic shock, reversal of shock requires administration of inotropic infusions. The phosophodiesterase inhibitor milrinone is the classic choice in heart failure, as it reduces afterload in addition to augmenting contractility. Such patients also benefit from preload reduction in the form of diuresis or dialysis (depending on a patient's renal function) to decrease myocardial strain. In cases of reversible ventricular failure refractory to inotropes, an intra-aortic balloon pump decreases afterload, improves myocardial perfusion, and may serve as a life-saving bridge to definitive therapy.

Unlike the case of ventricular failure, vasodilatory effects render milrinone a poor choice in sepsis-induced cardiomyopathy. In such scenarios, dobutamine is preferred [30]. Dopamine and epinephrine serve as second-line agents, as they induce tachyarrhythmias and increase the afterload.

15.3 Support of Oxygenation and Ventilation

Indications for intubation and mechanical ventilation in acute care surgery remain the same as for any critically ill patients: (1) hypoxemia, (2) hypercarbia, and/or (3) threatened airway.

15.3.1 Mechanical Ventilation

Mechanical ventilation of critically ill surgical patients should adhere to a lung protective ventilatory strategy. Lung protective ventilation stems from the ARDSnet research and aims to minimize lung injury by avoiding dramatic increases in airway pressure and alveolar overdistension [31]. Such a strategy applies to patients in shock and multiorgan failure; patients who are not systemically ill do not require ARDSnet settings, although in theory practitioners should highly prioritize avoidance of baro- and volutrauma in all situations.

ARDSnet settings call for low-tidal volumes (4–6 cc/kg), high PEEP, permissive hypercapnea, and monitoring of plateau pressures, with a goal of <30 mmHg. Although the original research employed volume control ventilation to achieve these parameters, pressure control modes can also meet these criteria. Patients with severe lung injury, as evidenced by PaO_2/FiO_2 ratio < 200, may require proning, neuromuscular blockade, and minimization of intravenous fluids, all which have correlated with improved outcomes in ARDS [4, 32, 33].

15.3.2 Noninvasive Positive Pressure Ventilation

Noninvasive ventilation, commonly known as continuous positive pressure (CPAP) or bilevel positive pressure (BiPAP), allows for administration of positive pressure without the morbidity of endotracheal intubation and mechanical ventilation. It serves as an appealing alternative method of ventilation support in the setting of rapidly reversible causes of respiratory distress, e.g., chronic obstructive pulmonary disease (COPD) exacerbation or congestive heart failure (CHF) exacerbation. Data also support judicious NIV use in select patients with community-acquired pneumonia, and with postoperative respiratory failure after abdominal surgery [34]. Surgeons should avoid the temptation, however, to use NIV in patients with ARDS or severe hypoxemic respiratory failure. Although NIV can delay mechanical ventilation in such cases, the failure rate is high, and in such scenarios NIV may confer additional lung injury secondary to aspiration pneumonitis.

References

1. Weil MH, Tang W. From intensive care to critical care medicine: a historical perspective. Am J Respir Crit Care Med. 2011;183(11):1451–3.
2. Ashbaugh DG, Bigelow DB, Pett TL, et al. Acute reespiratory distress in adults. Lancet. 1967;2:319–23.
3. Demling RH. The pathogenesis of respiratory failure after trauma and sepsis. Surg Clin North Am. 1980;60:1373–90.
4. Wiedemann HP, Wheeler AP, Bernard GR, et al. Comparison of two fluid-management strategies in acute lung injury. N Engl J Med. 2006;354(24):2564–75.
5. Maxwell RA, Fabian TC, Croce MA, et al. Secondary abdominal compartment syndrome: an underappreciated manifestation of severe hemorrhagic shock. J Trauma. 1999;47:995–9.
6. Madigan M, Kemp CD, Johnson JC, et al. Secondary abdominal compartment syndrome after severe extremity injury: are early, aggressive fluid resuscitation strategies to blame? J Trauma. 2008;64:280–5.
7. Hashim R, Frankel H, Tandon M, et al. Fluid resuscitation-induced cardiac tamponade. J Trauma. 2002;53:1183–4.
8. Cotton BA, Guy JS, Morris JA, et al. The cellular, metabolic, and systemic consequences of aggressive fluid resuscitation strategies. Shock. 2006;26:115–21.
9. Boyd JH, Forbes J, Nakada TA, et al. Fluid resuscitation in septic shock: a positive fluid balance and elevated central venous pressure are associated with increased mortality. Crit Care Med. 2011;39:259–65.
10. Monnet X, Rienzo M, Osman D, et al. Passive leg raising predicts fluid responsiveness in the critically ill. Crit Care Med. 2006;34(5):1402–7.

11. Michard F, Boussard S, Chemla D, et al. Relation between respiratory changes in arterial pulse pressure and fluid responsiveness in septic patients with acute circulatory failure. Am J Respir Crit Care Med. 2000;162(1):134–8.
12. Marik P, Cavallazzi R, Vasu T, et al. Dynamic changes in arterial waveform derived variables and fluid responsiveness in mechanically ventilated patients: a systematic review of the literature. Crit Care Med. 2009;37:2642–7.
13. Zhang Z, Lu B, Sheng X, et al. Accuracy of stroke volume variation in predicting fluid responsiveness: a systematic review and meta-analysis. J Anesth. 2011;25(6):904–16.
14. Reuter DA, Felbinger TW, Schmidt C, et al. Stroke volume variations for assessment of cardiac responsiveness to volume loading in mechanically ventilated patients after cardiac surgery. Intensive Care Med. 2002;28(4):392–8.
15. Belloni L, Pisano A, Natale A, et al. Assessment of fluid-responsiveness parameters for off-pump coronary artery bypass surgery: a comparison among LiDCO, transesophageal echocardiography, and pulmonary artery catheter. J Cardiothorac Vasc Anesth. 2008;22(2):243–8.
16. Barbier C, Jardin F, Vieillard-Baron A. Respiratory changes in inferior vena cava diameter are helpful in predicting fluid responsiveness in ventilated septic patients. Intensive Care Med. 2004;30:1740–6.
17. Feissel M, Michard F, Faller JP, et al. The respiratory variation in inferior vena cava diameter as a guide to fluid therapy. Intensive Care Med. 2004;30:1834–7.
18. Dipit A, Soucy Z, Surana A, et al. Role of inferior vena cava diameter in assessment of volume status: a meta-analysis. Am J Emerg Med. 2012;30(8):1414–9.
19. Marik PE, Cavallazzi R. Does the central venous pressure predict fluid responsiveness? An updated meta-analysis and a plea for some common sense. Crit Care Med. 2013;41(7):1774–81.
20. Walley PE, Walley KR, Goodgame B, et al. A practical approach to goal-directed echocardiography in the critical care setting. Crit Care. 2014;18:681–92.
21. Wilcox J, Elmer SR, Raja A. Massive tranfusion in traumatic shock. J Emerg Med. 2013;44(4):829–38.
22. Holcomb JB, Tilley BC, Baranuik S, et al. Transfusion of plasma, platelets, and red blood cells in a 1:1:1 vs a 1:1:2 ratio and mortality in patients with severe trauma: the PROPPR randomized clinical trial. JAMA. 2015;313(5):471–82.

23. Schöchl H, Voelckel W, Grassetto A, Schlimp CJ. Practical application of point-of-care coagulation testing to guide treatment decisions in trauma. J Trauma Acute Care Surg. 2013;74(6):1587–98.

24. Holcomb JB, Minei KM, Scerbo ML, et al. Admission rapid thrombo-elastography can replace conventional coagulation tests in the emergency department: experience with 1974 consecutive trauma patients. Ann Surg. 2012;256(3):476–86.

25. Johansson PI. Coagulation monitoring of the bleeding traumatized patient. Curr Opin Anaesthesiol. 2012;25(2):235–41.

26. Shakur H, Roberts I, Bautista R, et al. Effects of tranexamic acid on death, vascular occlusive events, and blood transfusion in trauma patients with significant haemorrhage (CRASH-2): a randomised, placebo-controlled trial. Lancet. 2010;376(9734):23–32.

27. Hauser CJ, Boffard KD, Dutton R, et al. Results of the CONTROL trial: efficacy and safety of recombinant activated Factor VII in the management of refractory traumatic hemorrhage. J Trauma. 2010;69(3):489–500.

28. Rizoli SB, Boffard KD, Riou B, et al. Recombinant factor VIIa as adjunctive therapy for bleeding control in severe trauma patients with coagulopathy: subgroup analysis from two randomized trials. Crit Care. 2006;10:R178.

29. Simpson E, Lin Y, Stanworth S, Birchall J, Doree C, Hyde C. Recombinant factor VIIa for the prevention and treatment of bleeding in patients without haemophilia. Cochrane Database Syst Rev. 2012;14(3):CD005011.

30. Dellinger RP, Levy MM, Rhodes A, et al. Surviving sepsis campaign: international guidelines for management of severe sepsis and septic shock: 2012. Crit Care Med. 2013;41:580–637.

31. The Acute Respiratory Distress Syndrome Network. Ventilation with lower tidal volumes as compared with traditional tidal volumes for acute lung injury and the acute respiratory distress syndrome. N Engl J Med. 2000;342(18):1301–9.

32. Lee JM, Bae W, Lee YJ, et al. The efficacy and safety of prone positional ventilation in acute respiratory distress syndrome: an updated study-level meta-analysis of 11 randomized controlled trials. Crit Care Med. 2014;42:1252–62.

33. Papazian L, Forel JM, Gacoin A, et al. Neuromuscular blockers in early acute respiratory distress syndrome. N Engl J Med. 2010;363(12):1107–16.

34. Ferrer M, Torres A. Noninvasive ventilation for acute respiratory failure. Curr Opin Crit Care. 2015;21:1–6.

Chapter 16
Septic Shock and Resuscitation Strategies

Shariq S. Raza and Marc de Moya

16.1 Introduction

Sepsis and its complications are a common cause of morbidity and mortality in the surgical intensive care unit (SICU). Its clinical burden is estimated to be approximately 700,000 cases per year in the United States [1], with further unquantifiable impact on reduced quality of life in survivors. Over 34,000 deaths are attributed to sepsis annually, making it the 10th most common cause of death in the United States [2], with its financial burden estimated at $26 billion per year [1]. Despite this significant burden and numerous recent advances in diagnostic and therapeutic modalities, sepsis remains a largely insurmountable disease entity owing to a less than ideal understanding of its pathophysiology and an unclear target for therapeutics.

S.S. Raza, MD • M. de Moya, MD, FACS (✉)
Division of Trauma, Emergency Surgery, and Surgical Critical Care,
Harvard Medical School, Massachusetts General Hospital,
165 Cambridge Street, Suite 810, Boston, MA 02114, USA
e-mail: ssraza@mgh.harvard.edu; mdemoya@mgh.harvard.edu

© Springer International Publishing Switzerland 2017
S. Di Saverio et al. (eds.), *Acute Care Surgery Handbook*,
DOI 10.1007/978-3-319-15341-4_16

16.2   Definitions

Sepsis is defined as a systemic inflammatory response syndrome (SIRS) in the setting of a known or presumed infection. Clinically, SIRS is defined by a set of agreed upon cut-off values for heart and respiratory rates, temperature, and leukocytosis, as listed in Table 16.1 [3]. As sepsis worsens, severe sepsis develops with hallmarks of organ dysfunction, hypoperfusion, or hypotension. Sepsis with persistent refractory hypotension, despite adequate fluid resuscitation, is defined as septic shock [4].

16.2.1   Third International Consensus Definitions for Sepsis and Septic Shock (Sepsis-3)

The definitions of sepsis and septic shock have been revised in 1991 and 2001. Despite considerable recent advances in the pathophysiology of sepsis, the epidemiology and management of sepsis remain hampered by an inadequate sensitivity and specificity of the SIRS criteria, and the limitations of having multiple unclear definitions for sepsis, septic shock, and organ dysfunction.

The Third International Consensus Definitions for Sepsis and Septic Shock (Sepsis-3) proposed at the 2016 45th Annual Meeting of the Society of Critical Care Medicine (SCCM) includes updated definitions for sepsis and septic shock, as summarized in Fig. 16.1 [5].

Sepsis is further defined as a life-threatening organ dysfunction caused by a dysregulated host response to infection. Organ dysfunction can be represented by an increase in the Sequential [Sepsis-Related] Organ Failure Assessment (SOFA) score of 2 points or more, which is associated with a higher risk of in-hospital mortality. These SOFA scores for major organ system are detailed in Table 16.2 [5].

Table 16.1 1991 ACCP/SCCM consensus definitions of sepsis and its complications

Infection	Inflammatory response to the presence of microorganisms or the invasion of those microorganisms into a host	
Bacteremia	Presence of viable bacteria in the blood	
Systemic infammatory response syndrome (SIRS)	The systemic inflammatory response to clinical insults and must meet ≥2 of the following	Temp >38 °C or <36 °C Heart rate >90 beats/min Resp rate >20 breaths/min or PaCO$_2$ <32 torr (<4.3 kPa) WBC >12,000 cells/mm^3, <4,000 cells/mm^3, or >10 % bands
Severe sepsis	Sepsis associated with organ dysfunction, hypoperfusion, or hypotension	
Septic shock	Sepsis with hypotension, despite adequate fluid resuscitation and presence of perfusion abnormalities (i.e., lactic acidosis, elevated base deficit, etc.)	
Hypotension	Systolic BP <90 mmHg	
Multiple organ dysfunction syndrome	Presence of altered organ function in an acutely ill patient such that homeostasis cannot be maintained without intervention	

Adapted from: *Crit Care Med*/Ref: 1991 ACCP/SCCM consensus definitions of sepsis and its complication

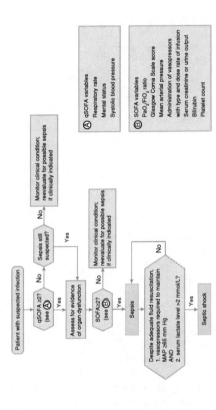

Fig. 16.1 Operationalization of clinical criteria identifying patients with sepsis and septic shock. The baseline Sequential [Sepsis-related] Organ Failure Assessment (SOFA) score should be assumed to be zero unless the patient is known to have preexisting (acute or chronic) organ dysfunction before the onset of infection. *qSOFA* indicates quick SOFA, *MAP* mean arterial pressure (From Singer et al. [5])

Table 16.2 Sequential [Sepsis-Related] Organ Failure Assessment score

System	Score				
	0	1	2	3	4
Respiration					
Pao_2/Fio_2, mmHg (kPa)	≥400 (53.3)	<400 (53.3)	<300 (40)	<200 (26.7) with respiratory support	<100 (13.3) with respiratory support
Coagulation					
Platelets, ×10³/μL	≥150	<150	<100	<50	<20
Liver					
Bilirubin, mg/dL (μmol/L)	<1.2 (20)	1.2–1.9 (20–32)	2.0–5.9 (33–101)	6.0–11.9 (102–204)	>12.0 (204)
Cardiovascular	MAP ≥70 mmHg	MAP <70 mmHg	Dopamine <5 or dobutamine (any dose)[a]	Dopamine 5.1–15 or epinephrine ≤0.1 or norepinephrine ≤0.1[a]	Dopamine >15 or epinephrine >0.1 or norepinephrine >0.1[a]
Central nervous system					
Glasgow Coma Scale score[b]	15	13–14	10–12	6–9	<6

(continued)

Table 16.2 (continued)

System	Score				
	0	1	2	3	4
Renal					
Creatinine, mg/dL (μmol/L)	<1.2 (110)	1.2–1.9(110–170)	2.0–3.4 (171–299)	3.5–4.9 (300–440)	>5.0 (440)
Urine output, mL/day				<500	<200

Adapted from Annane et al. [27]

From Singer et al. [5]

Abbreviations: *Fio2* fraction of inspired oxygen, *MAP* mean arterial pressure, *Pao2* partial pressure of oxygen

[a]Catecholamine doses are given as μg/kg/min for at least 1 h

[b]Glasgow Coma Scale scores range from 3 to 15; higher score indicates better neurological functions

Septic shock is defined as sepsis with particularly profound circulatory, cellular, and metabolic abnormalities that are associated with an even greater risk of in-hospital mortality. Patients with septic shock are clinically identified by a vasopressor requirement to maintain adequate hemodynamic and perfusion goals.

A new clinical score termed quickSOFA (qSOFA) is also proposed for adult patients outside of the intensive care unit (ICU) and with suspected infection. This score is largely based on tacchypnea, hypotension, and altered mentation, and is deemed a marker for poor outcomes [5].

16.3   Clinical Features and Diagnosis

The recognition of SIRS in a patient should prompt close monitoring for signs of development of sepsis and end organ dysfunction. Diagnosis of sepsis is dependent upon set criteria of signs, and more recently has been a subject of much debate.

16.3.1   Clinical Criteria Identifying Patients with Sepsis and Septic Shock

SIRS can manifest itself by the hallmark features of tachycardia, tachypnea, hyperthermia, and leukocytosis, among other traditionally accepted upon criteria outlined in Table 16.1 [3]. Where SIRS is presumed to be caused by a suspected or proven infection, the criteria for sepsis is considered to have been met.

It is vital to embark upon a search for rapid identification of a microbial cause as the source of infection. Patients should be promptly pan-cultured, with administration of broad-spectrum antimicrobial therapy in rapid succession. Even still, a microbial source is not clearly identified via cultures in up to one-third of sepsis cases [6]. Appropriate imaging modalities – including plain radiographs, computed tomography (CT), and ultrasound scans – should be utilized to search for the source of infection.

With worsening sepsis, hypoperfusion and hypotension may set in, leading to the development of end organ dysfunction. This rapidly deteriorating clinical state with persistent refractory hypotension despite adequate resuscitation is known as septic shock.

16.3.2 Sepsis-3 and SOFA Scores

According to the updated consensus definitions for sepsis and septic shock (Sepsis-3) proposed at the 45th Annual SCCM Meeting, sepsis is defined as a life-threatening organ dysfunction caused by a dysregulated host response to infection (see Fig. 16.1). Organ dysfunction is further defined by an increase in the SOFA score of 2 points or more (see Table 16.2).

Among ICU patients with suspected infection, SOFA scores signaling organ dysfunction are associated with a higher risk of in-hospital mortality, supporting its use in clinical criteria for sepsis [7].

16.3.3 Biomarkers of Sepsis

Identification of biomarkers for sepsis has been the topic of considerable research work. Despite a handful of biomarkers being proposed as possible markers of sepsis, at present time biomarkers are not routinely utilized for the diagnosis of sepsis, or to guide and assess response to therapy.

C-reactive protein (CRP) is a marker for generalized inflammation and it is markedly elevated in the setting of infection [8].

The persistence of elevated CRP levels past 36 h has been shown to be associated with worse outcomes in septic patients [9], while a decreasing CRP level over the first 48 h indicates effective antimicrobial therapy [10].

Generalized inflammation and infection also causes an elevation in the levels of procalcitonin (PCT). PCT assays have been shown to be a superior target biomarker than CRP in recent studies, with rising levels seen in worsening sepsis, and a decrease noted after institution of appropriate antimicrobial therapy [11–13]. A decreasing PCT level at day 3 of therapy has been associated with improved survival [14].

More recently, efforts are directed at identifying novel targets as biomarkers to differentiate SIRS from sepsis. Recent data suggest that one such target of measure is monocyte distribution width, where elevated monocyte distribution width in blood was shown to be a superior biomarker than any of the other volumetric cell parameters assessed in helping distinguish sepsis from uninfected patients with SIRS. For sepsis, the negative predictive value of normal monocyte distribution width was 98 % [15].

16.4 Management of Sepsis and Septic Shock

The Surviving Sepsis Campaign (SSC) has published clear guidelines for the treatment of sepsis and septic shock [16]. This has led to the development of sepsis bundles to streamline the application of therapy in many intensive care units, reducing morbidity, mortality, and health care costs associated with sepsis and septic shock [17–21]. Early recognition of signs of sepsis paired with prompt administration of appropriate therapy are cornerstones in reducing sepsis-associated mortality. The general principles of management of sepsis and septic shock include resuscitation, source control, monitoring, and supportive care.

16.4.1 Initial Resuscitation and Hemodynamic Support

In their seminal paper, Rivers et al. outline the endpoints of resuscitation that signal adequate tissue perfusion. Specific resuscitation parameters for MAP, CVP and ScvO2 are set forth as a goal to be achieved in the first 6 h of the onset of severe sepsis or septic shock (see Fig. 16.2) [22].

16.4.1.1 Fluids

While the SAFE trial demonstrated equivalent outcomes of either 4 % albumin or normal saline in the resuscitation of critically ill patients in the ICU [23], two large meta-analyses seemed to favor crystalloid over colloid especially in the trauma patient population [24, 25]. Fluid challenges should be utilized until hemodynamics fail to reflect overall improvement despite adequate cardiac filling pressures. The volume of resuscitation should be directed by either pressure, i.e., central venous pressure, monitoring, or by bedside ultrasound parameters. Bedside ultrasound can effectively determine volume responsiveness by directly observing inferior venal caval respiratory fluctuations. Greater than 16 % size variation suggests that the patient is hypovolemic and may warrant additional volume resuscitation. The volume of fluid must be judicious in order to avoid the adverse effects of excessive volume administration.

16.4.1.2 Oxygen Demand and Delivery/Blood Transfusions

The underlying principle of oxygen debt in sepsis is based on a mismatch between oxygen delivery and oxygen extraction

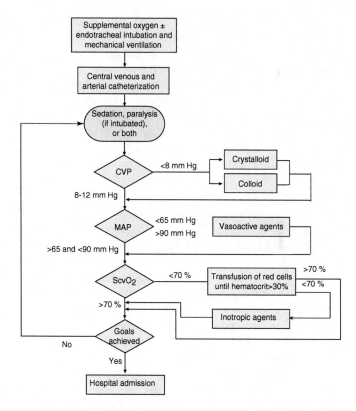

Fig. 16.2 Early goal-directed therapy in the treatment of severe sepsis and septic shock (From Rivers et al. [22])

in peripheral tissues. Assessment of oxygen debt and tissue hypoxia is paramount in monitoring for progression of sepsis and guiding therapy. This should be achieved not only by measuring mixed or central venous oxygen saturation, but also by arterial lactate concentration, base deficit, and pH [21]. If the measured central venous oxygen saturation is less than 70 %, transfusion of packed red blood cells should be considered to achieve a hematocrit of ≥30% and optimize arterial oxygen content. Through their TRICC trial, Hébert et al. demonstrated that utilization of a restrictive transfusion strategy (hemoglobin concentration between 7–9 g/dL and 10–12 g/dL) in critically ill patients was associated with significantly lower mortality [26].

After achieving an adequate MAP goal, oxygen delivery can be further affected by raising the cardiac output by preferentially using dobutamine or norepinephrine, per the Surviving Sepsis Campaign guidelines [16].

16.4.1.3 Vasopressors and Inotropes

If central venous oxygen saturation remains less than 70% despite meeting the aforementioned parameters of resuscitation having already utilized fluids and blood transfusions, it is recommended to initiate inotropic support. The preferred inotrope for resuscitation in severe sepsis and septic shock is dopamine followed by norepinephrine. Antidiuretic hormone (ADH), also known as vasopressin, is a frequently utilized adjunct given its central mode of action on V1a vasopressin receptor resulting in peripheral vasoconstriction. The dose of vasopressin is physiologic at 0.04 units/min; however, there appears to be a state of suppression during states of septic shock. The use of vasopressin is complementary and can improve effect of other pressors, i.e., norepinephrine.

16.4.2 Corticosteriods

The use of corticosteroids in septic patients refractory to high-dose vasopressors despite being adequately resuscitated remains the subject of many studies. Contradictory evidence has been shown in recent studies citing both an increase (Cochrane Review) [27, 28] and a decrease (PROGRESS registry) [29] in mortality associated with the use of low-dose exogenous corticosteroids therapy in patients with sepsis and septic shock.

Recent data from Sprung et al. suggest an earlier resolution of shock with low-dose hydrocortisone treatment for 5 days, followed by a 6-day taper, despite no clear mortality benefit [30].

It is our recommendation that low-dose (<300 mg/day) hydrocortisone be administered in poorly responsive patients without administering any ACTH stimulation test. We further recommend continuing this therapy for duration of 7 days, with the addition of a fludrocortisone dose of 50 µg per day for provision of its mineralocorticoid benefits [31].

16.4.3 Source Control and Antibiosis

Infection is a leading cause of sepsis requiring admission to the SICU, with respiratory tract, bloodstream, urinary tract and abdomen being the most frequent sites of infection [32]. Many of these sources of infection are surgically treatable and all attempts must be made to control these sources within 6 h of admission to the SICU. Line sepsis and *Clostridium difficile* colitis remain another frequent source of morbidity in patients with a prolonged stay in the SICU [33, 34].

SSC guidelines recommend early initiation of appropriate antimicrobial therapy directed by the suspected or known source of infection. It calls for blood cultures to be drawn and broad-spectrum antibiotics to be administered ideally within the first hour and preferably in that order [16]. Once the inciting organism is definitely identified, these antibiotics should be properly tailored to the sensitivities expressed.

16.4.4   Glycemic Control

Hyperglycemia is frequently encountered in diabetic and non-diabetic patients presenting with sepsis and infection. Intensive insulin therapy via continuous insulin infusion to maintain blood glucose levels between 80 and 110 mg/dL has been shown to be associated with a marked reduction in overall in-hospital mortality [35] More recently, the NICE-SUGAR study compared an intensive insulin group (target blood glucose 80–110 mg/dL) to a more conventional group (target blood glucose <180 mg/dL) and showed a significant decrease in mortality along with a decrease in the number of hypoglycemic events in the conventional group [36]. The most commonly agreed upon approach is to utilize intravenous administration of insulin to achieve a target blood glucose concentration between 120 and 180 mg/dL.

16.4.5   Recombinant Human Activated Protein C

Endogenous protein C plays an important role in regulating inflammation, cell death, and protecting the permeability of endothelium in humans. Owing to these cytoprotective effects, recombinant human activated protein C (APC) has been utilized in septic patients, with the PROWESS study demonstrating a decrease in mortality with its use in high-risk (APACHE II score ≥ 25, or multi-organ failure) patients [37]. This mortality benefit however was not carried over in the ADDRESS study when APC was utilized in low-risk (APACHE II score < 25, or single-organ failure) patients [38].

Additionally protein C is also a major component in the anti-coagulation pathway, and its use has been associated with an increase in the number of bleeding episodes in surgical patients. Given this side effect profile, we recommend judicious use of APC only in the high-risk subset of septic patients.

16.4.6 Supportive ICU Care

The care of the septic patient involves many other aspects of carefully orchestrated supportive adjuncts. These include stress ulcer prophylaxis preferably with proton pump inhibitors, deep vein thrombosis prophylaxis, and early enteral or parenteral nutritional support.

Mechanical ventilation and renal replacement therapy can be instituted to maximize oxygenation, reduce work of breathing, and reduce the burden of fluid overload and toxins. The specifics of exact application of these modalities remain beyond the scope of this discussion.

References

1. Martin GS, Mannino DM, Eaton S, et al. The epidemiology of sepsis in the United States from 1979 through 2000. N Engl J Med. 2003;348(16):1546–54.
2. Heron M, Hoyert DL, Murphy SL, et al. Deaths: final data for 2006. National vital statistics report, vol. 57, no. 14. National Center for Health Statistics; 2009.
3. Bone RC, Balk RA, Cerra FB, et al. American College of Chest Physicians/Society of Critical Care Medicine Consensus Conference: definitions for sepsis and organ failure and guidelines for the use of innovative therapies in sepsis. Crit Care Med. 1992;20:864–74.
4. Levy MM, Fink MP, Marshall JC. 2001 SCCM/ESICM/ACCP/ATS/STS/SIS International sepsis definitions conference. Crit Care Med. 2003;31:1250–6.
5. Singer M, Deutschman CS, Seymour CW, Shankar-Hari M, Annane D, Bauer M, Bellomo R, Bernard GR, Chiche JD, Coopersmith CM, Hotchkiss RS, Levy MM, Marshall JC, Martin GS, Opal SM, Rubenfeld GD, van der Poll T, Vincent JL, Angus DC. The third international consensus definitions for sepsis and septic shock (Sepsis-3). JAMA. 2016;315:801–10.
6. Sands KE, Bates DW, Lanken PN, et al. Epidemiology of sepsis syndrome in 8 academic medical centers. JAMA. 1997;278:234–40.

7. Seymour CW, Liu VX, Iwashyna TJ, et al. Assessment of clinical criteria for sepsis: for the third international consensus definitions for sepsis and septic shock (Sepsis-3). JAMA. 2016;315:762–74.

8. Vigushin DM, Pepys MB, Hawkins PN. Metabolic and scintigraphic studies of radioiodinated human C-reactive protein in health and disease. J Clin Invest. 1993;91:1351–7.

9. Lobo SM, Lobo FR, Bota DP, et al. C-reactive protein levels correlate with mortality and organ failure in critically ill patients. Chest. 2003;123(6):2043–9.

10. Schmidt X, Vincent JL. The time course of blood c-reactive protein levels in relation to the response to initial antimicrobial therapy in patients with sepsis. Infection. 2008;36:213–9.

11. Becker KL, Snider R, Nylen ES. Procalcitonin assay in systemic inflammation, infection and sepsis: clinical utility and limitations. Crit Care Med. 2008;36:941–52.

12. Assicot M, Gendrel D, Carsin H, et al. High serum procalcitonin concentrations in patients with sepsis and infection. Lancet. 1993;341:515–8.

13. Uzzan B, Cohen R, Nicolas P, et al. Procalcitonin as a diagnostic test for sepsis in adults after surgery or trauma: a systematic review and meta-analysis. Crit Care Med. 2006;34:1996–2003.

14. Charles PE, Tinel C, Barbar S, et al. Procalcitonin kinetics within the first days of sepsis: relationship with the approproateeness of antubiotic therapuy and the outcomes. Crit Care. 2009;13:R38.

15. A feasibility trial to detect sepsis in the emergency department based upon blood monocyte volume variability. In: Crouser E, Parrillo J, Angus D, et al. 45th critical care congress, Society of Critical Care Medicine, Orlando; 2016.

16. Dellinger RP, et al. Surviving sepsis campaign: international guidelines for management of severe sepsis and septic shock. Crit Care Med. 2008;36:296–327.

17. Levy MM, Dellinger RP, Townsend SR, et al. The surviving sepsis campaign: results of an international guideline-based performance improvement program targeting severe sepsis. Crit Care Med. 2010;38:367–74.

18. Gao F, Melody T, Daniels DF, et al. The impact of compliance with 6-hour and 24-hour sepsis bundles on hospital mortality in patients with severe sepsis: a prospective observational study. Crit Care. 2005;9:R764–70.

19. Ferrer R, Artigas A, Suarez D, et al. Effectiveness of treatments for severe sepsis: a prospective, multicenter, observational study. Am J Respir Crit Care Med. 2009;180:861–6.

20. Castellanos-Ortega A, Suberviola B, Garcia-Astudillo LA, et al. Impact of the surviving sepsis campaign protocols on hospital length of stay and mortality in septic shock patients: results of a three-year follow-up quasi-experimental study. Crit Care Med. 2010;38:1036–43.
21. Rivers E, et al. Early goal-directed therapy in the treatment of severe sepsis and septic shock. N Engl J Med. 2001;345:1368–77.
22. Rivers E, Nguyen B, Havstad S, et al. Early goal-directed therapy in the treatment of severe sepsis and septic shock. N Engl J Med. 2001;345:19.
23. Finfer S, et al. A comparison of albumin and saline for fluid resuscitation in the intensive care unit. N Engl J Med. 2004;350:2247–56.
24. Choi PT, et al. Crystalloids vs. colloids in fluid resuscitation: a systematic review. Crit Care Med. 1999;27:200–10.
25. Schierhout G, Roberts I. Fluid resuscitation with colloid or crystalloid solutions in critically ill patients: a systematic review of randomised trials. BMJ. 1998;316:961–4.
26. Hébert PC, Wells G, Blajchman MA, et al. A multicenter, randomized, controlled clinical trial of transfusion requirements in critical care. N Engl J Med. 1999;340:409–17.
27. Annane D, Bellissant E, Bollaert PE, et al. Corticosteroids in the treatment of severe sepsis and septic shock in adults. JAMA. 2009;301:2362–75.
28. Annane D, Bellissant E, Bollaert P, et al. Corticosteroids for treating sepsis. Cochrane database of systematic reviews. 2015;12:CD002243. doi:10.1002/14651858.CD002243.pub3.
29. Baele R, Janes JN, Brunkhorst FM, et al. Global utilization of low-dose corticosteroids in severe sepsis and septic shock: a report from the PROGRESS registry. Crit Care. 2010;14:R102.
30. Sprung CL, Annane D, Keh D, et al. CORTICUS Study Group. Hydrocortisone therapy for patients with septic shock. N Engl J Med. 2008;358(2):111–24.
31. Annane D, Sébille V, Charpentier C, et al. Effect of treatment with low doses of hydrocortisone and fludrocortisone on mortality in patients with septic shock. JAMA. 2002;288(7):862–71.
32. Vincent JL, et al. International study of the prevalence and outcomes of infection in intensive care units. JAMA. 2009;302:2323–9.
33. Blot F, et al. Earlier positivity of central-venous versus peripheral-blood cultures is highly predictive of catheter-related sepsis. J Clin Microbiol. 1998;36:105–9.
34. Leclair MA, et al. Clostridium difficile infection in the intensive care unit. J Intensive Care Med. 2010;25:23–30.

35. van den Berghe G, Wouters P, Weekers F, et al. Intensive insulin therapy in critically ill patients. N Engl J Med. 2001;345(19):1359–67.
36. Finfer S, Chittock DR, Su SY, et al. NICE-SUGAR Study Investigators. Intensive versus conventional glucose control in critically ill patients. N Engl J Med. 2009;360(13):1283–97.
37. Bernard GR, Vincent JL, Laterre PF, et al. Efficacy and safety of recombinant human activated protein C for severe sepsis. N Engl J Med. 2001;344:699–709.
38. Abraham E, Laterre PF, Garg R, et al. Drotrecogin alfa (activated) for adults with severe sepsis and a low risk of death. N Engl J Med. 2005;353:1332–41.

Chapter 17
Antibiotic Management in Acute Care Surgery

Massimo Sartelli and Fikri M. Abu-Zidan

17.1 Introduction

Antibiotics are commonly used in the intensive care units. In critically ill patients, empirical antimicrobial therapy should be always administered when the suspected infection is serious. Avoiding unnecessary antibiotic use and optimizing the administration of antimicrobial agents may improve patient outcome and minimize risks for bacterial resistance.

Sepsis is the main condition encountered in acute care surgery that needs appropriate antibiotics. This condition is complex and multifactorial. It is usually secondary to infection,

M. Sartelli (✉)
Department of Surgery, Macerata Hospital, Macerata, Italy
e-mail: massimosartelli@gmail.com

F.M. Abu-Zidan, MD, FACS, FRCS, PhD, DAST
Department of Surgery, College of Medicine and Health Sciences, UAE University, Al-Ain, UAE
e-mail: fabuzidan@uaeu.ac.ae

© Springer International Publishing Switzerland 2017   309
S. Di Saverio et al. (eds.), *Acute Care Surgery Handbook*,
DOI 10.1007/978-3-319-15341-4_17

varies in severity, and may lead to functional impairment of vital organs [1].

Mortality rates were stabilized because of advancements in the management of the underlying infection and combined support of failing organs. Nevertheless, these death rates remain high [2] and dramatically increase in patients with severe sepsis and septic shock [3]. Aggressive treatment of these patients may improve outcomes [4].

In patients having severe sepsis and septic shock, appropriate antibiotic therapy with broad-spectrum antimicrobial agents should be started as soon as possible. It is important to promptly achieve and maintain an optimal exposure at the infection site, regardless of the origin of the infection.

Antibiotics are useful only when the source of infection is controlled. Antibiotics will support the treatable surgical causes only when proper radiological or surgical interventions have been performed (Fig. 17.1).

17.2   Antimicrobial Therapy in Critically Ill Patients

An insufficient or inadequate antimicrobial regimen is one of the variables strongly associated with unfavorable outcomes in critically ill patients [5].

Recent Surviving Sepsis Campaign guidelines for the management of severe sepsis and septic shock [6] included three important recommendations about antimicrobial therapy: (1) administration of effective intravenous antimicrobials within the first hour of recognition of septic shock and severe sepsis without septic shock as the goal of therapy; (2) initial empiric anti-infective therapy of one or more drugs that have activity against all likely pathogens that penetrate in adequate concentrations into tissues presumed to be the source of sepsis; (3)

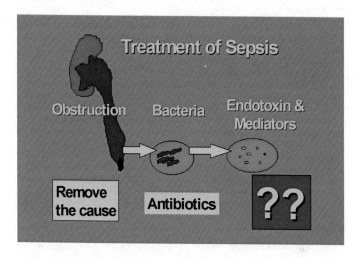

Fig. 17.1 Antibiotics therapy is useful only when the source of infection is controlled. Removing the ureteric obstruction in this scenario is essential for antibiotics to work. The search for new therapies targeting endotoxins and shock mediators once they adhere to receptors at end organs is still going on without real breakthroughs (Diagram drawn by Professor Fikri Abu-Zidan as part of his PhD defense "Role of platelet activating factor in sepsis and shock", Section of Trauma and Disaster Medicine, Department of Surgery, Linköping University, Sweden: October 1995)

antimicrobial regimen should be reassessed daily for potential de-escalation.

Some studies [7–8] showed that modifying an initial inadequate antibiotic therapy, according to microbiological results, in critically ill patients with ventilation aspiration pneumonia (VAP) does not translate into a better outcome. Therefore, the best approach for reducing infection-related mortality in critically ill patients seems to be the initial institution of an adequate and broad-spectrum antibiotic regimen, which should be de-escalated when culture results are available and clinical status can be better assessed, 48–72 h after initiation of empiric therapy. The concept of de-escalation strategy can easily be translated to all critically ill patients. If the empiric therapy is administered in a timely manner by using appropriate agents that lead to rapid bacterial killing, this strategy can minimize the emergence of resistance, optimizing antimicrobial treatment.

We should decide the optimal dosage when starting antimicrobial therapy considering the "dilution effect," also called the third spacing phenomenon. Low plasma antimicrobial levels can lead to low antimicrobial concentrations in the peritoneal fluid with potentially reduced antimicrobial delivery to the target tissues when administering hydrophilic agents. This includes β-lactams, aminoglycosides, and glycopeptides, which are selectively distributed to the extracellular space. Therefore, higher than standard loading doses of these drugs should be administered to ensure optimal exposure at the infection site whenever treatment is begun in patients with severe sepsis or septic shock [9].

Once appropriate initial treatment is started, it is mandatory to reassess the antimicrobial regimen daily, because the pathophysiological changes of the critically ill patients, may significantly affect drug distribution. Lower than standard dosages of renally excreted drugs should be administered in the presence of impaired renal function. Higher than standard dosages of renally excreted drugs may be needed for optimal exposure in patients with glomerular hyperfiltration [9].

This is crucial for hydrophilic antimicrobials (β-lactams, aminoglycosides, and glycopeptides) and for moderately lipophilic antimicrobials (ciprofloxacin and levofloxacin).

Table 17.1 shows the recommended dosing regimens of the most frequently used renally excreted antimicrobials according to renal function [10].

In the last years, the relevance of pharmacokinetic-pharmacodynamic relationships in optimizing drug exposure has been progressively highlighted in critically ill patients [11]. Different approaches should be pursued according to the mechanism of antimicrobial activity exhibited by each antibiotic [12].

Two patterns of bactericidal activity have been identified: time-dependent activity (where the time that the plasma concentration persists above the minimum inhibitory concentration [MIC] of the etiological agent is considered the major determinant for efficacy) and concentration-dependent activity (where the efficacy is mainly related to the plasma peak concentration in relation to the MIC of the microorganism).

Concentration-dependent antibiotics, such as aminoglycosides and quinolones, are more effective at higher concentrations. These agents show an associated concentration-dependent postantibiotic effect, and bactericidal action continues for a period of time after the antibiotic level falls below the MIC [9]. Concentration-dependent agents administered in high dosage, short-course, once-a-day treatment regimens may promote more rapid and efficient bactericidal action and prevent the development of resistant strains and antibiotic toxicity.

Time-dependent antibiotics, such as β-lactams and glycopeptides, demonstrate optimal bactericidal activity when drug concentrations are maintained above the MIC. The efficacy of time-dependent antibacterial agents in critically ill patients is based on the constant maintenance of suprainhibitory drug concentrations [13] and should be administered in multiple doses per day or in continuous infusion. For these antibiotics the use of intravenous continuous infusion, which ensures the highest steady-state concentration under the same total daily dosage, may be the most effective way of maximizing pharmacodynamic exposure [12]

17.3 Biomarkers to Discontinue Antimicrobial Therapy in Critically Ill Patients

The duration of antimicrobial therapy is based on the clinical response of the patient to the treatment and should be shortened

Table 17.1 Recommended dosing regimens of the most frequently used renally excreted antimicrobials according to renal function

	Renal function			
Antibiotic	Increased	Normal	Moderately impaired	Severely impaired
Piperacillin/ tazobatam	16/2 g q24 h CI or 3.375 q6 h EI over 4 h	4/0.5 g q6 h	3/0.375 g q6 h	2/0.25 g q6 h
Imipenem	500 mg q4 h or 250 mg q3 h over 3 h CI	500 mg q6 h	250 mg q6 h	250 mg q12 h
Meropenem	1 g q6 h over 6 h CI	500 mg q6 h	250 mg q6 h	250 mg q12 h
Ertapenem	ND	1 g q24 h	1 g q24 h	500 mg q24 h
Gentamycin	9–10 mg/kg q24 h	7 mg/kg q24 h	7 mg/kg q36–48 h	7 mg/kg q48–96 h
Amikacin	20 mg/kg q24 h	15 mg/kg q24 h	15 mg/kg q36–48 h	15 mg/kg q48–96 h
Ciprofloxacin	600 mg q12 h or 400 mg q8 h	400 mg q12 h	400 mg q12 h	400 mg q24 h
Levofloxacin	500 mg q12 h	750 mg q24 h	500 mg q24 h	500 mg q48 h
Vancomycin	30 mg/kg q24 h CI	500 mg q6 h	500 mg q12 h	500 mg q24–72 h
Teicoplanin	LD 12 mg/kg q12 h for 3–4 doses; MD 6 mg/kg q12 h	LD 12 mg/kg q12 h for 3–4 doses; MD 4–6 mg/kg q12 h	LD 12 mg/kg q12 h for 3–4 doses; MD 2–4 mg/kg q12 h	LD 12 mg/kg q12 h for 3–4 doses; MD 2–4 mg/kg q24 h

Table 17.1 (continued)

Antibiotic	Renal function			
	Increased	Normal	Moderately impaired	Severely impaired
Tigecycline	LD 100 mg; MD 50 mg q12 h	LD 100 mg; MD 50 mg q12 h	LD 100 mg; MD 50 mg q12 h	LD 100 mg; MD 50 mg q12 h

Reproduced with permission from Sartelli et al. [10]
CI continuous infusion, *LD* loading dose

to prevent antimicrobial resistance. However, the high death rates of sepsis and septic shock require maintaining a high index of clinical suspicion for these conditions.

Septic patients should be monitored carefully with inflammatory response markers. The most widely used biomarkers in clinical settings are C reactive protein (CRP) and procalcitonin (PCT). CRP is a protein found in blood plasma, synthesized, and released by the liver. CRP production is part of the nonspecific acute-phase response to most forms of inflammation, infection, and tissue damage [14]. Currently, CRP is used as a clinical marker to assess the presence of infection [15]. Numerous studies have reported the high sensitivity and specificity of CRP for the diagnosis of sepsis [16]. Nevertheless, CRP levels are not indicative of antibiotics discontinuation.

PCT is a 116 amino acid protein with a molecular weight of 13 kDa and is a precursor of calcitonin produced by C-cells of the thyroid gland, which is intracellularly cleaved by proteolytic enzymes into the active hormone [14]. PCT was first described for the diagnosis of sepsis in 1993 [17].

PCT algorithms for antibiotic treatment decisions have been studied in adult patients from primary care, emergency department, and intensive care unit (ICU) settings, suggesting that procalcitonin-guided therapy may reduce antibiotic exposure without increasing the mortality rate [18].

Procalcitonin guidance for antimicrobial duration appears to safely decrease antibiotics use in critically ill patients and may decrease the length of stay in the ICU (Fig. 17.2) [19].

17.4   Antibiotic Stewardship in Critical Care Surgery Patients

Antimicrobial resistance has emerged as an important determinant of outcome for patients in the intensive care units [20].

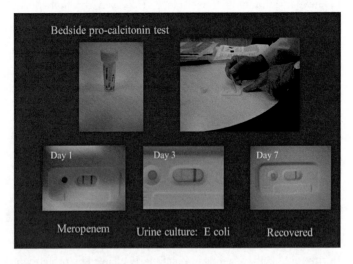

Fig. 17.2 A 70-year-old hypertensive, nondiabetic woman presented to the hospital confused and irritable. She had no fever, abdominal pain, or dysuria. Her abdomen was soft and lax. Point-of-care procalcitonin test was positive. The patient was empirically started on meropenem. Urine culture was positive for *Escherichia coli*. The patient gradually improved. Procalcitonin test became weakly positive on day 3 and became completely normal on day 7. The patient has clinically recovered on day 7 (Courtesy of Professor Fikri Abu-Zidan, Al-Ain Hospital, Al-Ain, UAE.)

Optimal antibiotic use is crucial in the critical care setting, especially in an era of rising antibiotic resistance and lack of new antimicrobial development. Local guidelines and recommendations should be developed in each hospital and community depending on their own bacterial flora and resistance pattern. Using international regimens without looking into the local setting may have side effects [21].

Selection of appropriate antibiotics and their prescription at appropriate doses are important in order to optimize empirical therapy and minimize antimicrobial resistance.

However, appropriate antibiotic stewardship in intensive care units includes not only rapid identification and optimal treatment of bacterial infections in critically ill patients, based on pharmacokinetic-pharmacodynamic characteristics, but also improving clinician's ability to avoid administering unnecessary broad-spectrum antibiotics and shortening the duration of treatment. If clinicians will not be able to implement such a policy, patients will face an uncontrollable surge of very difficult-to-treat pathogens.

Important Learning Points

- Antibiotics are useful only when the source of infection is controlled.
- In patients having severe sepsis and septic shock, appropriate antibiotic therapy with broad-spectrum antimicrobial agents should be started as soon as possible.
- A de-escalation of the antimicrobial therapy is possible when culture results are available and clinical status can be better assessed, 48–72 h after initiation of empiric therapy.
- It is important to promptly achieve and maintain an optimal exposure at the infection site, regardless of the origin of the infection.
- Although most surgeons are aware of the problem of antimicrobial resistance, most underestimate the degree of resistance in their own hospital.

- Optimal antibiotic use is crucial in the critical care setting, especially in an era of rising antibiotic resistance and lack of new antimicrobial development.

References

1. Levy MM, Fink MP, Marshall JC, Abraham E, Angus D, Cook D, Cohen J, Opal SM, Vincent JL, Ramsay G. SCCM/ESICM/ACCP/ATS/SIS international sepsis definitions conference. Crit Care Med. 2001;2003(31):1250–6.
2. Angus DC, van der Poll T. Severe sepsis and septic shock. N Engl J Med. 2013;369(9):840–51.
3. Bone RC, Balk RA, Cerra FB, Dellinger RP, Fein AM, Knaus WA, Schein RM, Sibbald WJ. American College of Chest Physicians/Society of Critical Care Medicine Consensus Conference: definitions for sepsis and organ failure and guidlines for the use of innovative therapies in sepsis. Chest. 1992;101:1644–55.
4. Esteban A, Frutos-Vivar F, Ferguson ND, Peñuelas O, Lorente JA, Gordo F, Honrubia T, Algora A, Bustos A, García G, Diaz-Regañón IR, de Luna RR. Sepsis incidence and outcome: contrasting the intensive care unit with the hospital ward. Crit Care Med. 2007;35(5):1284–9.
5. Shani V, Muchtar E, Kariv G, Robenshtok E, Leibovici L. Systematic review and meta-analysis of the efficacy of appropriate empiric antibiotic therapy for sepsis. Antimicrob Agents Chemother. 2010;54(11):4851–63.
6. Dellinger RP, Levy MM, Rhodes A, Annane D, Gerlach H, Opal SM, Sevransky JE, Sprung CL, Douglas IS, Jaeschke R, Osborn TM, Nunnally ME, Townsend SR, Reinhart K, Kleinpell RM, Angus DC, Deutschman CS, Machado FR, Rubenfeld GD, Webb S, Beale RJ, Vincent JL, Moreno R. Surviving sepsis campaign guidelines committee including the pediatric subgroup. Surviving sepsis campaign: international guidelines for management of severe sepsis and septic shock, 2012. Intensive Care Med. 2013;39(2):165–228.
7. Höffken G, Niederman MS. Nosocomial pneumonia: the importance of a de-escalating strategy for antibiotic treatment of pneumonia in the ICU. Chest. 2002;122:2183–96.
8. Alvarez-Lerma F. Modification of empiric antibiotic treatment in patients with pneumonia acquired in the intensive care unit: ICU-

Acquired Pneumonia Study Group. Intensive Care Med. 1996;22:387–94.

9. Pea F, Viale P. Bench-to-bedside review: appropriate antibiotic therapy in severe sepsis and septic shock–does the dose matter? Crit Care. 2009;13(3):214.

10. Sartelli M, Viale P, Catena F, Ansaloni L, Moore E, Malangoni M, Moore FA, Velmahos G, Coimbra R, Ivatury R, Peitzman A, Koike K, Leppaniemi A, Biffl W, Burlew CC, Balogh ZJ, Boffard K, Bendinelli C, Gupta S, Kluger Y, Agresta F, Di Saverio S, Wani I, Escalona A, Ordonez C, Fraga GP, Junior GA, Bala M, Cui Y, Marwah S, et al. 2013 WSES guidelines for management of intra-abdominal infections. World J Emerg Surg. 2013;8(1):3. doi:10.1186/1749-7922-8-3.

11. Pea F, Viale P. The antimicrobial therapy puzzle: could pharmacokinetic-pharmacodynamic relationships be helpful in addressing the issue of appropriate pneumonia treatment in critically ill patients? Clin Infect Dis. 2006;42(12):1764–71.

12. Sartelli M, Viale P, Koike K, Pea F, Tumietto F, van Goor H, Guercioni G, Nespoli A, Tranà C, Catena F, Ansaloni L, Leppaniemi A, Biffl W, Moore FA, Poggetti R, Pinna AD, Moore EE. WSES consensus conference: guidelines for first-line management of intra-abdominal infections. World J Emerg Surg. 2011;6:2. doi:10.1186/1749-7922-6-2.

13. McKenzie C. Antibiotic dosing in critical illness. J Antimicrob Chemother. 2011;66 Suppl 2:ii25–31.

14. Biron BM, Ayala A, Lomas-Neira JL. Biomarkers for sepsis: what is and what might be? Biomark Insights. 2015;10 Suppl 4:7–17.

15. Pepys MB, Hirschfeld GM. C-reactive protein: a critical update. J Clin Invest. 2003;111(12):1805–12.

16. Orati JA, Almeida P, Santos V, Ciorla G, Lobo SM. Serum C-reactive protein concentrations in early abdominal and pulmonary sepsis. Rev Bras Ter Intensiva. 2013;25(1):6–11.

17. Prkno A, Wacker C, Brunkhorst FM, Schlattmann P. Procalcitonin-guided therapy in intensive care unit patients with severe sepsis and septic shock–a systematic review and meta-analysis. Crit Care. 2013;17(6):R291.

18. Agarwal R, Schwartz DN. Procalcitonin to guide duration of antimicrobial therapy in intensive care units: a systematic review. Clin Infect Dis. 2011;53(4):379–87.

19. Kollef MH, Fraser VJ. Antibiotic resistance in the intensive care unit. Ann Intern Med. 2001;134(4):298–314.

20. Luyt CE, Bréchot N, Trouillet JL, Chastre J. Antibiotic stewardship in the intensive care unit. Crit Care. 2014;18(5):480.

21. Abu-Zidan FM, McAteer E, Elhag KM. Selective decontamination of the digestive tract in Kuwait. Crit Care Med. 1989;17:1364.

Chapter 18
Nutrition in Sepsis and Acute Surgical Patients

Brodie Parent and Ronald V. Maier

18.1 Introduction

Malnutrition is defined as the imbalance between dietary intake and underlying energy requirements. Malnutrition is common globally in the acute care hospital setting, and various studies estimate a prevalence of 25–50 % in US hospitals [1–3]. Myriad studies have shown that malnutrition during an inpatient hospital stay is associated with poor outcomes [4]. Patients who undergo major operations or experience sepsis are uniquely at risk for malnutrition, mainly because their physiology is characterized by hyper-metabolism, inflammation, and catabolism [5]. Indeed, these patients have resting energy needs that can increase by up to 40 % in the first hospital week, and by over 100 % in the second week [6]. Moreover, surgical patients have frequent periods of starvation prior to procedures and secondary

B. Parent, MD (✉) • R.V. Maier, MD, FACS, FRCS Ed (Hon)
Department of Surgery, University of Washington, Harborview Medical Center, Seattle, WA, USA
e-mail: bparent@uw.edu; ronmaier@uw.edu

© Springer International Publishing Switzerland 2017
S. Di Saverio et al. (eds.), *Acute Care Surgery Handbook*,
DOI 10.1007/978-3-319-15341-4_18

to perioperative complications such as ileus and inability to tolerate feeding [7–9]. Acute malnutrition during an inpatient stay can have dire effects in these patients, particularly if they have preexisting malnutrition, advanced age or chronic disease.

The American Society for Parenteral and Enteral Nutrition (ASPEN) states that the goals of nutrition therapy are to preserve lean body mass, maintain immune function, avoid metabolic complications, and ameliorate the oxidative stress of critical illness [10]. The surgical critical-care literature is replete with studies showing that targeted nutrition therapy and supplementation are associated with decreased infections, duration of mechanical ventilation, length of stay (LOS) and mortality in critically ill patients in the intensive care unit (ICU) [11]. This chapter will summarize these findings and offer a systematic approach to nutrition therapy in septic and acute surgical patients.

18.2 Metabolism in Sepsis, Surgery, and Trauma

Inflammation and oxidative stress characterize the physiologic state following trauma, surgery, and sepsis. Oxidative stress occurs when a biologic system generates reactive oxygen species (ROS) in a quantity that overwhelms the endogenous capacity to detoxify [12]. This creates a systemic ROS imbalance, and these species go on to damage cell membranes, enzymes, mitochondria, and DNA, leading to a cascade of metabolic derangements. Indeed, oxidative stress from an excessive proinflammatory immune response is directly linked to catabolism, insulin resistance, systemic acidosis, and coagulopathy [5, 6].

Malnutrition exacerbates the metabolic derangements of the septic and postoperative state. Malnutrition is associated with prolonged oxidative stress, immunosuppression, and delayed wound healing, which all increase the risk for disseminated infection and multiple organ failure [5, 13]. Moreover, catabolism associated with malnutrition and oxidative stress causes deconditioning and muscle atrophy, which likely contributes to prolonged mechanical ventilation [4]. Finally, the intestine is also affected by malnutrition and starvation, with mucosal atrophy and malabsorption occurring early in the hospital course. Gut-associated lymphoid tissue is diminished, increasing the risk for disseminated infection [14]. Enteral nutrition (EN) ameliorates many of the aforementioned metabolic derangements in septic and postoperative patients. EN maintains the gut mucosal barrier function, enhances immunity and IgA secretion, decreases systemic inflammation and oxidative injury, and prevents muscle atrophy [14, 15].

18.3 General Nutrition Approach and Algorithm

Critical care nutrition guidelines are designed for patients who are anticipated to be in the ICU for ≥2 days or who are anticipated to lack spontaneous enteral intake for ≥7 days [10]. Recently, clinical scoring systems have been developed which can help identify patients that will most benefit from artificial nutrition therapy. The "Nutrition Risk in Critically ill" (NUTRIC) score is a contemporary example [16] (Table 18.1).

The use of structured protocols and algorithms to manage nutrition support in the ICU is backed by high-level evidence and is associated with improved patient outcomes [17, 18]. An example of such a feeding algorithm is found in Fig. 18.1. Moreover, nutrition therapy is optimized by the use of multidisciplinary nutrition support teams, dietitians [19], and nurse-driven protocols [10].

Table 18.1 The "Nutrition Risk in Critically Ill" (NUTRIC) score

Character istic	Age	APACHE II[a]	SOFA[b] score	Number of comorbidities	Inpatient floor stay prior to ICU[c] admit?	IL-6[d]
Points	$\geq$50=1, $\geq$75=2	$\geq$15=1 $\geq$20=2 $\geq$28=3	$\geq$6=1 $\geq$10=2	$\geq$2=1	Yes=1	$\geq$400=1

$\geq$5 points is deemed "high risk"
[a]Acute Physiology and Chronic Health Evaluation II score
[b]Sepsis-Related Organ Failure Assessment score
[c]Intensive-care unit
[d]Interleukin-6

18.4 Calculating Energy Requirements

Depending on the characteristics of the patient and their illness severity, resting energy requirements can vary substantially between individuals. Current tools to capture this variation and characterize "nutrition status" are limited [20]. This is mainly because traditional biochemical indices for nutrition status (albumin, prealbumin, and transferrin) are not valid in the ICU setting. These markers, rather than reflecting calorie intake or underlying "nutritional reserve," more likely reflect the presence of vascular permeability and hepatic synthetic reprioritization during acute illness [10]. Moreover, other methods like calorimetry, nitrogen balance, and anthropometry are labor intensive and imprecise, and have not been associated with improved outcomes [20]. Common formulas such as the Harris-Benedict equation can help assess calorie needs, but these formulas were not designed and validated in a critical-care population. Therefore, determination of calorie targets in the critically ill is a blend of art and science, where the provider must utilize existing imperfect methods combined with their clinical judgment and consultation with nutrition support teams.

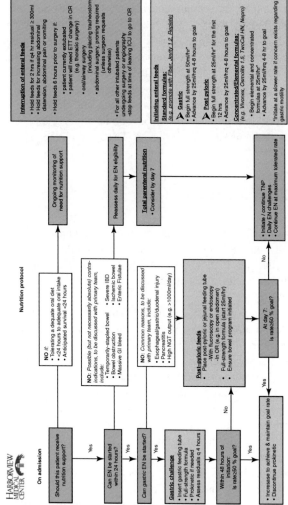

Fig. 18.1 Illustrative example of an intensive-care-unit nutrition protocol. *EN* enteral nutrition, *ETT* endotracheal tube, *ICU* intensive-care-unit, *OR* operating room

With these caveats in mind, a simple (albeit imprecise) method is to use weight-based estimates of calorie requirements. In the ICU, the recommended range for calorie intake is 20–40 kcal/kg/day, with 1.5–2 g/kg/day of protein. Obesity requires a special consideration: for BMI 30–50, the recommended calorie intake is 11–14 kcal/kg/day *actual* body weight, while for BMI > 50, the recommended intake is 22–25 kcal/kg/day *ideal* body weight [10]. These estimates must be adjusted upward for "high-risk" patients (those who are elderly, have severe injury, or significant traumatic brain injury [TBI], are previously malnourished, or have a NUTRIC score ≥5).

18.5 Enteral Nutrition (EN)

EN therapy is the preferred primary nutrition therapy and has several advantages over parenteral nutrition (PN) therapy. Multiple trials and meta-analyses have demonstrated that relative to PN, EN reduces overall complications, infections, cost, and LOS [1, 10].

However, known risks of EN include gut ischemia, vomiting, and aspiration pneumonia. The critical-care surgeon should always be aware of the potential for gut ischemia and necrosis with EN therapy and must consider this in the setting of distension, diarrhea, or acidosis. Basic essential practices that lower the risks for aspiration pneumonia include head of bed elevation, oropharyngeal decontamination, and continuous rather than bolus feeding. Monitoring gastric residual volumes may not be clinically meaningful; about 20 % of patients with "low" residual volumes (<150 cc) still have aspiration events and those with high residual volumes (up to 300 cc) do not appear to have any higher aspiration risk [21–23].

Contraindications to EN therapy are few and include gastrointestinal discontinuity and hemodynamic instability. EN in a patient with persistent hypotension and/or vasopressor use increases the risk for bowel ischemia in the setting of an already compromised intestinal microcirculation. Relative contraindications for EN include irritable bowel disease (IBD) acute flares, enteric fistulae, and gastrointestinal bleeding.

Diarrhea is a common problem facing the ICU patient on EN, and should not automatically lead to cessation of feeds. Generally, if the patient has >300 mL/day or >4 loose stools/day, a *Clostridium difficile* toxin assay should be sent, and other infectious sources should be considered. Once infection is ruled out, adding 10–20 g soluble fiber and/or switching to elemental formula may help decrease diarrhea [17]. If the problem persists, consider use of supplemental PN (see next section).

There are some special circumstances related to feeding route. Postpyloric feeding tubes should be considered if the patient has (a) signs of gastric intolerance, (b) high aspiration risk, or (c) injury to the esophagus, stomach, or duodenum. Placement of postpyloric tubes in pancreatitis has recently been called into question and is no longer clinically indicated [10]. Surgical feeding tubes are associated with a decreased risk for aspiration relative to nasogastric or orogastric tubes [23] and should be considered in patients anticipated to require EN beyond 14 days.

Recommendations continue to evolve regarding timing for EN calorie delivery. Early enteral nutrition, given in the first 24–48 h of ICU admission, has consistently been associated with reduced infections and mortality in several observational cohorts [10, 24]. However, most of these studies are subject to residual confounding by indication (patients who are less ill tend to be successfully fed earlier). Adequately powered randomized trials are needed to more definitively address the issue of timing.

Optimal calorie goals are an ongoing controversy in nutrition science. Recent literature indicates that trophic feeds ("trickle feeds" at a rate of 10–20 ml/h) may be equivalent to full goal calorie feeds [25], and in some cases, achieving 100% of the daily calorie goal may actually increase infection rates, days of mechanical ventilation, and LOS, when compared to trophic feeding [26, 27]. Practically speaking, trophic feeding or hypo-caloric feeding is a reasonable strategy for low-risk patients in the first 7 days of ICU stay, but high-risk patients (e.g., a NUTRIC score ≥ 5) should probably still reach ≥80% goal calorie and protein intake as quickly as possible [10]. Strategies to minimize "nil-per-os" periods should be employed, including allowing some intubated patients to continue EN up until the time of transfer to the operating room, or continued through select operations [9].

18.6   Parenteral Nutrition (PN)

PN should be initiated only after a trial of all enteral routes. EN is generally preferred over PN because several randomized con-trolled studies have demonstrated that PN decreases immune function, increases the risk of infections, and prolongs hospital LOS, when compared to EN [10, 14]. PN use has generally declined over the past decade due to a growing recognition of its associated morbidity [28]. Some subpopulations of patients may still benefit from PN therapy, but these patients are often the most metabolically and medically complex. For this reason, a multidisciplinary nutrition support team with dietitian support provides essential assistance in these nuanced and difficult treat-ment decisions [19, 29].

PN should be considered in patients with absolute or relative contraindications for EN, or for those who are EN "intolerant." For "low-risk" patients (NUTRIC score <5) who are unable to achieve goal calories via an enteral route, trophic feeding should continue *without* attempting to "supplement" calorie intake with PN. In the "low-risk" enteral-intolerant patient, good quality evidence indicates that starting supplemental PN prior to hospital day 7 is associated with prolonged length of stay, increased days of mechanical ventilation, and increased infections [30, 31]. However, starting PN before day 7 may benefit "high-risk" (NUTRIC score >5/preexisting malnutrition) enteral-intolerant patients. PN should also be considered for patients who continue to fail in enteral therapy beyond 7 days [32].

For those patients who have a contraindication to any early enteral intake (including tropic feeding), PN therapy may have some benefit. In this population, PN therapy appears to cause no additional morbidity or infections, and may even improve lean body mass and total vent free days [33]. These findings are particularly relevant for surgical patients, since many perioperative patients have contraindications to enteral intake. A summary of an evidence-based approach to EN and PN is given in Table 18.2.

Of note, PN (either exclusive or supplemental) is contraindicated in patients who are in the acute phases of sepsis or septic shock. Available observational studies indicate that PN in this context increases mortality [10].

18.7   Immunonutrition

Immunonutrition is defined by the administration of enteral formulas, which reduce oxidation and inflammation and improve immune function. Therapy with vitamins, antioxidants, and other pharmaconutrients has the potential to decrease complications and increase survival, particularly for surgical patients [34].

Certain subpopulations of patients with systemic inflammation have proven benefits from immunonutrition. In particular, therapy with antioxidants and vitamins (vitamin C, E, zinc, and selenium) appears to decrease rates of multiple organ failure, days of mechanical ventilation, and ICU LOS in patients with

Table 18.2 Evidence-based priorities for enteral nutrition (EN) and parenteral nutrition (PN) in the first 7 days of intensive care unit stay

---

Start EN within 24–48 h. Titrate to goal calorie intake

If *unable* to achieve goal enteral calorie intake:

    In "low risk"[a] patient: maintain trophic feeds up to 7 days *without* supplemental PN

    In "high risk"[a] patient: consider starting supplemental PN within 48 h

If contraindication[b] to *all* enteral intake anticipated beyond 72 h, start early PN

---

[a]High risk = preexisting malnutrition, advanced age, multiple comorbidities, and/or frailty. "Nutrition Risk in Critically ill" (NUTRIC) score ≥5 also indicates high risk

[b]Special populations with EN contraindications who may be recommended for PN therapy:

    1. Malnourished patients prior to a scheduled operation

    2. Patients with acute "flare" of irritable bowel disease, bowel discontinuity, or high-output enterocutaneous fistulas

    3. Patients with short gut physiology, as a bridge to definitive therapy

burns >30 % and multisystem trauma [35]. In addition, formulations containing arginine and omega-3 fatty acids are thought to reverse T-cell suppression and decrease inflammation. These nutrients likely decrease infections and improve recovery time for patients with traumatic brain injury and for perioperative patients [10, 36, 37]. Finally, glutamine has been shown to increase expression of HLA-DR on monocytes and to improve phagocytosis. However, the literature on glutamine does not demonstrate consistent benefits for ultimate outcomes in critically ill patients [38], and some studies have actually shown harm [39].

The literature on immunonutrition is limited by lack of dosing standards, varying study quality, heterogeneous populations of interest, mixed interventions, and inconsistently defined outcomes. For all these reasons, immunonutrition continues to be an evolving field in need of more rigorous standards and higher-quality research.

18.8   Conclusion

A targeted and systematic approach to nutrition therapy is essential to improve outcomes in septic and surgical patients. This population is particularly vulnerable to the effects of catabolism, mounting energy debt, prolonged starvation, and malnutrition. Available tools to evaluate "nutrition status" and calculate calorie needs are limited, and research into novel methods is needed. Early enteral nutrition is the preferred therapy in the ICU, while indications for parenteral nutrition are becoming more limited. Ongoing research is needed to evaluate the role for immunonutrition in critically ill septic and surgical patients.

References

1. McClave SA, Martindale RG, Vanek VW, et al. Guidelines for the provision and assessment of nutrition support therapy in the adult critically Ill patient: Society of Critical Care Medicine (SCCM) and American Society for Parenteral and Enteral Nutrition (A.S.P.E.N.). JPEN J Parenter Enteral Nutr. 2009;33(3):277–316.
2. Binnekade JM, Tepaske R, Bruynzeel P. Daily enteral feeding practice on the ICU: attainment of goals and interfering factors. Crit Care (London, England). 2005;9(3):R218–25.
3. Reid C. Frequency of under- and overfeeding in mechanically ventilated ICU patients: causes and possible consequences. J Hum Nutr Diet Off J Br Diet Assoc. 2006;19(1):13–22.
4. Giner M, Laviano A, Meguid MM, Gleason JR. In 1995 a correlation between malnutrition and poor outcome in critically ill patients still exists. Nutrition. 1996;12(1):23–9.
5. Keel M, Trentz O. Pathophysiology of polytrauma. Injury. 2005;36(6):691–709.
6. Plank LD, Hill GL. Sequential metabolic changes following induction of systemic inflammatory response in patients with severe sepsis or major blunt trauma. World J Surg. 2000;24(6):630–8.

7. Heyland DK, Murch L, Cahill N, et al. Enhanced protein-energy provision via the enteral route feeding protocol in critically ill patients: results of a cluster randomized trial. Crit Care Med. 2013;41(12):2743–53.

8. Chung CK, Whitney R, Thompson CM, Pham TN, Maier RV, O'Keefe GE. Experience with an enteral-based nutritional support regimen in critically ill trauma patients. J Am Coll Surg. 2013;217(6):1108–17.

9. Parent B, Mandell S, Maier R, Minei J, Sperry J, Moore E, O'Keefe G. Safety of Minimizing Pre-operative Starvation in Critically-ill and Intubated Trauma Patients. J Trauma Acute Care Surg. 2016;80(6):957–63.

10. McClave SA, Taylor BE, Martindale RG, et al. Guidelines for the provision and assessment of nutrition support therapy in the adult critically Ill patient: Society of Critical Care Medicine (SCCM) and American Society for Parenteral and Enteral Nutrition (A.S.P.E.N.). JPEN J Parenter Enteral Nutr. 2016;40(2):159–211.

11. Huynh D, Chapman MJ, Nguyen NQ. Nutrition support in the critically ill. Curr Opin Gastroenterol. 2013;29(2):208–15.

12. Grune T, Berger MM. Markers of oxidative stress in ICU clinical settings: present and future. Curr Opin Clin Nutr Metab Care. 2007;10(6):712–7.

13. Motoyama T, Okamoto K, Kukita I, Hamaguchi M, Kinoshita Y, Ogawa H. Possible role of increased oxidant stress in multiple organ failure after systemic inflammatory response syndrome. Crit Care Med. 2003;31(4):1048–52.

14. Marik PE, Zaloga GP. Meta-analysis of parenteral nutrition versus enteral nutrition in patients with acute pancreatitis. BMJ (Clinical research ed). 2004;328(7453):1407.

15. McClave SA, Heyland DK. The physiologic response and associated clinical benefits from provision of early enteral nutrition. Nutr Clin Pract Off Publ Am Soc Parenter Enter Nutr. 2009;24(3):305–15.

16. Rahman A, Hasan RM, Agarwala R, Martin C, Day AG, Heyland DK. Identifying critically-ill patients who will benefit most from nutritional therapy: Further validation of the "modified NUTRIC" nutritional risk assessment tool. Clin Nutr (Edinburgh, Scotland). 2016;35(1):158–62.

17. Doig GS, Simpson F, Finfer S, et al. Effect of evidence-based feeding guidelines on mortality of critically ill adults: a cluster randomized controlled trial. JAMA. 2008;300(23):2731–41.

18. Jain MK, Heyland D, Dhaliwal R, et al. Dissemination of the Canadian clinical practice guidelines for nutrition support: results of a cluster randomized controlled trial. Crit Care Med. 2006;34(9):2362–9.

19. Parent B, Shelton M, Nordlund M, Aarabi S, O'Keefe G. Parenteral nutrition utilization after implementation of multidisciplinary nutrition support team oversight: a prospective cohort study. JPEN J Parenter Enteral Nutr. 2015.

20. Ferrie S, Allman-Farinelli M. Commonly used "nutrition" indicators do not predict outcome in the critically ill: a systematic review. Nutr Clin Pract Off Publ Am Soc Parenter Enter Nutr. 2013;28(4):463–84.

21. Elke G, Felbinger TW, Heyland DK. Gastric residual volume in critically ill patients: a dead marker or still alive? Nutr Clin Pract Off Publ Am Soc Parenter Enter Nutr. 2015;30(1):59–71.

22. Reignier J, Mercier E, Le Gouge A, et al. Effect of not monitoring residual gastric volume on risk of ventilator-associated pneumonia in adults receiving mechanical ventilation and early enteral feeding: a randomized controlled trial. JAMA. 2013;309(3):249–56.

23. McClave SA, Lukan JK, Stefater JA, et al. Poor validity of residual volumes as a marker for risk of aspiration in critically ill patients. Crit Care Med. 2005;33(2):324–30.

24. Artinian V, Krayem H, DiGiovine B. Effects of early enteral feeding on the outcome of critically ill mechanically ventilated medical patients. Chest. 2006;129(4):960–7.

25. Rice TW, Mogan S, Hays MA, Bernard GR, Jensen GL, Wheeler AP. Randomized trial of initial trophic versus full-energy enteral nutrition in mechanically ventilated patients with acute respiratory failure. Crit Care Med. 2011;39(5):967–74.

26. Arabi YM, Haddad SH, Tamim HM, et al. Near-target caloric intake in critically ill medical-surgical patients is associated with adverse outcomes. JPEN J Parenter Enteral Nutr. 2010;34(3):280–8.

27. Singer P, Anbar R, Cohen J, et al. The tight calorie control study (TICACOS): a prospective, randomized, controlled pilot study of nutritional support in critically ill patients. Intensive Care Med. 2011;37(4):601–9.

28. Rhee P, Hadjizacharia P, Trankiem C, et al. What happened to total parenteral nutrition? The disappearance of its use in a trauma intensive care unit. J Trauma. 2007;63(6):1215–22.

29. Trujillo EB, Young LS, Chertow GM, et al. Metabolic and monetary costs of avoidable parenteral nutrition use. JPEN J Parenter Enteral Nutr. 1999;23(2):109–13.

30. Casaer MP, Mesotten D, Hermans G, et al. Early versus late parenteral nutrition in critically ill adults. N Engl J Med. 2011;365(6):506–17.

31. Dissanaike S, Shelton M, Warner K, O'Keefe GE. The risk for bloodstream infections is associated with increased parenteral caloric intake

in patients receiving parenteral nutrition. Crit Care (London, England). 2007;11(5):R114.

32. Singer P, Pichard C. Reconciling divergent results of the latest parenteral nutrition studies in the ICU. Curr Opin Clin Nutr Metab Care. 2013;16(2):187–93.

33. Doig GS, Simpson F, Sweetman EA, et al. Early parenteral nutrition in critically ill patients with short-term relative contraindications to early enteral nutrition: a randomized controlled trial. JAMA. 2013;309(20):2130–8.

34. Torgersen Z, Balters M. Perioperative nutrition. Surg Clin North Am. 2015;95(2):255–67.

35. Nathens AB, Neff MJ, Jurkovich GJ, et al. Randomized, prospective trial of antioxidant supplementation in critically ill surgical patients. Ann Surg. 2002;236(6):814–22.

36. Drover JW, Dhaliwal R, Weitzel L, Wischmeyer PE, Ochoa JB, Heyland DK. Perioperative use of arginine-supplemented diets: a systematic review of the evidence. J Am Coll Surg. 2011;212(3):385–99, 399.e381.

37. Barker LA, Gray C, Wilson L, Thomson BN, Shedda S, Crowe TC. Preoperative immunonutrition and its effect on postoperative outcomes in well-nourished and malnourished gastrointestinal surgery patients: a randomised controlled trial. Eur J Clin Nutr. 2013;67(8):802–7.

38. Tan HB, Danilla S, Murray A, et al. Immunonutrition as an adjuvant therapy for burns. Cochrane Database Syst Rev. 2014;(12):CD007174.

39. Heyland D, Muscedere J, Wischmeyer PE, et al. A randomized trial of glutamine and antioxidants in critically ill patients. N Engl J Med. 2013;368(16):1489–97.

Chapter 19
Point-of-Care Ultrasound in Critically Ill Patients

Fikri M. Abu-Zidan and Ashraf F. Hefny

19.1   Introduction

The use of point-of-care (POC) ultrasound has dramatically expanded during the last two decades. Using bedside ultrasound by non-radiologists as a critical decision-making tool in the management of life-threatening conditions proved to be very useful. More acute care physicians are currently eager to learn and practice POC ultrasound.

POC ultrasound is a non-invasive, quick, and accurate bedside diagnostic tool that can be performed even on unstable patients. It can be done repeatedly without the risk of radiation. Furthermore, it is less expensive than CT scanning and MRI. We will try in this concise book chapter to give a general overview

F.M. Abu-Zidan, MD, FACS, FRCS, PhD (✉)
Department of Surgery, College of Medicine and Health Sciences, UAE University, PO Box 17666, Al-Ain, UAE
e-mail: fabuzidan@uaeu.ac.ae

A.F. Hefny, MS, MRCS, FACS
Department of Surgery, Al Rahba Hospital, Abu Dhabi, UAE

© Springer International Publishing Switzerland 2017   335
S. Di Saverio et al. (eds.), *Acute Care Surgery Handbook*,
DOI 10.1007/978-3-319-15341-4_19

on the common uses of diagnostic POC ultrasound in critically ill patients that can be performed bedside by non-radiologists.

19.2   Basic Physics

It is essential to understand the basic physics of ultrasound in order to make accurate bedside critical decisions using POC ultrasound. Ultrasound machines generate and receive ultrasound waves. These waves have high frequencies (2–15 MHz) [1, 2]. The brightness mode (B mode) is the most common used ultrasound mode [2]. This mode produces two-dimensional (2D) black and white images having a thickness of 1 mm slices.

Ultrasound waves pass through different body tissues having different densities (ranging from fluid to solid material). Reflection of ultrasound waves will depend on the tissue density. Wave reflection will create an ultrasound image [3]. The denser the tissue, the whiter it is on the image. In general, fluid will be black (anechoic), soft tissue will be grey, fibrous tissue will be white without a shadow, while bones and stones will be white with a shadow (Fig. 19.1) [4]. Air is a strong ultrasound reflector. It gives a very shiny white (hyperechoic image) image which is difficult to see behind [5].

There are different ways in which an ultrasound image can be modified including the frequency of the wave, the size and shape of the ultrasound probe, and the timing in which the waves are emitted [6, 7]. Abdominal examination in obese adults and deeper structures needs lower frequency probes (2–5 MHz) having deep penetration. In contrast, probes of high frequency (10–12 MHz) have better resolution and less depth of penetration. They should be used for superficial structures [2]. Ultrasound waves are generated perpendicular to the surface of the probe. Bending the surface of the probe will widen its field and reduce its resolution at depth (convex array transducers). Flat probes will give a rectangular image with good resolution

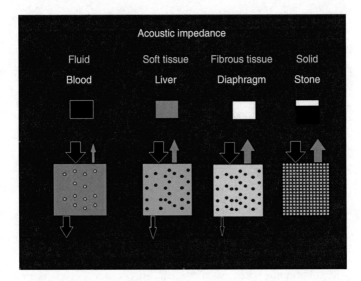

Fig. 19.1 The denser the material is the more it reflects the sonographic waves. Fluid (like *blood*) transmits ultrasound waves and have minimum waves reflected back. This yields a black "anechogenic" image. Soft tissues (like the *liver*) yield different grey colour scales. Fibrous tissue will be white without a shadow (like the *diaphragm*). Stones yield white images (hyperechoic) with a shadow behind them (Reproduced with permission from Abu-Zidan et al. [7])

in the whole image (linear array transducers). Small print ultrasound probes are needed for imaging thoracic structures using the sonographic windows between the ribs [8].

19.3   Detection of Intra-peritoneal and Chest Fluid

Ultrasound is very sensitive in detecting fluid in the peritoneum and pleura [9]. Detection of intra-peritoneal and pleural fluid is a simple skill that can be easily learnt by surgeons, or emergency physicians, if they were properly trained [10, 11]. Fresh blood is generally hypoechoic on ultrasound. Nevertheless, clotted blood will be echogenic and can be missed. Ultrasonography cannot differentiate between different types of fluid including blood, urine, bile, lymph, transudate, or exudate [12]. The nature of the fluid can be known if correlated with the clinical picture or if tapped. Intra-peritoneal fluid in a hypotensive patient is most probably blood.

Currently, ultrasonography is the modality of choice in detection of haemoperitoneum in blunt trauma patients (Fig. 19.2). Ultrasound has replaced the diagnostic peritoneal lavage in the majority of patients. Performing a secondary ultrasound examination, even in stable patients, increases the sensitivity of ultrasound in detecting intra-peritoneal free fluid [13].

Intra-peritoneal fluid is likely to collect in the most dependent areas. These include hepatorenal space (Morison's pouch), left subphrenic space or splenorenal recess, and pelvis (retro-uterine pouch or retrovesical pouch) [14, 15]. The site where maximum fluid is collected depends on the position of the patient. Fluid will accumulate in the hypochondria in the Trendelenburg position while it will accumulate in the pelvis in the anti-Trendelenburg position. We usually examine the patient in the horizontal position because that is required for measuring the IVC diameter during resuscitation. Fluid in the pericardial sac can be detected in the subxiphoid or parasternal views while pleural fluid can be detected in the coronal sonographic view of the hypochondria [16].

19.4   Echocardiography

Echocardiography is a very useful diagnostic modality in life-threatening conditions. It can also guide interventional procedures like aspiration of the pericardial effusion. We usually use a small

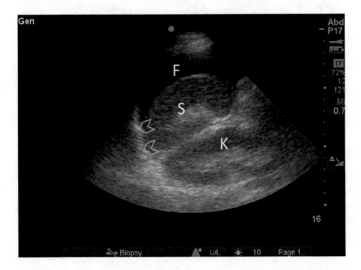

Fig. 19.2 A 36-year-old front seat male passenger, who was not wearing a seatbelt, was involved with a front impact collision and was ejected through the front wind screen. He was haemodynamically stable but had tenderness and guarding all over the abdomen. Surgeon-performed POC ultrasound of the abdomen showed free intra-peritoneal fluid (*F*) between the spleen (*S*) and diaphragm (*arrowheads*). The patient had a laparotomy. He had extensive mesenteric tears with small bowel and sigmoid colon injuries without solid organ injuries (Sonographic study was performed by Professor Fikri Abu-Zidan, Department of Surgery, Al-Ain Hospital, Al-Ain, UAE)

print probe having 2–5 MHz. We start always by the subxiphoid and four-chamber apical views [17, 18]. These are usually enough to get the information needed in the acute care setting to make critical decisions. Severe obesity, distended stomach, sub-cutaneous emphysema, lung inflation due to chronic obstructive airway disease, or chest deformity may limit the access to these windows. Long parasternal and short parasternal views are used when other windows are difficult to obtain.

As acute care surgeons, we always keep the marker of the probe to the right (contrary to cardiologist who keep it to the left). This is important because echocardiography will be performed as an extension of the abdominal examination especially in shocked patients. The setting of the machine will not be changed, and the right ventricle will be on the right side of the screen. The subxiphoid four-chamber view can be obtained by placing the probe left to xiphoid process with the beam directed towards the left shoulder. The apical four-chamber view can be obtained by placing the probe on the heart apex beat (fifth intercostal space at midclavicular line). The beam should be directed towards the right shoulder [17, 18].

In focused echocardiography, simple questions are usually answered. These include: (1) Are the heart ventricles contracting properly? (2) Is there pericardial fluid? (3) What is the volume of each ventricle: Is it enlarged, normal, or reduced in volume. The answers to these simple questions can lead to very important information.

The subxiphoid view is the best to diagnose pericardial effusion around the right ventricle and the right atrium as it shows a hypoechoic area between the liver and the heart [19] (Fig. 19.3). Pericardial effusion on the left side of the heart is easier to differentiate on long parasternal view as it will show as a hypoechoic area anterior to the aorta compared to pleural effusion which will be behind the aorta. The pressure of the pericardial fluid on the heart causes a tamponade effect. Compression of the right ventricle is easier to observe during early diastole while compression of the right atrium is easier to observe during late diastole. IVC diameter will increase and will lose the inspiratory collapse. Occasionally, you may see a thrombus in the ventricle or atrium.

Massive pulmonary embolism will increase the resistance to the flow from the right ventricle. The volume of the right ventricle will be enlarged and the interventricular septum will be

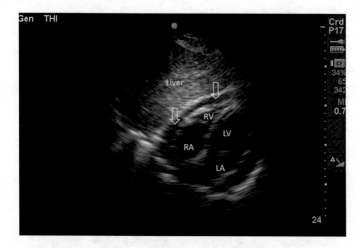

Fig. 19.3 A 36-year-old male driver who was involved with a front impact road traffic collision. He had chest trauma treated by bilateral chest tubes in another hospital, then transferred to our hospital 2 weeks later. He was haemodynamically stable. POC ultrasound of the heart using a subxiphoid approach showed moderate amount of pericardiac fluid (*arrows*) not affecting the function of the heart. The patient was treated conservatively. *RA* right atrium, *RV* right ventricle, *LV* left ventricle, *LA* left atrium (Sonographic study was performed by Professor Fikri Abu-Zidan, Department of Surgery, Al-Ain Hospital, Al-Ain, UAE)

pushed towards the left ventricle [19] (Fig. 19.4). This changes the shape of the right ventricle in the short axis view from a C shape to a D shape. In severe sepsis without hypovolemia, the volume of both ventricles will be dilated and their contractility will be reduced due to the cardiac inhibition caused by endotoxins. In severe bleeding or hypovolemia, the heart will be tachycardic and the ventricles will be empty [18]. Echocardiography is very useful during resuscitation as it can accurately diagnose the pulseless electrical activity when there is no contractility of the heart.

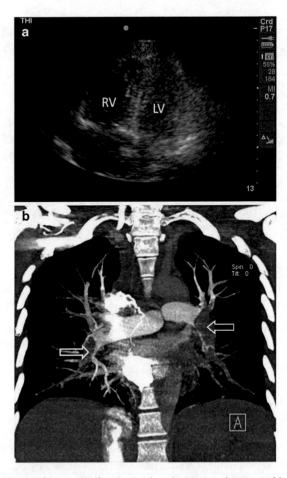

Fig. 19.4 A 35-year-old female developed syncope, shortness of breath, and shock following a 9 h air flight. POC ultrasound shows a dilated right ventricle (*RV*), which was larger than the left ventricle (*LV*). The RV was not properly contracting (**a**). CT angio showed the presence of massive bilateral pulmonary embolism (*arrows*) (**b**) (Sonographic study was performed by Professor Fikri Abu-Zidan, Department of Surgery, Al-Ain Hospital, Al-Ain, UAE)

19.5 Measuring IVC Diameter

The value of measuring the IVC diameter in shocked patients is debatable [20, 21]. We advocate imaging the IVC directly between the ribs at the right midclavicular line at the lower chest wall so as to locate the IVC in its longitudinal section. For this we use a small print convex array probe having a frequency of 3–5 MHz. We use the longitudinal B mode to evaluate the gross collapsibility of the IVC while we use the M mode to calculate the percentage of changes in IVC diameter both longitudinally and transversely [22].

The technique to measure the IVC should be standardized. The ultrasound beam should be vertical to the IVC section. Common pitfalls encountered in measuring the IVC diameter include sectioning the IVC peripherally or obliquely (Fig. 19.5). We found that relative visual changes of the IVC are more useful than absolute calculated numbers. Combining these two approaches will increase the value of IVC measurement in evaluating shocked patients. If the operator defines the area in which he repeatedly measures the IVC for a specific patient, then the results will be more reliable.

Common pitfalls that falsely increase the IVC diameter include increased right atrial pressure during artificial ventilation, severe sepsis without hypovolemia causing increased resistance of the pulmonary circulation (Fig. 19.6), or by pulmonary embolism [23]. In contrast, increased intra-abdominal pressure in abdominal compartment syndrome will cause direct pressure on the IVC and give false small IVC diameter [24]. The measurement of IVC diameter should be correlated with the findings of echocardiography and the clinical picture as a whole.

19.6 Lung Ultrasound

Understanding the reverberation artefact is central for the interpretation of lung ultrasound [6, 7]. This artefact is the normal

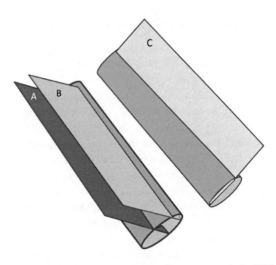

Fig. 19.5 A figure demonstrating the technique to measure the IVC diameter longitudinally. The ultrasound cross section should be vertical to the IVC (*A*). Common pitfalls in measurement include measuring the IVC peripherally (*B*) or obliquely (*C*) (Reproduced with permission from Abu-Zidan [22])

pattern of the lung. Both visceral and peripheral pleura are fibrous tissue that are white in colour. Since they are moving during inspiration, pleural sliding will be clearly demonstrated. The pleura are strong ultrasound reflectors. When ultrasound is emitted from the ultrasound probe, it will be reflected from the pleura. Nevertheless, some waves repeatedly bounce between the ultrasound probe and the pleura [6, 7]. As the reflected waves are gradually picked up by the ultrasound probe, the bouncing waves become gradually less. The ultrasound machine receives these waves as parallel white horizontal lines with gradual decrease in density and equal distance between them. These are called A lines (Fig. 19.7).

Abolished lung sliding and A lines can been seen in any lung that does not move [25]. This can be possibly a pneumothorax or

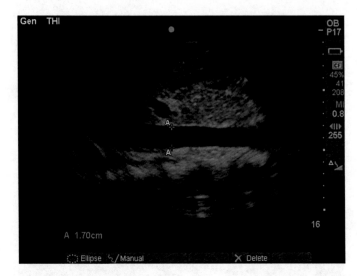

Fig. 19.6 A 30-year-old 10 weeks pregnant women presented with fever, abdominal pain, and vaginal discharge of 7 days duration. When seen in the ICU, she was ventilated, having a blood pressure of 50/30 mmHg and a pulse of 130 bpm. Her abdomen was distended. POC ultrasound showed an intrauterine dead fetus and minimal intra-peritoneal fluid. Both cardiac ventricles were dilated and weakly contracting. The IVC was grossly dilated (1.7 cm) which ruled out hypovolemia. The POC ultrasound were highly suggestive of septic shock caused by infected abortion. The uterus was evacuated from its contents under general anaesthesia. The patient survived and went home in good condition (Sonographic study was performed by Professor Fikri Abu-Zidan, Department of Surgery, Al-Ain Hospital, Al-Ain, UAE)

alternatively a lung collapse caused by a plug or contralateral tracheal intubation. Presence of lung sliding rules out pneumothorax [25]. Nevertheless, ultrasound will only inform us that the lung is not moving and this should be correlated with the clinical picture to know the cause. The only accepted pathognomonic sign for a pneumothorax is the presence of the *lung point* (the dynamic change of the edge of the lung sliding) [25].

The air in the lung is very reflective and does not permit ultrasound waves to be transmitted. Nevertheless, when there are some alveoli with scattered fluid in the alveolus or around it, then shiny vertical lines that pass through the whole ultrasound image are present. These are called B lines [25]. Any fluid may cause these lines including pulmonary oedema, pneumonia, aspiration, or lung contusion. The number of B lines and extent involved in the chest area will reflect the severity of the pathology. The B lines represent white areas on the chest X-ray. Accordingly, both lungs can be mapped by ultrasound (Fig. 19.8). Complete collapse of the lung will be clearly seen on ultrasound similar to a liver tissue because there is no or little air in the alveoli.

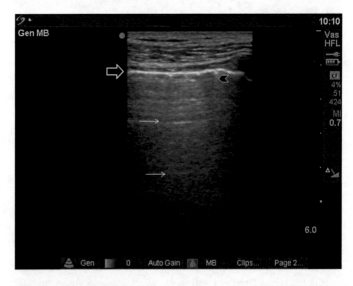

Fig. 19.7 Reverberation artefact of the lung occurs as ultrasound waves bounce between the transducer and the pleura. The pleura is shown as a hyperdense white line (*black arrow*). The reverberation lines (*white arrows*) represent repetition of the pleural line. The distance between these lines are equal. A comet tail artefact is also shown (*black arrowhead*) (Reproduced with permission from Abu-Zidan et al. [7])

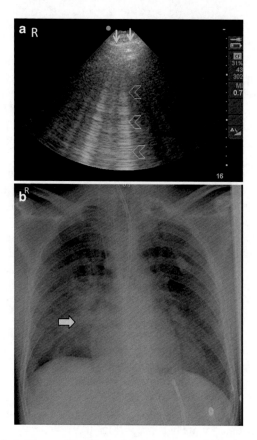

Fig. 19.8 A 26-year-old man who fell from 3 m high. He sustained open fracture of the left tibia and spine fracture. He suddenly developed hypoxia in the ward without a clear cause and was transferred to the ICU. Pulmonary embolism was suspected. POC ultrasound of the right lung using a portable ultrasound machine and a small print convex array probe with a frequency of 3–5 MHz demonstrated extensive B lines in the right lung (*arrowheads*) indicating the source of hypoxia (**a**). Chest X-ray confirmed the findings (*yellow arrow*) (**b**). The patient was successfully treated for aspiration of the right lung

19.7 Scanning the Aorta

The aorta should be surveyed by ultrasound in any patient having unexplained shock. Sonography is recommended as an accurate diagnostic test in that situation [26]. Abdominal probe having a frequency of 2.5–3.5 MHz is used [26, 27]. The aorta is located to the left of the midline. The aorta will be pulsatile and the coeliac axis and superior mesenteric arteries will be seen stemming from the aorta anteriorly in the longitudinal section. Turn the probe 90° with the marker pointing to the right and see the transverse section of the aorta. Scan the aorta starting from the epigastrium and follow it distally till the bifurcation where the two common iliac arteries are seen.

The outer diameter should be included in the measurement. A diameter larger than 3 cm or more than 1.5 times of the proximal uninvolved diameter of the aorta should be considered abnormal [26, 28]. A thrombus may be seen within the aortic lumen. Flow or Colour Doppler can be used to study the flow within the aneurysm. Finding free intra-peritoneal fluid is very serious as it may indicate a ruptured aortic aneurysm. It may be difficult to visualize the abdominal aorta from the anterior abdominal approach because of presence of gas or obesity. Gentle compression may be needed to move the bowel gas away from the view. Try to visualize the aorta from the left lateral side through the retroperitonium if you encounter difficulty while using the anterior approach [27] (Fig. 19.9).

19.8 Diagnosis of Deep Vein Thrombosis

Ultrasound is a sensitive and specific tool for the assessment of patients suspected to have lower limb deep vein thrombosis (DVT) [29]. A fresh clot may appear anechoic and difficult to be recognized by visual inspection resulting in a false negative study

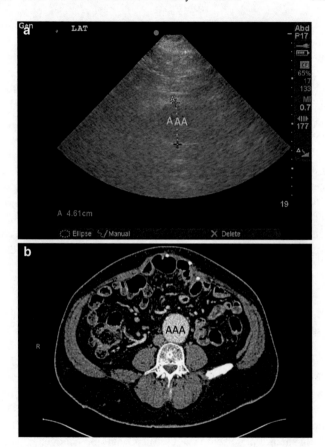

Fig. 19.9 A 65-year-old obese male presented to the Emergency Department complaining of a painful upper abdominal incisional hernia. The hernia was reducible. A pulsatile mass was felt above the umbilicus. Scanning of the aorta by a portable ultrasound machine using a small print convex array probe with a frequency of 3–5 MHz and a lateral abdominal approach demonstrated an abdominal aortic aneurysm (*AAA*) having a diameter of 4.61 cm (**a**). CT with intravenous contrast has confirmed the diagnosis (**b**) (Sonographic study was performed by Professor Fikri Abu-Zidan, Department of Surgery, Al-Ain Hospital, Al-Ain, UAE)

[30]. Compression ultrasonography at two points (common femoral vein and popliteal vein) is a simple, accurate, and commonly used first choice imaging modality in suspected DVT [29].

A high-frequency linear array probe gives better results. We usually perform the study bedside in the ICU while the patient is in the supine position. We need to flex the knee to be able to examine the popliteal vein from the back of the knee. The probe should be perpendicular to the skin surface in a transverse position. Apply firm compression to achieve complete collapse of the vein. The common femoral artery and vein should be identified at the groin slightly below the inguinal ligament. The vein is the most medial structure followed by the artery and then femoral nerve. The femoral nerve bundles will show as hyperechoic small structures packed together. The artery is pulsatile and non-compressible compared with the vein. You can use the colour Doppler if in doubt as the colour of the femoral vein and artery will be different (blue or red). The colour depends on the direction of the blood flow (with or against the probe). So both the artery and vein may be red or blue depending on the direction of the flow. At the popliteal fossa, the veins lie superficial to the artery and are compressible.

Exclusion of venous clot by complete compressibility of the vein with downward pressure of the ultrasound probe is the main sonographic finding. Compared with the artery, the vein is easily compressed under external force. However, if its lumen was obstructed by a thrombus, probe pressure will fail to compress the vein (Fig. 19.10). Incomplete or partial compressibility is considered abnormal. The clot itself may be echogenic. The older and more chronic the clot is, the more visible it will be on ultrasound [31].

19.9   The RUSH Protocol

The value of POC ultrasound in the diagnosis and management of shocked patients using specific protocols is well-established.

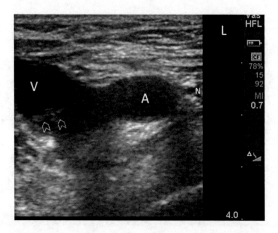

Fig. 19.10 An 83-year-old oncological patient suddenly developed unexplained shock. Compression ultrasound test of the left groin by a portable ultrasound machine using a linear probe with a frequency of 10–12 MHz showed non-compressible femoral vein (*V*) with a deep vein thrombus (*arrowheads*). *A* femoral artery, *N* femoral nerve. The patient was directly started on anticoagulation therapy (Sonographic study was performed by Professor Fikri Abu-Zidan, Department of Surgery, Al-Ain Hospital, Al-Ain, UAE)

This includes a focused study to look for fluid in the pericardium, pleural, and peritoneal cavities, measuring the IVC diameter, and evaluating the heart contractility. Our group follows the Rapid Ultrasound in Shock (RUSH) protocol which examines the pump (heart), tubes (great vessels), and reservoir (free intraperitoneal or intra-thoracic fluid) [32]. The simple logic of this protocol is that if you have no water at home, then either there is no fluid in the reservoir (loss of blood, plasma, or fluid), there is a problem with the electrical pump (myocardiac infarction, pericardiac tamponade, pulmonary embolism, or tension pneumothorax), or there is a problem in the tubes (aortic aneurysm or DVT) (Fig. 19.11). There is another clinical possibility which is that the tubes dilate or do not constrict (spinal shock, anaphylactic shock, or adrenal crisis). We found that this thinking

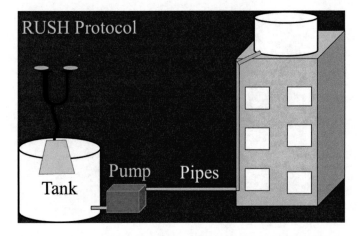

Fig. 19.11 The Rapid Ultrasound in Shock (*RUSH*) protocol examines the reservoir, pump, and the tubes. if there is no water at home, then either there is no fluid in the reservoir (loss of blood, plasma, or fluid), there is a problem with the electrical pump (myocardiac infarction, pericardiac tamponade, pulmonary embolism, or tension pneumothorax), or there is a problem in the tubes (aortic aneurysm or DVT) (Drawn by Professor Fikri Abu-Zidan, Department of Surgery, College of Medicine and Health Sciences, UAE University, Al-Ain, UAE)

approach is very logical and gives us an organised plan to follow. Actually, the RUSH protocol includes the Extended FAST (EFAST) exam. EFAST consists of examining eight sonographic points (8 p's) to detect fluid in the *P*eri-hepatic, *P*eri-splenic, *P*elvic, *P*eri-cardiac, right *P*leural recess, and left *P*leura recess areas, and to detect right *P*neumothroax and left *P*neumothorax [10, 33].

19.10   Free Intra-peritoneal Air

POC ultrasound examination is of great help to diagnose intra-peritoneal free air (IFA) [34, 35]. Even small amounts of IFA can be detected by ultrasound [36, 37]. The sonographic appearance of IFA results from scattering of the ultrasound waves at the interface of soft tissue and air. This results in increased echogenicity of a peritoneal stripe accompanied by reverberation echoes that hide the moving bowels behind it [38, 39]. This image can be changed by changing the patient's position. Reverberation may not be seen in small air collections. When a large volume of IFA is present, it may obscure the underlying abdominal organs [37]. We use the linear transducer in detecting IFA because it has a high resolution in the near field where air accumulates [37]. We usually examine the patient in supine position. We look for air behind the linea alba at midline of the abdomen, between the abdominal wall and the liver, and at the subhepatic region. Trapped air in subhepatic localized fluid may produce echogenic foci moving within the fluid collection [35, 40].

The peristaltic bowel and the hyperechoic gas within it will move with inspiration. IFA will be located just under the fascia of the abdominal wall and will not move with inspiration (Fig. 19.12). The intraluminal gas is seen inside a bowel loop having visible peristalsis and a normal wall thickness [37]. We advise clinicians to practice detecting IFA in the early post-laparotomy period so that they can be familiar with it in pathological conditions. We found it a very useful and easy skill to gain with experience. In suspected cases of IFA, repeating the abdominal ultrasound examination is essential as more free air will accumulate overtime and become more evident [35].

19.11   Post-operative Ileus

The differentiation between post-operative ileus and mechanical intestinal obstruction can be challenging. A Gastrografin follow-through study may be used. Nevertheless, it is time-consuming and poorly tolerated by patients. Sonography is a

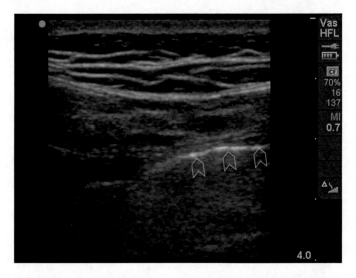

Fig. 19.12 Surgeon-performed POC ultrasound of the abdomen of the same patient shown in Fig. 19.2. The study was performed using a linear probe (10–12 MHz) located at the abdominal midline. The image shows a hyperechoic dense line behind the abdominal fascia and outside the bowel (*arrowheads*). This line did not move with respiration indicating the presence of significant free intra-paritoneal air. The patient had a laparotomy. He had extensive mesenteric tears with small bowel and sigmoid colon injuries without solid organ injuries (Sonographic study was performed by Professor Fikri Abu-Zidan, Department of Surgery, Al-Ain Hospital, Al-Ain, UAE)

very useful tool in this situation [41, 42]. It can evaluate bowel movement and wall thickness [43]. We usually start with general abdominal sonography examination using a 3–5 MHz curvilinear abdominal transducer followed by a higher frequency linear transducer (10–12 MHz) to study the small bowel in more detail [44, 45].

The small bowel diameter is 3–4 cm [42, 46]. Normally, the bowel appears as a single circular hypoechoic layer (muscle layer) surrounding hyperechoic bowel contents of gas and food particles. The normal thickness of the small bowel during contraction is 2–3 mm. Graded abdominal compression by the transducer slowly moves the air away and helps detect bowel wall pathology [45]. The sonographic findings of an obstructed bowel include dilated fluid-filled bowel loops and hyperechoic gas spots moving within them. Dilated loops may show thickened wall and increased to-and-fro motion of the bowel contents [46].

Real-time sonography may differentiate between mechanical intestinal obstruction and ileus. In paralytic ileus, the bowel will not move if observed for few minutes [42]. The movement of the mechanically obstructed bowel will initially increase. Subsequently, it will decrease with prolonged obstruction or development of bowel ischemia [47, 48]. Serial ultrasound examinations are safe and can be used to evaluate the progress of mechanical intestinal obstruction in patients who are treated conservatively [42].

19.12 Optimizing the Use of Ultrasound

The quality of ultrasound images depend on the patient's body build, the operator's experience, and the quality of the ultrasound machine. Ultrasound images are sometimes difficult to gain in obese patients because of poor tissue penetration. Furthermore, air in the subcutaneous tissue or distended bowel may limit the sonographic window to visualise the intra-abdominal organs. Ultrasound cannot accurately define the nature of intra-abdominal fluid [12].

Training and credentialing is a major pillar for the successful use of POC ultrasound in making critical decisions [49, 50]. The training period will be shortened when the operator uses the focused approach [10]. Surgeons should be very familiar with the control of their ultrasound machine and their transducers. They should be particularly knowledgeable of the basic physics of ultrasound including its artefacts. These artefacts are sometimes useful in ruling out pneumothorax or confirming the presence of free intra-peritoneal air [6, 7].

It is very important that POC ultrasound should be simplified by asking simple binary questions that should be answered by yes or no without performing a detailed radiological study [49, 50]. For example: Does the pleura of a patient with a chest stab wound move? This is actually the greatest advantage of POC ultrasound when performed by the treating surgeon. POC ultrasound will be used as a timely decision-making tool in critically ill patients. In fact, this approach will change POC ultrasound to become as an extension of the clinical examination [51]. Furthermore, POC ultrasound evaluates the pathophysiology and not only the anatomy when performed by surgeons. Accordingly surgeons are capable to instantaneously correlate the sonographic findings with the clinical findings and make timely critical decisions that may save the life of a patient. We have actually seen this repeatedly in our hands to a stage that ultrasound is always accompanying us on our surgical on calls and rounds.

References

1. Wells PNT. Physics and bioeffects. In: McGahan JP, Goldberg BB, editors. Diagnostic ultrasound, a logical approach. Philadelphia: Lppincott-Raven Publishers; 1998. p. 1–19.
2. Hangiandreou NJ. AAPM/RSNA physics tutorial for residents. Topics in US: B-mode US: basic concepts and new technology. Radiographics. 2003;23:1019–33.
3. Rose JS. Ultrasound physics and knobology. In: Simon BC, Snoey ER, editors. Ultrasound in emergency and ambulatory medicine. St Louis: Mosby-Year book Inc.; 1997. p. 10–38.
4. Rose JS, Bair AE. Fundamentals of ultrasound. In: Cosby KS, Kendall JL, editors. Practical guide to emergency ultrasound. Philadelphia: Lippincott Willaims and Wilkins; 2006. p. 27–41.

5. Schuler A. Image artifacts and pitfalls. In: Mathis G, editor. Chest sonography. 2nd ed. New York: Springer; 2008. p. 175–82.

6. Abu-Zidan FM. Basic ultrasound physics, instrumentation, and knobology. In: Zago M, editor. Essential US for trauma: E-FAST. 1st ed. Milan: Springer-Verlag Italia; 2014. p. 1–13.

7. Abu-Zidan FM, Hefny AF, Corr P. Clinical ultrasound physics. J Emerg Trauma Shock. 2011;4:501–3.

8. Whittingham TA. Medical diagnostic applications and sources. Prog Biophys Mol Biol. 2007;93:84–110.

9. Harris T, Davenport R, Hurst T, Jones J. Improving outcome in severe trauma: trauma systems and initial management: intubation, ventilation and resuscitation. Postgrad Med J. 2012;88:588–94.

10. Mohammad A, Hefny AF, Abu-Zidan FM. Focused Assessment Sonography for Trauma (FAST) training: a systematic review. World J Surg. 2014;38:1009–18.

11. McKenney MG, McKenney KL, Compton RP, Namias N, Fernandez L, Levi D, Arrillaga A, Lynn M, Martin L. Can surgeons evaluate emergency ultrasound scans for blunt abdominal trauma. J Trauma. 1998;44:649–53.

12. Radwan MM, Abu-Zidan FM. Focussed Assessment Sonograph Trauma (FAST) and CT scan in blunt abdominal trauma: surgeon's perspective. Afr Health Sci. 2006;6:187–90.

13. Rajabzadeh Kanafi A, Giti M, Gharavi MH, Alizadeh A, Pourghorban R, Shekarchi B. Diagnostic accuracy of secondary ultrasound exam in blunt abdominal trauma. Iran J Radiol. 2014;11:e21010.

14. Dittrich K, Abu-Zidan FM. Role of ultrasound in mass-casualty situations. Int J Dis Med. 2004;2:18–23.

15. Abu-Zidan FM, Al-Zayat I, Sheikh M, Mousa I, Behbehani A. Role of ultrasonography in blunt abdominal trauma, aprospective study. Eur J Surg. 1996;162:361–5.

16. Smith J. Focused assessment with sonography in trauma (FAST): should its role be reconsidered? Postgrad Med J. 2010;86:285–91.

17. Snoey ER. Echocardiography. In: Simon BC, Snoey ER, editors. Ultrasound in emergency and ambulatory medicine. St Louis: Mosby-Year book Inc.; 1997. p. 221–49.

18. Lichtenstein DA. Simple emergency cardiac sonography. In: Lichtenstein DA, editor. Whole body ultrasonography in the critically ill. 1st ed. Berlin/Heidelberg: Springer; 2010. p. 211–21.

19. Noble VE, Nelson B, SutingcoAN. Echocardiography. In: Noble VE, Nelson B, SutingcoAN, editors. Emergency and critical care ultrasound. 1st ed. Cambridge University Press: Cambridge, UK; 2007. p. 53–84.

20. Corl K, Napoli AM, Gardiner F. Bedside sonographic measurement of the inferior vena cava caval index is a poor predictor of fluid

responsiveness in emergency department patients. Emerg Med Australas. 2012;24:534–9.

21. Dipti A, Soucy Z, Surana A, Chandra S. Role of inferior vena cava diameter in assessment of volume status: a meta-analysis. Am J Emerg Med. 2012;30:1414–9.

22. Abu-Zidan FM. Optimizing the value of measuring inferior vena cava diameter in shocked patients. World J Crit Care Med. 2016;5(1):7–11.

23. Seif D, Mailhot T, Perera P, Mandavia D. Caval sonography in shock: a noninvasive method for evaluating intravascular volume in critically ill patients. J Ultrasound Med. 2012;31:1885–90.

24. Abu-Zidan FM, Idris K. Sonographic Measurement of the IVC Diameter as an Indicator for Fluid Resuscitation: Beware of the Intra-abdominal Pressure. World J Surg. 2015;39:2608–9.

25. Lichtenstein DA. Pneumothorax. In: Lichtenstein DA, editor. Whole body ultrasonography in the critically ill. 1st ed. Berlin/Heidelberg: Springer; 2010. p. 163–79.

26. Frazee BW. The abdominal aorta. In: Simon BC, Snoey ER, editors. Ultrasound in emergency and ambulatory medicine. St Louis: Mosby-Year book Inc.; 1997. p. 190–202.

27. Noble VE, Nelson B, SutingcoAN. Abdominal aortic aneurysm. In: Noble VE, Nelson B, Sutingco AN, editors. Emergency and critical care ultrasound. 1st ed. Cambridge University Press: Cambridge, UK; 2007. p. 105–18.

28. Lichtenstein DA. Aorta. In: Lichtenstein DA, editor. Whole body ultra-sonography in the critically ill. 1st ed. Berlin/Heidelberg: Springer; 2010. p. 83–8.

29. Lensing AW, Prandoni P, Brandjes D, Huisman PM, Vigo M, Tomasella G, Krekt J, Wouter Ten Cate J, Huisman MV, Büller HR. Detection of deep-vein thrombosis by real-time B-mode ultrasonography. N Engl J Med. 1989;320:342–5.

30. Cronan JJ, Dorfman GS. Advances in ultrasound imaging of venous thrombosis. Semin Nucl Med. 1991;21:297–312.

31. Tan M, van Rooden CJ, Westerbeek RE, Huisman MV. Diagnostic management of clinically suspected acute deep vein thrombosis. Br J Haematol. 2009;146:347–60.

32. Perera P, Mailhot T, Riley D, Mandavia D. The RUSH exam: rapid ultrasound in SHock in the evaluation of the critically ill. Emerg Med Clin North Am. 2010;28:29–56.

33. Zago M. Introduction and focused questions. In: Zago M, editor. Essential US for trauma: E-FAST. 1st ed. Milan: Springer-Verlag Italia; 2014. p. 15–8.

34. Coppolino F, Gatta G, Di Grezia G, Reginelli A, Iacobellis F, Vallone G, Giganti M, Genovese E. Gastrointestinal perforation: ultrasonographic diagnosis. Crit Ultrasound J. 2013;5 Suppl 1:S4.
35. Hefny AF, Abu-Zidan FM. Sonographic diagnosis of intraperitoneal free air. J Emerg Trauma Shock. 2011;4:511–3.
36. Chen SC, Wang HP, Chen WJ, Lin FY, Hsu CY, Chang KJ, Chen WJ. Selective use of ultrasonography for the detection of pneumoperitoneum. Acad Emerg Med. 2002;9:643–5.
37. Chadha D, Kedar RP, Malde HM. Sonographic detection of pneumoperitoneum: an experimental and clinical study. Australas Radiol. 1993;37:182–5.
38. Blaivas M, Kirkpatrick AW, Rodriguez-Galvez M, Ball CG. Sonographic depiction of intraperitoneal free air. J Trauma. 2009;67:675.
39. Kim SY, Park KT, Yeon SC, Lee HC. Accuracy of sonographic diagnosis of pneumoperitoneum using the enhanced peritoneal stripe sign in Beagle dogs. J Vet Sci. 2014;15:195–8.
40. Grassi R, Romano S, Pinto A, Romano L. Gastro-duodenal perforations: conventional plain film, US and CT findings in 166 consecutive patients. Eur J Radiol. 2004;50:30–6.
41. Jang TB, Schindler D, Kaji AH. Bedside ultrasonography for the detection of small bowel obstruction in the emergency department. Emerg Med J. 2011;28:676–8.
42. Ogata M, Mateer JR, Condon RE. Prospective evaluation of abdominal sonography for the diagnosis of bowel obstruction. Ann Surg. 1996;223:237–41.
43. Roccarina D, Garcovich M, Ainora ME, Caracciolo G, Ponziani F, Gasbarrini A, Zocco MA. Diagnosis of bowel diseases: the role of imaging and ultrasonography. World J Gastroenterol. 2013;19:2144–53.
44. Nylund K, Ødegaard S, Hausken T, Folvik G, Lied GA, Viola I, Hauser H, Gilja OH. Sonography of the small intestine. World J Gastroenterol. 2009;15:1319–30.
45. Lim JH. Ultrasound examination of gastrointestinal tract diseases. J Korean Med Sci. 2000;15:371–9.
46. Silva AC, Pimenta M, Guimarães LS. Small bowel obstruction: what to look for. Radiographics. 2009;29:423–39.
47. Grassi R, Romano S, D'Amario F, Giorgio Rossi A, Romano L, Pinto F, Di Mizio R. The relevance of free fluid between intestinal loops detected by sonography in the clinical assessment of small bowel obstruction in adults. Eur J Radiol. 2004;50:5–14.

48. Hefny AF, Corr P, Abu-Zidan FM. The role of ultrasound in the management of intestinal obstruction. J Emerg Trauma Shock. 2012;5:84–6.

49. Abu-Zidan FM, Dittrich K, Czechowski J, Kazzam E. Establishment of a "Focused Assessment Sonography for Trauma" (FAST) Course. Saudi Med J. 2005;26:806–11.

50. Abu-Zidan FM, Freeman P, Mandivia D. The first Australian workshop on bedside ultrasound in the emergency department. N Z Med J. 1999;112:322–4.

51. Abu-Zidan FM. Point-of-care ultrasound in critically ill patients: where do we stand? J Emerg Trauma Shock. 2012;5:70–1.

Chapter 20
Interventional Radiology for Nontraumatic Acute Thoraco-Abdominal Bleeding

Nicola Montanari and Antonio Affinita

20.1 Introduction

Thoraco-abdominal nontraumatic/gastrointestinal bleeding emergencies that can be treated by interventional radiology are relatively rare. Among this heterogeneous group of pathologies, the most frequent is definitely massive hemoptysis.

Thoracic and abdominal nontraumatic aortic rupture endovascular treatment, although considered first-line therapy, is restricted to centers with cardiovascular surgery and elevated skills in EndoVascular Aortic Repair (EVAR) [1].

An emerging pathology in the last decade is spontaneous bleeding in patients treated with anticoagulant therapy and they account for the second-most frequent request for angioembolization.

N. Montanari (✉) • A. Affinita
Radiology Department, RADOM, Ospedale Maggiore,
Largo Nigrisoli, 2, Bologna 40133, Italy
e-mail: montanari.nicola@gmail.com; antonio.affinita@ausl.bologna.it

© Springer International Publishing Switzerland 2017   361
S. Di Saverio et al. (eds.), *Acute Care Surgery Handbook*,
DOI 10.1007/978-3-319-15341-4_20

Finally, massive spontaneous bleeding can occasionally originate from a wide range of pathologies: neoplasms, chronic inflammations, arterovenous malformations, aneurysm. An interventional radiologist is often called in to manage these bleeding as surgery does not maintain the tamponade of the hematoma and bleeding identification and control is often difficult [2].

This chapter will cover massive hemoptysis and anticoagulant-related spontaneous ematomas. A brief mention of EVAR will also be made.

20.2   Massive Hemoptysis

Massive hemoptysis is one of the most dreaded of all respiratory emergencies and can have a variety of underlying causes. In 90 % of cases, the source of massive hemoptysis is the bronchial circulation.

Massive hemoptysis is usually defined as coughing up 600 mL or more of blood within 24 h [3].

Conservative management of massive hemoptysis carries a mortality rate of 50–100 % [4].

Surgery for massive hemoptysis has a mortality rate that ranges from 7.1 to 18.2 %, while, if performed in emergency, it increases up to 40 % [5].

BAE is now an established procedure and the first-line treatment in the management of massive and recurrent hemoptysis [6].

When an increased need of oxygenated blood occurs (like in inflammatory disorders, systemic hypoxemia, pulmonary infarction, alveolar hypoxia) bronchial arteries undergo smooth muscle wall hypertrophy or dilate. Intercostal, internal mammary, and inferior phrenic arteries are also involved in chronic pulmonary ischemia.

The total systemic cardiac output to the bronchial arteries may increase from 1 to 18–30 %.

In Western countries, bronchogenic carcinoma and chronic inflammatory lung diseases (due to bronchiectasis, aspergillosis, and cystic fibrosis) are the most prevalent causes.

In the non-Western world, the most common underlying cause of hemoptysis is pulmonary tuberculosis and particularly tuberculosis bronchiectasis [4].

After a chest radiograph and flexible bronchoscopy, a contrast CT scan of the chest may be helpful to detect the underlying pathology and abnormal bronchial arteries: in adults, normal bronchial arteries have a diameter less than 1.5 mm; a bronchial artery more than 2 mm in diameter at CT is considered pathologic (Fig. 20.1a).

Before of BAE, the bronchial artery number and origin must be carefully evaluated.

Always, other vessels that can be involved in hemoptysis must be investigated: intercostals, subclavian, phrenic, and mammary arteries.

The decision of which arteries need embolization is carried out on the base of CT, bronchoscopic and angiographic findings.

The most used embolic material in BAE is polyvinyl alcohol particles, usually 350–500 μm in diameter, as they are nonreadsorbable (Fig. 20.1c). Smaller particles can lead to pulmonary infarction as bronchopulmonary anastomosis of 325 μm are demonstrated in human lung [7].

Gelatin sponge may lead to recanalization and therefore is less used than particles.

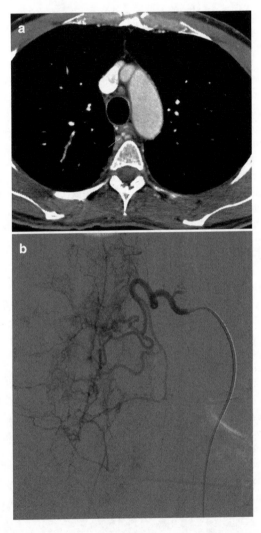

Fig. 20.1 Massive hemoptysis (**a**) CT Scan shows a bronchial artery of 2.3 mm in diameter (*arrow*). (**b**) Angiogram of the pathologic bronchial arteries in a chronic inflammatory disease. (**c**) Angiogram after emboliza-tion with particles

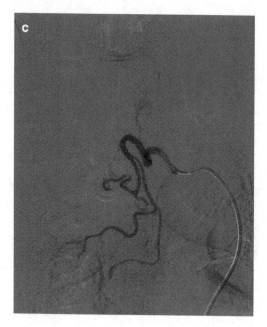

Fig. 20.1 (continued)

Coils are indicated in mammary artery and in bronchial artery aneurysm.

Isobutyl-2 cyanoacrylate could be used in neovascularization and AV malformation.

BAE is very effective in acute massive hemoptysis. Long-term recurrence rate, however, has been reported to be from 10 to 52 % [8]. Recurrence of bleeding is more frequent in tuberculosis, aspergilloma, and neoplasms.

Complications of BAE are usually transient: more frequent complications are chest pain and dysphagia. The prevalence of spinal cord ischemia is reported to be 1.4–6.5 % and embolization, when Adamkiewicz is visualized at angiogram of target vessel, must be avoided.

20.3   Anticoagulation-Related Soft Tissue Spontaneous Hemorrhages

In the last decade, the widespread use of anticoagulation therapy in elder patients has led to an increase in soft tissue spontaneous hemorrhage [9, 10].

While conservative management (anticoagulation withdrawal or reversal, volume expansion, transfusion of fresh frozen plasma and packed RBCs, and vasoactive drugs) is recommended in hemodynamically stable patients [11], the treatment of life-threatening hemorrhage is endovascular embolization [12].

Embolization preserves the tamponade effects, if in a muscular compartment, of the already developed hematoma, is repeatable and allows selective closure of target vessel.

A CT is normally performed before embolization: usually, if there is an active bleeding, the vessel where hemorrhage originates can be identified (Fig. 20.2a).

The embolization materials in these cases are mainly gelatin sponge, as adsorbable material allows the recovery of vascularization after the coagulopathy is solved.

Precautionary embolization with readsorbable materials of arteries feeding tha anatomical region of the hematoma should be performed also if absence of active bleeding at angiography: bleeding is often intermittent and to restrict embolization to angiographic evident blush leads to more frequent reintervention needs.

20.4   Aorta

Acute rupture of the thoracic and abdominal aorta (AAR) is a life-threatening condition that had an extremely high mortality rate before the introduction of thoracic and abdominal

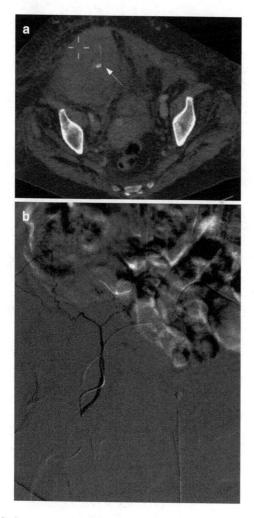

Fig. 20.2 Spontaneous rectus sheet bleeding: (**a**) CT scan shows large hematoma and contrast media blush (*arrow*); (**b**) selective angiogram of the inferior epigastric artery in the same patient

endovascular aortic repair (TEVAR/EVAR). Emergency surgical repair of the aorta consisted of thoracotomy or laparotomy, replacement of the diseased aorta, and interposition of a prosthetic graft.

Despite advances in perioperative management, conventional aortic surgery in patients presenting with rupture still has a significant risk of mortality [13].

TEVAR has emerged as an alternative to open surgery for AAR [14]. AAR was defined as disruption of the aortic wall with concomitant extravasation of fresh blood outside the adventitia of the aorta or concomitant hemomediastinum, hemothorax, or hemoperitoneum, as documented by preoperative MDCT.

Surgery is associated with mortality rates approaching 33–45 %.

TEVAR is considered the preferred treatment option over open surgery in patients with ruptured aneurysms of the descending aorta due to lower mortality rates ranging from 0 to 17.4 %. The major goal of endovascular repair in an emergency setting is to achieve immediate control of the bleeding due to complete exclusion of the aneurysm from the systemic circulation, including the tear site.

References

1. Botsios S, Frömke J, Walterbusch G, et al. Endovascular treatment for nontraumatic rupture of the descending thoracic aorta: long-term results. J Card Surg. 2014;29:353–8.
2. Dohan A, Sapoval M, Chousterman BG, et al. Spontaneous soft-tissue hemorrhage in anticoagulated patients: safety and efficacy of embolization. AJR Am J Roentgenol. 2015;204:1303–10.
3. Shigemura N, Wan IY, Yu SC, et al. Multidisciplinary management of lifethreatening massive hemoptysis: a 10-year experience. Ann Thorac Surg. 2009;87(3):849–53.

4. Najarian KE, Morris CS. Arterial embolization in the chest. J Thorac Imaging. 1998;13:93–104.

5. Fernando HC, Stein M, Benfield JR, Link DP. Role of bronchial artery embolization in the management of hemoptysis. Arch Surg. 1998;133:862–6.

6. Wholey MH, Chamorro HA, Rao G, Ford WB, Miller WH. Bronchial artery embolization for massive hemoptysis. JAMA. 1976;236:2501–4.

7. Pump K. Distribution of bronchial arteries in human lung. Chest. 1972;62:447–51.

8. Katoh O, Kishikawa T, Yamada H, Matsumoto S, Kudo S. Recurrent bleeding after arterial embolization in patients with hemoptysis. Chest. 1990;97:541–6.

9. Alla VM, Karnam SM, Kaushik M, Porter J. Spontaneous rectus sheath hematoma. West J Emerg Med. 2010;11:76–9.

10. Cherry WB, Mueller PS. Rectus sheath hematoma: review of 126 cases at a single institution. Medicine (Baltimore). 2006;85:105–10.

11. Landefeld CS, Beyth RJ. Anticoagulant-related bleeding: clinical epidemiology, prediction, and prevention. Am J Med. 1993;95:315–28.

12. Zissin R, Gayer G, Kots E, Ellis M, Bartal G, Griton I. Transcatheter arterial embolisation in anticoagulant- related haematoma: a current therapeutic option—a report of four patients and review of the literature. Int J Clin Pract. 2007;61:1321–7.

13. Bozinovski J, Coselli JS. Outcomes and survival in surgical treatment of descending thoracic aorta with acute dissection. Ann Thorac Surg. 2008;85:965–70.

14. Jonker FH, Verhagen HJ, Lin PH, et al. Open surgery versus endovascular repair of ruptured thoracic aortic aneurysms. J Vasc Surg. 2011;53(5):1210–6.

Chapter 21
Percutaneous Techniques for Management of Intra-abdominal Abscesses

Francesco Cinquantini, Alice Piccinini, Nicola Montanari, Andrea Biscardi, Gregorio Tugnoli, and Salomone Di Saverio

21.1 Pathophysiology

Intra-abdominal abscesses are localized collections of pus confined in the peritoneal cavity or in the retroperitoneal space by an inflammatory wall. This barrier may include the omentum, inflammatory adhesions, or contiguous viscera. The abscesses usually contain a mixture of aerobic and anaerobic bacteria, coming from the gastrointestinal tract.

Bacteria in the peritoneal cavity, in particular those arising from the large intestine, stimulate the arriving of acute inflammatory cells. The omentum and viscera tend to localize the site

F. Cinquantini, MD • N. Montanari, MD (✉)
Department of Radiology, Interventional Radiology Unit, C A Pizzardi
Maggiore Hospital, Bologna, Italy
e-mail: montanari.nicola@gmail.com

A. Piccinini, MD • A. Biscardi, MD • G. Tugnoli, MD • S. Di Saverio, MD, FACS, FRCS
Department of Emergency and General Surgery and Trauma Surgery Unit, C A Pizzardi Maggiore Hospital Trauma Center, Bologna, Italy

© Springer International Publishing Switzerland 2017
S. Di Saverio et al. (eds.), *Acute Care Surgery Handbook*,
DOI 10.1007/978-3-319-15341-4_21

of infection, producing a phlegmon. The resulting hypoxia in the area facilitates the growth of anaerobes and impairs the bactericidal activity of granulocytes. The phagocytic activity of these cells degrades cellular and bacterial debris, creating a hypertonic milieu that expands and enlarges the abscess cavity in response to osmotic forces.

If untreated, the process continues until bacteremia develops, which then progresses to generalized sepsis with shock.

21.2 Etiology

Although multiple causes of intra-abdominal abscesses exist, the following are the most common:

- Perforation of bowels, which includes peptic ulcer perforation
- Perforated appendicitis and diverticulitis
- Gangrenous cholecystitis
- Pancreatitis or pancreatic necrosis progressing to pancreatic abscess

Other causes include untreated penetrating trauma to the abdominal viscera with missing HVI and postoperative complications, such as anastomotic leakage [1, 2] or missed gallstones during laparoscopic cholecystectomy (Fig. 21.1).

21.3 Percutaneous Treatment

The first studies on the percutaneous abscess drainage have been published around 30 years ago as an alternative to the more invasive surgical treatments [3–5] and have since then become the standard of care.

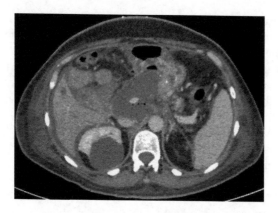

Fig. 21.1 Post-duodenocefalopancreasectomy collection

The drainage of abdominal fluid collection can be performed with a diagnostic or therapeutic purpose.

Diagnostic

- Characterization of the abdominal fluid collection (pus, bile, blood, urine, lymph, pancreatic juice)
- Differentiate infected from noninfected collections and characterization of the responsible microorganism

Therapeutic

- To treat abscesses that can be fully drained
- Adjuvant measure in the cases of multiple incompletely drainable abscesses or in critical patients

21.4 Indications

The main indications of the percutaneous drain placement are the presence of an abdominal infected collection. The abscess size is usually bigger than 4 cm. For the management of smaller (<3 cm) collections, most authors advocate a trial of antibiotics alone with consideration given to needle aspiration to hone antibiotic coverage for persistent cases [6, 7].

Symptoms such as pain or pressure from a large noninfected fluid collection, or obstruction of the bowel or ureter, are also indications for drainage.

The only absolute contraindications to perform a percutaneous drainage are the lack of a safe access or when the access can be impaired by the interposition of organs of vascular structures.

However, in most cases the absence of a safe way to reach the collection can be resolved by changing decubitus or by using curved needles or choosing alternative approaches: transgluteal (Fig. 21.2), transvaginal, or transperineal paths are used for

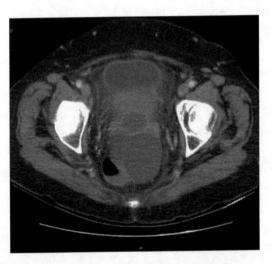

Fig. 21.2 A 69-year-old woman with diverticolitis and pelvic collection. After endovenous mdc subministration, it is possible to clearly differentiate the collection from the free fluid in the Douglas pouch

pelvic collections and transhepatic to reach the epiploon and peripancreatic cavities.

If the way of access is covered by a small bowel loop or the stomach, the drainage can be done relatively safely through those organs via a needle. However, it is not recommended to pass a needle through the colon.

Coagulopathy, transpleurical pass, echinococcal cyst, and asymptomatic sterile fluid collections are relative contraindication.

The presence of coagulation disorders have to be corrected before the procedure by the administration of fresh frozen plasma or platelets.

Transpleural passage should be avoided as much as possible because it is painful and can cause a pleuric effusion or a secondary infection of the pleural space.

The drainage of echinococcal cysts is not therapeutic and can be complicated by anaphylactic shock and spreading of the disease. Percutaneous treatment of such cysts can be, however, achieved using the so-called PAIR technique (puncture, aspiration, alcohol injection, re-aspiration) [8] with low rate of recurrence and complications.

The drainage of an asymptomatic sterile fluid collection is not recommended, and if it is done, the catheter should be left in place for the shortest possible time, to avoid possible secondary infections.

21.5 Imaging Guidance

Ultrasound and CT are the modalities used most of the times to guide the drainage procedures. Fluoroscopy is sometimes needed in addition to the sonography to monitor the drainage and the eventual presence of fistulas by iodinated contrast injection.

Ultrasound is the most useful way to visualize intra-abdominal abscesses. The main advantages of this technique are:

- The possibility to follow the needle pathway in real time, thus allowing the rapid execution of the drainage
- The possibility to perform this technique in the same patient's room (e.g., in cases of patients in intensive care unit)
- The easy availability of the equipment

Limitations of ultrasound are deep-located collections (retroperitoneum, pelvis, peripancreatic region) or when there is an overlapping structure (e.g., a bowel loop) impairing the ultrasounds guide.

CT is the preferred choice when a reasonably safe pathway cannot be found using ultrasonography. The main advantage of CT is the perfect visualization of all the anatomic structures and thus the possibility to track particularly difficult and/or deep paths. Another benefit of CT is that, through the administration of EV contrast media, it is possible to further improve the visualization of the fluid collection (Figs. 21.2 and 21.3).

The drawbacks of CT are the length of the procedure, the limited access to the equipment, the lack of real-time needle visualization during the procedure, the difficulty in following nonorthogonal paths, and the exposition to x-rays.

21.6 Patient Preparation

- Coagulative tests: $PT < 15$ s; $INR < 1,5$; platelet $> 75,000$
- Test of the kidneys functionality if an intravenous contrast is foreseen.
- Fasting
- Venous access
- Informed consent
- Monitoring

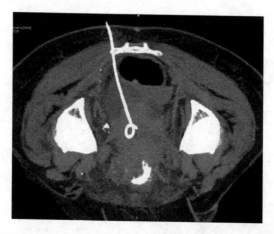

Fig. 21.3 MIP oblique reconstruction of the control scan after positioning of drainage catheter in the collection: 30 ml of pus were aspirated. During the multistep procedure of the needle insertion, a sample of the free fluid in the Douglas space was aspirated and cultured and it resulted negative for infection

21.7 Punction Technique and Other Technical Issues

The first common steps of the procedure are the study of the preliminary imaging to determine the optimal approach, the disinfection and preparation of the skin, a sterile work field large enough to place the guides and catheter and an adequate local anesthesia.

Seldinger Technique
- Choose the material. Chiba needles are preferable, having a good echogenicity and being relatively atraumatic.
- Position the needle in the collection (Fig. 21.4a). This phase can be done in one step if US-guided, or in more steps when using CT guidance. Using US we have a real time vision of the needle path while with CT, after each step, it will be

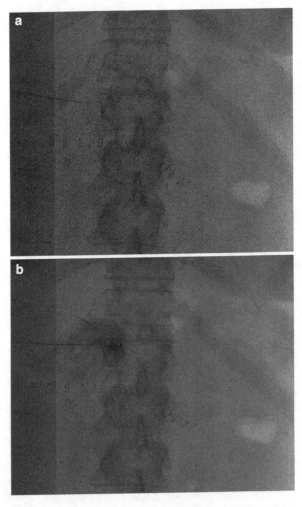

Fig. 21.4 Step of Seldinger technique, (**a**) puncture of the collection, (**b**) 0.018 nitinol guidewire and coaxial introducer in the opacificated collection, (**c**) 0.035 guidewire in the collection, (**d**) drainage catheter final positioning

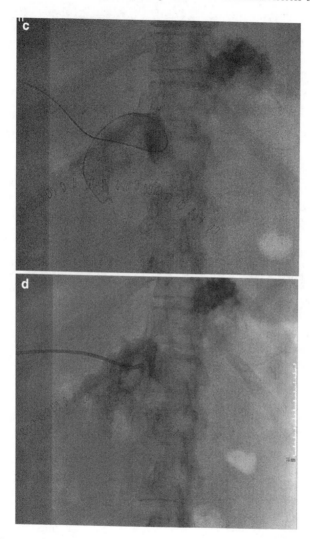

Fig. 21.4 (continued)

necessary to monitor the correct needle direction through repeated scans limited to the specific area of interest.

- Once the collection is reached, a sample of fluid will be collected and submitted for culture test and eventually laboratory analyses.
- A guide will be passed through the needle cannula and the cannula is withdrawn (Fig. 21.4c).
- The drain will be inserted over the wire to reach the correct position (Fig. 21.4d).

If the access is difficult, it is possible to use a fine needle (20–22G) through which can be inserted a 0.018 guide (Fig. 21.4b). Further to this, with specific coaxial kits it will be possible to place a larger guide (0.035–0.038), allowing the insertion of dilators and ultimately the drainage (usually 8–12f).

If the access is easier, it is possible to reach the collection area with an 18G needle that can allow to pass a larger guide and thus avoid the need of using a coaxial kit.

After the removal of the needle, with the guide only in place, a small cutaneous cut with the scalpel tip is performed to allow an easier insertion of dilators and catheter. At this stage, as the guide could be displaced or looped if it is not firmly kept in tension, caution should be taken.

Trocar Technique

When collections are superficial and large, Trocar catheters could be used, a faster and more simple procedure. Trocars are made up of a metallic sharp obturator, a cannula, and a seal. After skin cut with the scalpel tip, the trocar is advanced in one-step maneuver, under US real-time guide or CT guide, until it reaches the collection.

After drainage catheter positioning and guidewire removal, if the procedure is performed in a US-radiological suite, a small injection of iodine contrast media allows to study the abscess morphology and eventually the presence of fistulas (Fig. 21.5).

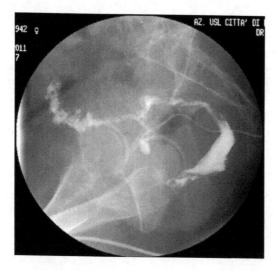

Fig. 21.5 Same patient as in Fig. 21.1. Iodinated contrast subministration via the catheter: a fistula with the sigma was depicted

Then drainage catheter is secured to the patient skin and covered with sterile gauzes taking care to avoid kinking and connected to collection pouch.

Once the catheter is in place, the cannula/catheter is attached to a drainage bag through a three-way stopcock. The cavity should be aspirated until there is no more return or the aspirate becomes blood stained. The cavity should then be irrigated with small volumes of saline solution (10–20 ml) and then re-aspirated until all particulate material is removed.

21.8   Complications

Complication rate is ranging between 2.5 and 10.4 % [9, 10]; major and minor complications can be distinguished.

Hemorrhage, septicemia, shock, enteric fistula, peritonitis, and hemopneumothorax account for major complications.

Accidental injury of an artery may lead to severe hemorrhage requiring blood transfusion or surgical repair. It is therefore mandatory to monitor vital signs after the procedure to identify an occult bleeding.

Particularly with US guide, the passage of the catheter through a bowel can be neglected in the beginning but can lead to enteric fistula, peritonitis, and occlusion. A CT scan with injection through the drainage catheter of diluted iodine contrast media is mandatory when bowel accidental puncture is suspected. Surgical repair is often required in such an event, particularly if a colon lesion is seen due to contaminated content, while gastric lesions usually are self-healing.

Minor complications include local pain and tenderness, cutaneous inflammation, self-limiting bleeding, catheter displacement, and pericatheter leak.

Pericatheter leak, if resulted by catheter malfunctioning, for instance kinking or obstruction, requires catheter unblock or replacement.

21.9 Success Rates

Drainage catheter should be kept in place until complete draining of the cavity and until vital signs are gone back to normal. Premature removal could lead to abscess recurrence.

When the output of the collected fluid is below 20 ml/die, usually the catheter could be removed.

If no clinical improvements occur, or an abrupt decrease or not satisfactory volume of fluid collected are seen, an imaging study is recommended.

If the drainage collects more than 50 ml of fluids after 4–5 days, a fistula should be suspected; in such an event, a prolonged period of drainage (4–6 weeks) or surgical repair is required.

The overall failure rate of the percutaneous drainage was 9 % in two studies [11, 12]. Simple unilocular abscesses are managed almost always by percutaneous drainage; more complicated abscesses, such as those with enteric fistulas (e.g., diverticular abscess) or pancreatic abscesses, have cure rates ranging from 65 to 90 % [13]. Percutaneous catheter change over a wire is the preferred intervention in cases of undrained abscess fluid despite technically adequate catheter placement, with 66 % of success [14].

Risk factors associated with failure of the drainage procedure are the complexity of the abscess cavity (septation, multiloculation, or clotted blood) and the presence of a fistula between the abscess and the bowel, biliary tree, or bladder.

Fibrinolysis of complex, multi-septated fluid collections refractory to PCD by intracavitary instillation of fibrinolytic agents has been reported to be safe and showed a reduction in hospital stay, drainage duration, and overall cost of treatment [15].

21.10 Conclusions

As recommended from the Surgical Infection Society and the Infectious Disease Society of America, where feasible, percutaneous drainage of abscesses and other well-localized fluid collections is preferable to surgical drainage with a level of evidence (B-II) [16]. Open surgical techniques are likely required for poorly localized, loculated, complex, or diffuse fluid collections and necrotic tissue, high-density fluid, or percutaneously unaccessible collections (guidelines).

Acute peritonitis is better treated surgically rather than with percutaneous drainage.

References

1. Eberhardt JM, Kiran RP, Lavery IC. The impact of anastomotic leak and intra-abdominal abscess on cancer-related outcomes after resection for colorectal cancer: a case control study. Dis Colon Rectum. 2009;52(3):380–6.

2. Yang YM, Tian XD, Zhuang Y, Wang WM, Wan YL, Huang YT. Risk factors of pancreatic leakage after pancreaticoduodenectomy. World J Gastroenterol. 2005;11(16):2456–61.

3. Haaga JR, Alfidi RJ, Havrilla TR, et al. CT detection and aspiration of abdominal abscesses. AJR Am J Roentgenol. 1977;128:465–74.

4. Gerzof SG, Robbins AH, Birkett DH, Johnson WC, Pugatch RD, Vincent ME. Percutaneous catheter drainage of abdominal abscesses guided by ultrasound and computed tomography. AJR Am J Roentgenol. 1979;133:1–8.

5. Haaga JR, Weinstein AJ. CT-guided percutaneous aspiration and drainage of abscesses. AJR Am J Roentgenol. 1980;135:1187–94.

6. Kumar RR, Kim JT, Haukoos JS, et al. Factors affecting the successful management of intra-abdominal abscesses with antibiotics and the need for percutaneous drainage. Dis Colon Rectum. 2006;49(2):183–9.

7. Siewert B, Tye G, Kruskal J, et al. Impact of CT-guided drainage in the treatment of diverticular abscesses: size matters. AJR Am J Roentgenol. 2006;186(3):680–6.

8. Filice C, Brunetti E, Bruno R, Crippa FG. Percutaneous drainage of echinococcal cysts (PAIR—puncture, aspiration, injection, reaspiration): results of a worldwide survey for assessment of its safety and efficacy. Gut. 2000;47(1):156–7.

9. Shahnazi M, Khatami A, Jamzad A, Shohitavi S. Safety and efficacy of percutaneous CT-guided drainage in the management of abdominopelvic abscess. Iran J Radiol. 2014;11(3):e20876.

10. vanSonnenberg E, Wing VW, Casola G, et al. Temporizing effect of percutaneous drainage of complicated abscesses in critically ill patients. AJR Am J Roentgenol. 1984;142:821–6.

11. Lambiase RE, Deyoe L, Cronan JJ, Dorfman GS. Percutaneous drainage of 335 consecutive ab- scesses: results of primary drainage with 1-year follow-up. Radiology. 1992;184:167–79.

12. Akinci D, Akhan O, Ozmen MN, et al. Percutane- ous drainage of 300 intraperitoneal abscesses with long-term follow-up. Cardiovasc Intervent Radiol. 2005;28:744–50.

13. vanSonnenberg E, Wittich GR, Goodacre BW, Casola G, D'Agostino HB. Percutaneous abscess drainage: update. World J Surg. 2001;25:362–9.

14. Michael S, Gee MS, Kim JY, Gervais DA, Hahn PF, Mueller PR. Management of abdominal and pelvic abscesses that persist despite satisfactory percutaneous drainage catheter placement. AJR Am J Roentgenol. 2010;194:815–20.
15. Laborda A, De Gregorio MA, Miguelena JM, et al. Percutaneous treatment of intrabdominal abscess: urokinase versus saline serum in 100 cases using two surgical scoring systems in a randomized trial. Eur Radiol. 2009;19(7):1772–9.
16. Solomkin JS, et al. Diagnosis and management of complicated intra-abdominal infection in adults and children: guidelines by the Surgical Infection Society and the Infectious Diseases Society of America. Clin Infect Dis. 2010;50(2):133–64.

Chapter 22
Damage Control Surgery for Emergency General Surgery

Dieter G. Weber and Cino Bendinelli

22.1 Introduction

Damage control surgery is an established and validated operative strategy, indicated for a select minority of trauma patients that present in physiological extremis and require immediate surgical control of haemorrhage and contamination [1–5]. Traditionally, surgeons aimed for primary definitive care, an operative strategy that aimed to achieve complete anatomical restoration in one intervention. While this approach served the majority of trauma patients well, patients with severe

D.G. Weber, MBBS (Hons.), FRACS (✉)
Trauma and General Surgeon, Royal Perth Hospital, The University of Western Australia, The University of Newcastle,
197 Wellington St, Perth, WA 6000, Australia
e-mail: dietergweber@gmail.com; Dieter.Weber@health.wa.gov.au

C. Bendinelli, MD, FRACS
Trauma, Endocrine and General Surgeon, John Hunter Hospital,
The University of Newcastle, Newcastle, Australia
e-mail: Cino.Bendinelli@hnehealth.nsw.gov.au

© Springer International Publishing Switzerland 2017
S. Di Saverio et al. (eds.), *Acute Care Surgery Handbook*,
DOI 10.1007/978-3-319-15341-4_22

physiological derangements were at times unable to tolerate the additional physiological stressors of surgery. This subgroup, defined by their state of shock and physiological compromise, was not optimally served by this primary definitive care approach, and was in need of an alternative treatment modality.

In recognition of the poor outcomes of primary definitive surgical care among the trauma patients in physiological extremis, several trauma centres began to experiment with abbreviated surgeries, aimed, in the first instance, at controlling blood loss and contamination in the abdomen, with a greater focus on simultaneous resuscitation of the patient's physiology, and with a delay of anatomical restoration to a later stage, until after the physiological derangements had been normalised [1–5]. The success of this approach was documented in several retrospective case series, demonstrating improved survival of these critically ill trauma patients, when compared with historic cohorts of patients undergoing primary definitive surgical manoeuvres [6–9]. Drawing analogy with the military processes of the navy, where the term 'damage control' had been used to summarise the behaviour of a ship's crew if their ship became damaged at sea, Rotondo introduced the term 'damage control' into everyday surgical parlance [6].

From its beginning in abdominal trauma surgery, the damage control modality of surgical care has been extended into other surgical fields. For example, orthopaedic damage control surgery is now well established. With the evolution of the field of acute care surgery, and subspecialisation of emergency general surgery, general surgeons practising in these fields have also sought to extend the lessons learnt in the subspecialty of trauma to non-traumatic abdominal emergencies [10–12]. This chapter reviews the damage control concept, with a focus on the evidence for its application in non-traumatic abdominal emergencies.

22.2 The Damage Control Strategy

Seriously injured patients who present in severe traumatic shock poorly tolerate further physiological stress from the protracted surgical insult necessary for definitive anatomical repair [1–5, 10–12]. However, surgical haemorrhage control may be unavoidable, and is an integral part of the acute resuscitative manoeuvres. In such patients, the goal of surgery is the treatment of the shock, rather than necessarily the restoration of the anatomical continuity.

Five phases of damage control surgery are identified: first, the appropriate patients for this treatment modality need to be identified; second, a rapid, targeted, surgical intervention is performed to arrest the cause of the shock (usually to stop haemorrhage and minimise contamination); third, the patient is reassessed, and judgement exercised to decide if the damage control strategy is still appropriate; fourth, the patient's physiology is resuscitated and restored, typically in the intensive care environment; and finally, definitive anatomical restoration of the injury is performed on the optimised patient [5]. Table 22.1.

Trauma patients differ pathophysiologically from patients with non-traumatic abdominal catastrophes [10, 11]: in trauma, the shock ensues from tissue injury, its associated inflammatory cascades, usually in combination with poor organ perfusion caused by the haemorrhage; in non-traumatic intra-abdominal emergencies, patients typically demonstrate either haemorrhagic shock in the absence of tissue injury (e.g. from a duodenal ulcer), or septic shock (e.g. from a perforated viscus). These fundamental pathophysiological differences require adaptations of precise clinical handling, and cannot be managed identically to trauma patients. For example in the case of septic shock, the initial, preoperative, resuscitation, and the administration of antibiotics are now both well established [13, 14]. As a result, we have proposed [10] the need for an additional phase (called

Table 22.1 Phases of damage control for non-traumatic abdominal emergencies

Haemorrhagic shock		Septic shock
Preoperative Haemostatic resuscitation	Phase 0	Preoperative resuscitation with fluids and vasoconstrictors
Hypothermia correction		Hypothermia correction
		Antibiotic administration
Identification of the patient: pathology and physiology	Phase 1	Identification of the patient: pathology and physiology
Haemorrhage control	Phase 2	Decontamination
		Sepsis source control
Reassessment during surgery	Phase 3	Reassessment during surgery
Physiological restoration in intensive care	Phase 4	Physiological restoration in intensive care
Optimisation of haemodynamics		Optimisation of haemodynamics
Correction of acidosis, hypothermia and coagulopathy		Correction of acidosis, hypothermia and coagulopathy
Optimisation and support of vital organs		Optimisation and support of vital organs
Intra-operative reassessment	Phase 5	Intra-operative reassessment
Definitive repair		Definitive repair
Abdominal wall closure		Abdominal wall closure

this Phase 0), in the damage control surgery phases, which precedes the classic five phases of damage control surgery for trauma described above. Phase 0 focuses on preoperative resuscitation, and may be considered what is described as 'damage control resuscitation' elsewhere.

22.3 Evidence for Damage Control Strategies in Abdominal Emergencies

Relatively minimal, direct, evidence has been published to support the application of the damage control strategy to patients with critical intra-abdominal emergencies. The literature is all Level III and IV data, and is largely on the basis of retrospective case series, which at times are referenced to historic or non-randomised cohorts or data-sets [10]. The progress in this field has been largely driven by instinctive recognition of potential benefits in this treatment modality by experienced trauma, acute care and general surgeons, which are involved in the current management of both trauma and general surgery patients. This intuitively transfer of the lessons learnt from the trauma cohort, to their other critically ill patients with non-traumatic intra-abdominal emergencies, continues to require further study. In particular, the precise indications and nature of the interventions offered will undoubtedly continue to evolve. Further clarification between varying definitions and clinical systems in these studies is also required. Table 22.2 summarises the currently available studies reporting on damage control in general surgical abdominal emergencies (case reports have been excluded) [15–32].

22.4   Patient Selection

Patient selection remains key for the realisation of benefit of the damage control strategy; inappropriate use (both over- and under-use) may lead to harm [2–6, 10]. Among trauma patients only a minority of trauma laparotomies (usually less than 30 %) require a damage control strategy. The precise rate varies greatly depending on a number of factors, including the trauma centre's injury patterns, the patient cohort, and the treatment systems, among others. While the potential harm from overuse was initially not emphasised, this has been brought into discussion more recently [33]. The authors have estimated that it is unlikely that more than a few percent of all abdominal emergencies would benefit from the damage control strategy [10].

Table 22.2 Studies reporting on damage control surgery in non-traumatic abdominal emergencies

Lead author	Year	Study design	Level of evidence	Number of cases	Pathology	Comparison cohort
Finlay et al. [15]	2003	Prospective comparative study	III	14	9 Intra-abdominal sepsis 2° visceral perforation 3 Ruptured abdominal aortic aneurysm 1 Post-operative bleed 1 Retroperitoneal bleed	POSSUM[a] P-POSSUM[b]
Freeman and Graham [16]	2004	Retrospective comparative study	III	3	Acute mesenteric ischaemia	Non-randomised concurrent patients
Banieghbal and Davies [17]	2004	Prospective series	IV	27	Neonatal generalised necrotising enterocolitis	–
Tamijmarane et al. [18]	2006	Retrospective series	IV	25	Complicated elective pancreatic surgery	–
Stawicki et al. [19]	2008	Retrospective comparative study	III	16	6 Sepsis 5 Intra-operative bleeding 3 Ischaemia 2 Necrotising pancreatitis	APACHE II[c] POSSUM[a]

Person et al. [20]	2009	Retrospective comparative series	III	31	15 Peritonitis 10 Mesenteric ischaemia 3 Bleeding 2 Obstruction 1 Other	Non-randomised concurrent patients
Ball et al. [21]	2010	Retrospective series	IV	6	Haemorrhage at pancreatic necrosectomy	—
Filicori et al. [22]	2010	Retrospective comparative study	III	8	Intra-abdominal haemorrhage	APACHE II[c]
Gong et al. [23]	2010	Retrospective series	IV	15	Acute mesenteric ischaemia	—
Morgan et al. [24]	2010	Retrospective series	IV	8	Complicated elective pancreatic resections 4 intra-operative haemorrhage 2 sepsis at reoperation 2 haemorrhage at reoperation	—
Perathoner et al. [25]	2010	Prospective comparative series	III	9	Complicated diverticulitis	Non-randomised concurrent patients

(continued)

Table 22.2 (continued)

Lead author	Year	Study design	Level of evidence	Number of cases	Pathology	Comparison cohort
Subramanian et al. [26]	2010	Retrospective series	IV	88	32 Planned relook[d], 26 Abdominal compartment syndrome, 29 Contamination, 15 Necrotising fasciitis, 14 Ischaemic bowel, 10 Haemodynamic instability	–
Tadlock et al. [27]	2010	Retrospective comparative series	III	13	Ruptured abdominal aortic aneurysm	Non-randomised concurrent patients
Kafka-Ritsch et al. [28]	2012	Prospective series	IV	51	Perforated diverticulitis	–
Khan et al. [29]	2013	Retrospective series	IV	42	13 Bowel ischaemia, 13 Haemorrhage, 10 Peritonitis, 6 Physiological instability	–

Goussous et al. [30]	2013	Retrospective series	IV	99	25 Bowel ischaemia 21 Bowel perforation 15 Haemorrhage 10 Anastomotic leak 7 Abdominal compartment syndrome 6 Incarcerated hernia 5 Ruptured abdominal aortic aneurysm 3 Enterocutaneous fistula 2 Necrotising pancreatitis 2 Necrotising fasciitis 3 Other	—
Liu et al. [31]	2015	Retrospective series	IV	6	6 Acute mesenteric ischaemia	—
Nentwich et al. [32]	2015	Retrospective series	IV	20	Completion of pancreatectomies after complicated Whipple's procedures	Non-randomised concurrent patients

[a] The physiological and operative severity score for the enumeration of mortality and morbidity

[b] The Portsmouth predictor equation for the physiological and operative severity score for the enumeration of mortality and morbidity

[c] Acute physiology and chronic health evaluation II

[d] Multiple indications for several patients

While specific trigger points for the application of a damage control strategy have been hypothesised and partially validated [2, 34], especially regarding physiological criteria, e.g. base excess <−8.0 or temperature <35 °C, the indications for damage control are not absolute and should not be considered as a discussion of isolated criteria. The various issues to consider as potential trigger points can be categorised into: patient factors; injury or disease factors; physiological factors; and treatment factors. These factors are summarised in Table 22.3.

The appropriate selection of a damage control strategy remains a complex, multifactorial decision, and represents a particular challenge for the judgement of surgeons operating on the critically ill. The appropriateness of the decision will depend on the precise situation of the day, incorporating the whole clinical picture, including the system caring for the patient, as well as what has gone before, and what is likely to happen in the patient's projected trajectory.

Table 22.3 Selection criteria for a damage control strategy in abdominal emergencies

Patient factors	Medical and surgical history
	Concurrent illness
	Medication
Injury/disease factors	Nature of pathology
	Severity of pathology
	Expected natural history
Physiological factors	Hypothermia
	Coagulopathy
	Organ dysfunction
	Haemodynamic instability
	Severity of the inflammation/sepsis
Treatment factors	Magnitude and quality of resuscitation
	Duration and physiological effect of surgery
	The magnitude of the definitive surgery

22.5 The Open Abdomen

The laparostomy is a useful technical manoeuvre that decompresses the abdominal compartment and facilitates recurrent access to the peritoneal cavity with relative ease. Either, or both, of these goals are often present in the treatment of intra-abdominal catastrophes, both in trauma and emergency general surgical pathologies [1, 5, 10, 35–39]. However, the damage control strategy per se does not mandate an open abdomen. The same clinical judgement required to decide on the polyfactorial decision on the indication of a damage control strategy is critical while making the decision whether or not to use a laparostomy [10].

The high morbidity and mortality rates associated with abdominal compartment syndromes advocate a relatively low threshold to use a laparostomy in association with a damage control strategy [39–43]. Complications associated with the open abdominal techniques, and in particular the difficulties with delayed closures, appear to have been reduced with the most recently described techniques and prostheses. While the reduced rates have been attributed to these advances, advances in modern intensive care, including fluid management, early nutritional therapies, and general advances in surgical care, have all also likely contributed to these improvements [44]. Paradoxically, these advances are likely reducing the need for the damage control strategy overall.

22.6 Clinical Application

Potential clinical application in general surgical emergencies is greatly varied [15–32], and may apply in the situation of the primary presentation of the pathology, or during the treatment of an operative complication. Pathologies fall into one of two causes of shock: haemorrhagic or septic. The patients purported to have benefited from the damage control strategies (Table 22.2) include bleeding duodenal and gastric ulcers, uncontrolled venous bleeding during pancreatic surgery (pack and return to finish the surgery after resuscitation), gastro-intestinal perforations with generalised peritonitis (source control, staple off/isolate the septic source, and return to theatre for reconstruction after resuscitation), acute mesenteric ischaemia (resect the toxic and ischaemic bowel, only reconstructing after revascularisation and resuscitation), toxic megacolon (resect for source control, temporise for resuscitation, and return to theatre to restore intestinal continuity, perhaps without stoma, after resuscitation), and acute cholecystitis (with the use of a operatively placed cholecystostomy in the severe example, delaying the definitive cholecystectomy to a secondary surgery). In each case, an abbreviated surgical procedure is utilised to assist the initial resuscitation and treatment of the cause of shock: either the haemorrhage is arrested or the sepsis source controlled. Only after the physiology is normalised, the patient is then returned to the operating theatre, for anatomical restoration or definitive surgery.

Disclosures The authors have no conflicts of interest to declare. This manuscript is entirely the work of the authors.

Funding
No funding was received.

References

1. Waibel BH, Rotondo MF. Damage control for intra-abdominal sepsis. Surg Clin N Am. 2012;92:243–57.
2. Chovanes J, Cannon JW, Nunez TC. The evolution of damage control surgery. Surg Clin N Am. 2012;92:859–75.

3. Waibel BH, Rotondo MMF. Damage control surgery: its evolution over the last 20 years. Rev Col Bras Cir. 2012;39:314–21.
4. Rotondo MF, Zonies DH. The damage control sequence and underlying logic. Surg Clin N Am. 1997;77:761–77.
5. Moore EE. Staged laparotomy for the hypothermia, acidosis, and coagulopathy syndrome. Am J Surg. 1996;172:405.
6. Rotondo MF, Schwab CW, McGonigal MD, et al. "Damage control": an approach for improved survival in exsanguinating penetrating abdominal injury. J Trauma. 1993;35:375–82.
7. Stone H, Strom P, Mullins R. Management of the major coagulopathy with onset during laparotomy. Ann Surg. 1983;194:532–5.
8. Ivatury R, Nallathambi M, Gunduz Y, et al. Liver packing in uncontrolled haemorrhage: a reappraisal. J Trauma. 1986;26:744–53.
9. Burch JM, Ortiz VB, Richardson RJ, et al. Abbreviated laparotomy and planned reoperation for critically injured patients. Ann Surg. 1992;215:476–84.
10. Weber DG, Bendinelli C, Balogh ZJ. Damage control surgery for abdominal emergencies. Br J Surg. 2014;101:e109–18.
11. Leppäniemi AK. Damage control – a paradigm change in trauma and emergency surgery. Pol Przegl Chir. 2010;82:484–8.
12. Leppäniemi AK. Physiology and emergency surgery. Scand J Surg. 2006;95:135.
13. Moore LJ, Moore FA. Early diagnosis and evidence-based care of surgical sepsis. J Intensive Care Med. 2013;28:107–17.
14. Dellinger P, Levy MM, Rhodes A, et al. Surviving sepsis campaign: international guidelines for management of severe sepsis and septic shock: 2012. Crit Care Med. 2013;41:580–637.
15. Finlay IG, Edwards TJ, Lambert AW. Damage control laparotomy. Br J Surg. 2004;91:83–5.
16. Freeman AJ, Graham JC. Damage control surgery and angiography in cases of acute mesenteric ischaemia. ANZ J Surg. 2005;75:308–14.
17. Banieghbal B, Davies MR. Damage control laparotomy for generalized necrotizing enterocolitis. World J Surg. 2004;28:183–6.
18. Tamijmarane A, Ahmed I, Bhati CS, et al. Role of completion pancreatectomy as a damage control option for post-pancreatic surgical complications. Dig Surg. 2006;23:229–34.
19. Stawicki SP, Brooks A, Bilski T, et al. The concept of damage control: extending the paradigm to emergency general surgery. Injury. 2008;39:93–101.
20. Person B, Dorfman T, Bahouth H, Osman A, Assalia A, Kluger Y. Abbreviated emergency laparotomy in the non-trauma setting. World J Emerg Surg. 2009;4:41–4.

21. Ball CG, Correa-Gallego C, Howard TJ, Zyromski NJ, Lillemoe KD. Damage control principles for pancreatic surgery. J Gastrointest Surg. 2010;14:1632–3.

22. Filicori F, Di Saverio S, Casali M, Biscardi A, Baldoni F, Tugnoli G. Packing for damage control of nontraumatic intra-abdominal massive hemorrhages. World J Surg. 2010;34:2064–8.

23. Gong JF, Zhu WM, Wu XJ, Li N, Li JS. Damage control surgery for acute mesenteric ischemia. Shonghua Vei Chang Wai Ke Za Zhi. 2010;13:22–5.

24. Morgan K, Mansker D, Adams DB. Not just for trauma patients: damage control laparotomy in pancreatic surgery. J Gastrointest Surg. 2010;14:768–72.

25. Perathoner A, Klaus A, Mühlmann G, Oberwalder M, Margreiter R, Kafka-Ritsch R. Damage control with abdominal vacuum therapy (VAC) to manage perforated diverticulitis with advanced generalized peritonitis – a proof of concept. Int J Colorectal Dis. 2010;25:767–74.

26. Subramanian A, Balentine C, Palacio CH, Sansgiry S, Berger DH, Awad SS. Outcomes of damage-control celiotomy in elderly non-trauma patients with intra-abdominal catastrophes. Am J Surg. 2010;200:783–9.

27. Tadlock MD, Sise MJ, Riccoboni ST, et al. Damage control in the management of ruptured abdominal aortic aneurysm: preliminary results. Vasc Endovascular Surg. 2010;44:638–44.

28. Kafka-Ritsch R, Birkfellner F, et al. Damage control surgery with abdominal vacuum and delayed bowel reconstruction in patients with perforated diverticulitis Hinchey III/IV. J Gastrointest Surg. 2012;16:1915–22.

29. Khan A, Hsee L, Mathur S, Civil I. Damage control laparotomy I nontrauma patients: review of indications and outcomes. J Trauma. 2013;75:365–8.

30. Goussous N, Jenkins DH, Zielinski MD. Primary fascial closure after damage control laparotomy: sepsis vs haemorrhage. Injury. 2014;45:151–5.

31. Liu K, Meng J, Yang S, et al. Transcatheter trhomolysis combined with damage control surgery for treatment of acute mesenteric venous thrombosis associated with bowel necrosis: a retrospective study. World J Emerg Surg. 2015;10:50.

32. Nentwich MF, El Gammal AT, Lemcke T, et al. Salvage completion pancreatectomies as damage control for post-pancreatic surgery complications: a single centre retrospective analysis. World J Surg. 2015;39:1550–6.

33. Higa G, Friese R, O'Keeffe T, et al. Damage control laparotomy: a vital tool once overused. J Trauma. 2010;69:53–9.

34. Paul J, Ridolfi TJ. A case study in intra-abdominal sepsis. Surg Clin N Am. 2012;92:1661–7.

35. Mughal MM, Bancewicz J, Irving MH. Laparostomy: a technique for the management of intractable abdominal sepsis. Br J Surg. 1986;73:253–9.

36. Schein M, Saadia R, Freinkel Z, Decker GAG. Aggressive treatment of severe diffuse peritonitis: a prospective study. Br J Surg. 1988;75:173–6.

37. Ivatury RR, Nallathambi M, Rao PM, Rohman M, Stahl WM. Open management of the septic abdomen: therapeutic and prognostic considerations based on APACHE II. Crit Care Med. 1989;17:511–7.

38. Schein M. Planned reoperations and open management in critical intra-abdominal infections: prospective experience in 52 cases. World J Surg. 1991;15:537–45.

39. Moore F, Moore LJ. Damage control Laparotomy in Surgical Sepsis. In: Moore LJ, Turner KL, Todd SR, editors. Common problems in acute care surgery. New York: Springer; 2013.

40. Diaz JJ, Cullinane DC, Dutton WD, et al. The management of the open abdomen in trauma and emergency general surgery: part 1 – damage control. J Trauma. 2010;68:1425–38.

41. Pick AW, Mackay J. Laparostomy: a technique for the management of severe abdominal sepsis. ANZ J Surg. 1993;63:888–93.

42. Balogh Z, McKinley BA, Holcomb JB, et al. Both primary and secondary abdominal compartment syndrome can be predicted early and are harberingers of multiple organ failure. J Trauma. 2003;54:848–59.

43. Balogh Z, McKinley BA, Cox Jr CS, et al. Abdominal compartment syndrome: the cause or effect of postinjury multiple organ failure. Shock. 2003;20:483–92.

44. Balogh ZJ, Yoshino O. Abdominal compartment syndrome. In: Moore LJ, Turner KL, Todd SR, editors. Common problems in acute care surgery. New York: Springer; 2013.

Chapter 23
The Abdominal Compartment Syndrome

Dieter G. Weber and Zsolt J. Balogh

23.1 Introduction

The abdominal compartment syndrome (ACS) is a challenging clinical condition that may develop in a wide variety of clinical settings and which is associated with significant morbidity and mortality. The clinical syndrome was researched and described over one century ago [1], though practical management strategies in surgical specialties appeared only recently: Paediatric surgeons recognised problems with intra-abdominal pressure

D.G. Weber, MBBS (Hons.), FRACS
Departments of Trauma and General Surgery, Royal Perth Hospital, The University of Western Australia and The University of Newcastle, Newcastle, Australia
e-mail: dieter.weber@health.wa.gov.au

Z.J. Balogh, MD, PhD, FRACS, FACS (✉)
Department of Traumatology, Division of Surgery, John Hunter Hospital, The University of Newcastle, Lookout Rd, New Lambton Heights, NSW 2305, Australia
e-mail: zsolt.balogh@hnehealth.nsw.gov.au

© Springer International Publishing Switzerland 2017
S. Di Saverio et al. (eds.), *Acute Care Surgery Handbook*,
DOI 10.1007/978-3-319-15341-4_23

after the forced closure of omphalocoeles [2, 3], vascular surgeons recognised this entity following emergency aortic aneurysm repairs [4] and trauma surgeons experienced a high incidence during the initial experiences with damage control laparotomies [5–8]. More recently, these experiences have been applied into the field of emergency general surgery [9, 10].

Consensus definitions of the ACS and associated entities were published in 2006, and revised in 2013, by the World Society of the Abdominal Compartment Syndrome [9]. The ACS is defined as a sustained intra-abdominal pressure >20 mmHg and which is associated with new organ dysfunction/failure. Sustained intra-abdominal pressures of ≥12 mmHg are considered to represent intra-abdominal hypertension, and graded (I: 12–15 mmHg, II: 16–20 mmHg, III: 21–25 mmHg, and IV: >25 mmHg) [9]. No organ dysfunction is present in the case of pure intra-abdominal hypertension [9].

For both research and applied clinical practice, measurement of intra-abdominal pressure has been standardised by manometry of the intravesical, bladder pressure. This is referenced at the level of the mid-axillary line, following maximal instillation of 25 mL of sterile saline, with the patient in the supine position, at end expiration, and in the absence of abdominal muscle contraction [9].

23.2   Aetiology and Risk Factors

An ACS may be of a primary or secondary cause: Primary ACS refers to the syndrome arising in the presence of an inciting condition associated with injury or disease in the abdomino-pelvic region, while secondary ACS occurs in conditions not originating in the abdomino-pelvic region. In secondary ACS, the pathophysiological processes in the abdominal cavity appear to be the consequence and result of events elsewhere [9, 11].

Patients affected by ACS are typically critically ill and admitted in an intensive care environment. While all such patients are potentially at risk of the syndrome, patients usually exhibit one or more of the following risk factors: (1) reduced abdominal compliance (e.g. major burns, trauma, intra-abdominal inflammation), (2) increased intraluminal contents (e.g. intestinal ileus), (3) increased intra-abdominal contents (e.g. intra-abdominal sepsis, ascites, etc.), (4) local or generalised oedema due to permeability changes secondary to inflammation and infection and (5) some potential iatrogenic effects from resuscitation, intensive therapy or surgical interventions [2]. In addition, age, obesity, abdominal surgery, certain patient positions, mechanical ventilation and other manoeuvres resulting in increased intra-thoracic pressure, bacteriaemia, sepsis, metabolic derangement and shock have all been linked with the development of ACS [9, 12]. A recent meta-analysis identified large volume crystalloid resuscitation, the respiratory status of the patient and shock as common risk factors for ACS among a heterogeneous group of inciting pathologies. In this review, obesity, sepsis, abdominal surgery, and large volume fluid resuscitation were risk factors achieving statistical significance.

23.3 Pathophysiology

Fundamental in the development of an ACS, both primary and secondary, is a complex cellular and tissue oedema and hypoxia [11]. In turn, organ dysfunction ensues. With the deteriorating organ function, a viscous cycle develops, further adding to the cellular injury and inflammatory response. Excessive and injudicious crystalloid resuscitation has been particularly implicated in further compounding this cycle [13, 14].

The effects of the ACS on the body are extensive and widespread [11]. In the brain, increased venous pressure is measured.

In the heart, reduced cardiac return due to *vena cava* compression in association with peripheral venous pooling in the lower extremities and torso is seen. Cardiac contractility is reduced by direct compression, and increased cardiac effort is required due to changes in afterload. The thoracic volume is reduced and pulmonary ventilation impaired. The precarious ventilator situation is further complicated by the high risk of an acute lung injury/adult respiratory distress syndrome. Hepatic dysfunction and renal impairment are the result of direct vascular and tissue compression, as well as the inflammatory organ crosstalk. Altered and dysfunctional neuro-hormonal axes are also implicated. In the kidney, the post-renal urinary obstruction does not completely account for the organ's dysfunction; ureteric stenting and renal pelvis decompression does not lead to major clinical improvement. In the intestine, numerous changes in blood flow, mucosal integrity and bacterial translocation are seen. All these changes by the ACS effectively perpetuate the viscous cycle responsible for the secondary ACS.

Most non-traumatic, emergency general surgical conditions leading to an ACS are of a primary nature (i.e. abdomino-pelvic pathological origin) [15]. The location of the primary stimulus necessitates effective source control and potential removal of pathological volume as well as the management of the ACS within the same anatomical region. Rapid attention to both these endeavours is critical to facilitate interruption of the futile cycle. Secondary ACS could present in acute general surgical cases when extra-abdominal bleeding or sepsis requires massive resuscitation.

23.4   Epidemiology

In initial studies, the incidence of ACS in major trauma patients was higher than one-third [16–18], though more recent experience suggests this has much reduced during the last two decades [11]. The combination of modern resuscitation strategies, management of coagulopathy, damage control surgical strategies and modern anaesthesia and intensive care has been credited with this reduction in incidence. However, while the incidence has reduced, if untreated, the condition remains highly lethal, with mortalities in excess of 50 % [8]. Reported reductions in the mortality rate of ACS reflect the more timely diagnosis and treatment.

Early studies during the 2000s, into the prevalence of ACS among non-traumatic emergencies (both abdominal and elsewhere), suggested the presence of intra-abdominal hypertension in greater than 50 % of intensive care patients, and ACS around 2–5 % of patients. Similar to trauma patients, a high mortality rate was reported [19, 20]. Approximately two-thirds of patients experienced a primary ACS [15]. While the benefits of modern critical care and resuscitative strategies may predict a reducing incidence in recent years, alarming reports of continued high prevalence may be found. A recent series from the Netherlands on pancreatitis reports all patients at their institution experiencing intra-abdominal hypertension, and almost half fulfilling the diagnostic criteria for an ACS [21], and almost equally high incidences were reported in a Belgian series on severe burns patients [22].

23.5 Clinical Presentation

As most patients developing an ACS are unable to communicate symptoms due to their critical illness, or sedation for ventilation, symptoms are rarely reported. On examination, most patients will have a distended abdomen, though the sensitivity and specificity of this sign is poor [23–25]. Signs of organ dysfunction, particularly of renal and pulmonary, are common. Imaging is largely unhelpful (though there may be evidence of the secondary effects of the increased intra-abdominal pressures: *vena cava* compression, renal compression, bowel oedema, abdominal wall herniation, lung atelectasis and reduced volume, etc.) [26].

An ACS may rapidly develop (over hours), and a high clinical level of suspicion is required for its timely diagnosis. Ideally, continuous screening on all patients at risk could be obtained; unless active screening for ACS is undertaken, the diagnosis will likely be missed early in its clinical course. Due to practical and operational constraints, most centres will rely on intermittent measurement, using the standardised technique of urinary bladder pressure, on patients clinically thought to be at risk. Abnormal measurement results must then trigger a timely clinical response. Regretfully, delayed decision-making and tardy decompression are common, and associated with poor outcomes [8].

The precise clinical course will vary depending on the underlying cause of the ACS. For example, the clinical course of an ACS that develops in the setting of severe acute pancreatitis is different to that seen if an ACS develops in the setting of a small bowel obstruction. In acute pancreatitis, the ACS may develop as a primary phenomenon due to the pancreatic phlegmon and oedema in the retroperitoneal tissues. It may also occur as a secondary ACS, due to the systemic inflammatory response that develops during the first day or so of severe acute pancreatitis, in combination with the chosen fluid resuscitation strategy. In an adhesive small bowel obstruction, an ACS may develop from critical distension, and provide an absolute surgical indication, even though the adhesive small bowel obstruction may have otherwise settled. As another example, a septic phlegmon from acute sigmoid diverticulitis may cause a primary ACS both from the inflammatory phlegmon, associated retroperitoneal oedema, potential space occupied by abscess formation, and from the possible large bowel obstruction, or due to secondary events due to injudicious fluid resuscitation, or an associated severe systemic inflammatory phenomenon. Each of these clinical cases is fundamentally different, and the early presentation will be dominated in the underlying pathology. However, in all cases, an acute deterioration occurs with the onset of physiologic compromise associated with the ACS. In all cases, an acute surgical indication to deal with the ACS develops, though in addition to the abdominal decompression, the patient will need a tailored strategy to address the underlying cause. In most cases, the patient's acute physiologic compromise will dictate a damage control operative strategy [10]. The type of abdominal closure will also depend on the clinical situation, and is influenced by the primary pathology and its treatment strategy, the severity (and success of treatment) of the ACS, as well as patient and situational factors.

23.6 Treatment

Surgical decompression of the abdomen is the ultimate definitive manoeuvre in the treatment of an ACS [9]. An immediate decrease in the abdominal pressures is realised, and the decompression correlates well with returned organ function [27–29]. However, the invasive procedure is associated with significant morbidity and mortality [9, 11, 28].

The surgical decompression of the peritoneal cavity is usually performed through a midline laparotomy. This incision may also serve treatment of the underlying cause of the compartment syndrome, such as control of a septic source control, evacuation of ascites or control of haemorrhage, depending on the situation. However, other incisions, such as subcostal and transverse, are also described. Furthermore, endoscopic release of the linea alba, with maintenance of skin integrity, has also been successfully described [29]. The intact skin may assist reducing septic complications from a formal laparostomy; this is of particular relevance in acute pancreatitis with otherwise exposed necrotic tissues.

In conjunction with surgical decompression, various supportive adjuncts deserve consideration [9]. These less invasive therapies may avoid the need for decompression in cases of mild intra-abdominal hypertension, and where the primary cause for the potential ACS can be rectified early in the clinical course. These therapies include: sedation and analgesia, neuromuscular blockade, body positioning, nasogastric and colonic decompression, evacuation of ascites or other intra-peritoneal fluids, promotility agents, enhanced ratios of plasma/packed cells during the resuscitation of major haemorrhage, and a fluid balance protocol to attempt to avoid positive cumulative balance. Each of these strategies has been suggested by the recent consensus guidelines [9]. Diuretics, renal replacement therapies and albumin administration are not sufficiently studied for a consensus recommendation [9]. Judicious and considered use of traditional intensive care interventions used to support organ dysfunction may minimise potentially deleterious effects of these therapies on the pathophysiological processes causing the compartment syndrome in the first place [30, 31].

For trauma, prophylactic use of a temporary laparostomy in conjunction with a damage control surgical strategy is relatively accepted [32, 33]. However, for non-traumatic, emergency general surgical laparotomies, consensus does not support such prophylactic application in the absence of specific concerns [9]. This approach reflects modern, tailored surgical strategy, balancing the aggressiveness of the index operation, the need for a subsequent surgical procedures and the strength of the indication for a damage control strategy, in light of the quality of the resuscitation and intensive medical care received, and the unique patient and situational factors that define the individual case.

The management of the open abdomen is challenging, complex, highly individualised and is beyond the scope of this chapter. Central in this management is the ability to achieve primary fascial closure; early closure may minimise many of the long-term complications seen with this technique. Negative pressure wound management systems, both proprietary and home-made, are associated with improved primary fascial closure rates, and appear well tolerated by both the patient and staff [34–36]. The negative pressure may facilitate removal of pro-inflammatory cytokines and fluids from the peritoneal space [34–37]. Unfortunately, some concerns regarding enteric fistulisation rates remain.

23.7 Conclusion

ACS is a highly lethal condition, typically encountered in critically ill surgical patients. The epidemiology of the disease continues to change, particularly regarding a reduced incidence attributable to the evolution of modern resuscitation practices, damage control surgical strategies and an increasing understanding of the entity. A high index of suspicion and associated accurate and timely diagnosis is critical in the management of the ACS. The lessons learnt from the clinical experiences in trauma surgery have extended into emergency general surgery, and are applicable to both primary and secondary ACS. In the situation of non-traumatic abdominal emergencies, the ACS is commonly primary in nature, and separate attention to address this pathology will be required; source control of sepsis, and/or haemorrhage control, is essential, and requires careful incorporation into the overall clinical strategy. Surgical decompression remains the ultimate therapeutic intervention.

Disclosures The authors have no conflicts of interest to declare. This manuscript is the work of the authors.

Funding
No funding was received.

References

1. Schein M. Historical background. In: Ivatury R, Cheatham M, Malbrain M, Sugrue M, editors. Abdominal compartment syndrome. Georgetown: Landes Biosciences; 2006. p. 1–07.

2. Wesley JR, Drongowski R, Coran AG. Intragastric pressure measurement: a guide for reduction and closure of the silastic chimney in omphalocele and gastroschisis. J Pediatr Surg. 1981;16:264–70.

3. Hershenson MB, Brouillette RT, Klemka L, Raffensperger JD, Poznanski AK, Hunt CE. Respiratory insufficiency in newborns with abdominal wall defects. J Pediatr Surg. 1985;20:348–53.

4. Fietsam R, Villalba M, Glover JL, Clark K. Intra-abdominal compartment syndrome as a complication of ruptured abdominal aortic aneurysm repair. Am Surg. 1989;55:396–402.

5. Kron IL, Harman PK, Nolan SP. The measurement of intra-abdominal pressure as a criterion for abdominal re-exploration. Ann Surg. 1984;199:28–30.

6. Burch JM, Ortiz VB, Richardson RJ, Martin RR, Mattox KL, Jordan GL. Abbreviated laparotomy and planned reoperation for critically injured patients. Ann Surg. 1992;215:476–83.

7. Stone HH, Strom PR, Mullins RJ. Management of the major coagulopathy with onset during laparotomy. Ann Surg. 1983;197:532–5.

8. Morris JA, Eddy VA, Blinman TA, Rutherford EJ, Sharp KW. The staged celiotomy for trauma. Issues in unpacking and reconstruction. Ann Surg. 1993;217:576–84.

9. Kirkpatrick AW, Roberts DJ, de Waele J, et al. Intra-abdominal hypertension and the abdominal compartment syndrome: updated consensus definitions and clinical practice guidelines form the World Society of the Abdominal Compartment Syndrome. Intensive Care Med. 2013;39:1190.

10. Weber DG, Bendinelli C, Balogh ZJ. Damage control surgery for abdominal emergencies. Br J Surg. 2014;101:e109.

11. Balogh ZJ, Lumsdaine W, Moore EE, Moore FA. Post injury abdominal compartment syndrome: from recognition to prevention. Lancet. 2014;384:1466.

12. Holodinsky JK, Roberts DJ, Ball CG, et al. Risk factors for intra-abdominal hypertension and abdominal compartment syndrome among adult intensive care unit patients: a systematic review and meta-analysis. Crit Care. 2013;17:R249.

13. Balogh Z, McKinley BA, Cocanour CS, et al. Secondary abdominal compartment syndrome is an elusive early complication of traumatic shock resuscitation. Am J Surg. 2002;184:538.

14. Balogh Z, McKinley BA, Holcomb JB, et al. Both primary and secondary abdominal compartment syndrome can be predicted early and are harbingers of multiple organ failure. J Trauma. 2003;54:848.
15. Reintam A, Parm P, Kitus R, et al. Primary and secondary intraabdominal hypertension – different impact on ICU outcome. Intensive Care Med. 2008;34:1624.
16. Ivatury RR, Porter JM, Simon RJ, Islam S, John R, Stahl WM. Intraabdominal hypertension after life-threatening penetrating abdominal trauma: prophylaxis, incidence, and clinical relevance to gastric mucosal pH and abdominal compartment syndrome. J Trauma. 1998;44:1016–21.
17. Offner PJ, de Souza AL, Moore EE, et al. Avoidance of abdominal compartment syndrome in damage-control laparotomy after trauma. Arch Surg. 2001;136:676–81.
18. Raeburn CD, Moore EE, Biffl WL, et al. The abdominal compartment syndrome is a morbid complication of post injury damage control surgery. Am J Surg. 2001;182:542–6.
19. Malbrain ML, Chiumello D, Pelosi P, et al. Incidence and prognosis of intraabdominal hypertension in a mixed population of critically ill patients: a multiple centre epidemiological study. Crit Care Med. 2005;33:315.
20. Malbrain ML, Chiumello D, Pelosi P, et al. Prevalence of intraabdominal hypertension in critically ill patients: a multicenter epidemiological study. Intensive Care Med. 2004;30:822.
21. Smit M, Buddingh KT, Bosma B, et al. Abdominal compartment syndrome and intra-abdominal ischemia in patients with severe acute pancreatitis. World J Surg. 2016;40:1454–61.
22. Wise R, Jacobs J, Pilate S, et al. Incidence and prognosis of intraabdominal hypertension and abdominal compartment syndrome in severely burned patients: pilot study and review of the literature. Anaesthesiol Intensive Ther. 2015;48:95–109.
23. Malbrain ML, Cheatham ML, Kirkpatrick A, et al. Results from the international conference of experts on intra-abdominal hypertension and abdominal compartment syndrome. I. Definitions. Intensive Care Med. 2006;32:1722.
24. Kirkpatrick AW, Brenneman FD, McLean RF, et al. Is clinical examination an accurate indicator of raised intra-abdominal pressure in critically injured patients? Can J Surg. 2000;43:207.
25. Sugrue M, Bauman A, Jones F, et al. Clinical examination is an inaccurate predictor of intraabdominal pressure. World J Surg. 2002;26:1428.
26. Pickhardt PJ, Shimony JS, Heiken JP, et al. The abdominal compartment syndrome: CT findings. AJR Am J Roentgenol. 1999;173:575.
27. De Waele J, Desender L, De Laet I, et al. Abdominal decompression for abdominal compartment syndrome in critically ill patients: a retrospective study. Acta Clin Belg. 2010;65:399.

28. De Waele JJ, Hoste EA, Malbrain ML. Decompressive laparotomy for abdominal compartment syndrome – a critical analysis. Crit Care. 2006;10:R51.

29. De Waele JJ, Kimball E, Malbrain M, et al. Decompressive laparotomy for abdominal compartment syndrome. Br J Surg. 2016;103:709.

30. Sugrue M, D'Amours S. The problems with positive end expiratory pressure (PEEP) in association with abdominal compartment syndrome (ACS). J Trauma. 2001;51:419.

31. Burch JM, Moore EE, Moore FAC, Franciose R. The abdominal compartment syndrome. Surg Clin North Am. 1996;76:833.

32. Kirkpatrick AW, Ball CG, D'Amours SK, Zygun D. Acute resuscitation of the unstable adult trauma patient: bedside diagnosis and therapy. Can J Surg. 2008;51:57.

33. Sugrue M, D'Amours SK, Joshipura M. Damage control surgery and the abdomen. Injury. 2004;35:642.

34. Dalfino L, Tullo L, Donadio I, et al. Intra-abdominal hypertension and acute renal failure in critically ill patients. Intensive Care Med. 2008;34:707.

35. Miller RP, Thompson JT, Faler BJ, et al. Late facial closure in lieu of ventral hernia; the next step in open abdomen management. J Trauma. 2002;53:843.

36. Miller RP, Meredith JW, Johnson JC, et al. Prospective evaluation of vacuum assisted fascial closure after open abdomen: planned ventral hernia rate is substantially reduced. Ann Surg. 2004;239:608.

37. Batacchi S, Matano S, Nella A, et al. Vacuum assisted closure device enhances recovery of critically ill patients following emergency surgical procedures. Crit Care. 2009;13:R194.

Chapter 24
Common Pediatric Surgical Emergencies

Andreas Fette

24.1 Head and Face

Caput Succedaneum   Cephalic swelling of the protruding part of the head caused by blood or lymphatic congestion. The swelling usually exceeds all sutures, and decreases within a few days and does not need any further treatment.

> *** Immediate emergency surgery/intervention
> ** Emergency surgery/intervention
> * Urgent surgery

A. Fette
Department of Pediatric and Adolescent Medicine and
Pediatric Surgery, Klinikstr. 11. 78052
Villingen-Schwenningen, Germany

University of Pécs, Medical School, Pécs, Hungary
e-mail: andreas.fette@gmx.de

© Springer International Publishing Switzerland 2017
S. Di Saverio et al. (eds.), *Acute Care Surgery Handbook*,
DOI 10.1007/978-3-319-15341-4_24

Galea Hematoma   Detachment injury of the periosteum or galea aponeurotica due to the shear forces happening during delivery. The swelling is always terminated by the sutures of the skull. In up to 50 % such a hematoma is associated with a skull fracture. The high blood loss into such a hematoma (in newborns) can cause anemia or even hemorrhagic shock requiring immediate *blood transfusion(s)***.

Hydrocephalus (Communicating or Noncommunicating)   The cardinal clinical features found in an infant with hydrocephalus are (i) accelerated head growth of the baby (head circumference charts!), (ii) full fontanelle and, separation of the skull sutures, and (iii) "sun setting" phenomena of the eyes. The two key diagnostics are an ultrasound scan via the (still) open fontanelle and a MRI. The classical surgical approach is implantation of a shunt system (= implantable silastic catheter with or without a pressure valve), where the central tip is placed inside the lateral ventricle, while the other end is placed in the peritoneal cavity (VP-shunt), the atrium of the heart (AV-shunt), and the pleural space or externally. An alternative (in noncommunicating) hydrocephalus is the endoscopic third ventriculotomy (ETV), where a fenestration by endoscope is made in the floor of the third ventricle to allow the cerebral spine fluid (CSF) to flow directly into the subarachnoidal space. Generally speaking, the "shunt" serves as an alternative pathway for the drainage of the (accumulated) CSF. The *timing of surgery* depends on the actual intracerebral/intraventricular pressure. Malfunction (due to blockage or dislocation/shortness of the tube) or infection is the most common problem seen after shunt insertion. That is why insertion under highly aseptic criteria and perioperative antibiotic prophylaxis is of key importance.

Nasal Bleeding/Epistaxis   Active nasal bleeding in children should be treated by *manual compression*** of the nostrils around the loci Kieselbachii, tamponade, and/or application of cold packs. In any case, put the child in an upright position to avoid aspiration. The most common cause is irritation of the mucosal vessels. If not the child should be transferred to an ENT specialist.

Foreign Bodies in the Nose or Ear   Following their behavioral instinct to explore everything by hand and mouth, infants and younger children do suffer such incidents quite frequently. Extraction by minimal invasive techniques (curved forceps, small speculas) is mandatory and possible in the majority of cases, if performed under general anesthesia or deep sedation, gently. In complicated cases ENT specialist's expertise might be useful.

Facial and Skull Cuts   Cuts of the skull are usually impressive, because of their excessive bleeding. This bleeding is controlled best by *firm digital compression on the wound margins**. Frazzled wound margins can be excised. These cuts are usually treated best *by deep bite layer sutures** in the galea and skin. A spray glue dressing is preferable to any other dressing because hairs sticking together cause pain during dressing changes and removals. In facial cuts wound margins should never be excised! If in need the margins should be refreshed only by gentle abrasion by a sharp scalpel blade. Suturing in the face should always be intracuticular using fine suture materials. To avoid removal of suture material, whenever possible, absorbable sutures should be used. To minimize scarring, esthetic plastic surgery techniques should be your first preference.

24.2 Neck

Foreign Bodies   Ingestion – esophagus (i.e., meat piece, button battery, coin); aspiration – trachea (i.e., peanut, pencil rubber, pin): "swallowing" usually happens during play, and since the majority of these patients are less than 6 years of age, every clinician must maintain a high index of suspicion. This is because parents and siblings would have noticed only "something" in the mouth of the children and together they would be able to give only a vague history of the incident. "Excessive salivation", "wheezing", and "chocking" are possible symptoms, but quite often the "swallows" are asymptomatic. Thus, if you suspect an ingestion or aspiration of a radio-opaque foreign body, an X-ray study (anteroposterior and lateral view), including the neck and nasopharynx, is recommended to localize it. *Esophageal foreign bodies*** will mainly be trapped in one of the three esophageal narrowings, while in the trachea-bronchial tree, they will mainly be trapped in the right mainstem bronchus. Especially, if located *in the trachea or the bronchial tree, immediate retrieval**** (by rigid/flexible scope) after visualization of the foreign object should be obtained. Aspirated peanuts can germinate and cause mycotic inflammatory reactions, besides hyperinflation, atelectasis, air trapping, shifting, and pneumonia. If the foreign body has already reached the stomach, it will be drained via the natural way in almost all cases. If it is still stuck into the esophagus, the foreign body should either be recovered transorally or gently pushed into the stomach for further "digestion". Extremely dangerous are retained ingested batteries or magnets since their current or acid leaking out can cause tissue damage like perforation, stricture, or fistulas.

Caustic Esophageal Injury   Acids and alkalis from household cleaners are mostly ingested by children <5 years of age or adolescent girls attempting to commit suicide. Strong alkalis tend to injure the proximal pharynx and esophagus and cause lesions with liquid necrosis. Strong acids, on the other hand, cause coagulation necrosis and result in more distal injuries of the esophagus and even stomach wall. More superficial mucosal injuries might resolve without any long-term sequelae. However, deeper lesions always heel by fibrosis and subsequent stricture formation. Every full thickness lesion even has the potential for perforation and fistula formation. Finally, such complications can require esophageal resection or even replacement. If you see a caustic ingestion the first step must be *to establish the patency of the airway***!* Because the resulting inflammatory swelling of the tissue can rapidly obstruct the airway, making emergency endotracheal intubation or even tracheostomy necessary to save the child. To induce vomiting is strictly contraindicated! This is because the (re-)regurgitation of the caustic substance bears the risk of reinjury to the mucosa and secondary aspiration pneumonia. *Endoscopic inspection*** is the second step. It is best done very gently within 24–48 h. A common endoscopic grading system is given: $0° =$ normal, $I° =$ mucosal edema with hyperemia, $IIa° =$ superficial lesion, $IIb° =$ sl + limited areas of deep or circumferential injury, $IIIa° =$ small (scattered) areas of necrosis, $IIIb° =$ extensive necrosis. A contrast study (with water soluble contrast media!!) is usually done 2–3 weeks after the incident to determine the presence and length of strictures. It should be done at first presentation as well, if a perforation is highly suspected. If the study shows free air, or the evidence of contrast media, either in the peritoneal or mediastinal cavity, *emergency surgical exploration*** is indicated.

Purulent Lymph Nodes/Abscess   Every child has at least one "palpable" cervical lymph node. By definition, any cervical lymph node is considered to be enlarged, if it is more than 1 cm at its longest diameter. Any palpable supraclavicular node is considered as abnormal per definition as well. The assessment of a child with lymphadenopathy requires a thorough history taking and physical examination; especially, the onset and duration of symptoms (e.g., recent animal bites or scratches, contact with infectious diseases, Epstein-Barr, cytomegalovirus, travel abroad, etc.) and the exact numbers of enlarged lymph nodes should be reported. On physical examination, hyperplastic lymph nodes in response to viral infections are small, discrete, mobile, nontender, and bilateral. Usually, they are not accompanied by cellulitis or periadenitis. Pyogenic nodes (caused by Staph aureus, Strept pyogenes infections), on the other hand, tend to be unilaterally large, warm, and tender with surrounding erythema and edema. Nodes associated with malignancy are generally firm or hard, discrete, and nontender. Staph aureus infections are most commonly seen in children between 1 and 4 years of age. Fluctuation occurs in one-fourth of patients. If fluctuation is present, antibiotics are administered and *purulence is drained surgically under general anesthesia**. Cat scratch disease (*Bartonella* species) is usually self-limiting, therefore, a surgical intervention is unnecessary.

Tongue Bites + Lip Cuts, Tooth Trauma   Fast hemostasis** in tongue bites is key. Then the wound is closed by interrupted, inverted, and fast absorbable sutures. Besides the hemostasis, the *exact reconstruction of the lip vermilion** is essential. In tooth trauma all pieces should be preserved and the child transferred to a dentist.

Tracheal Stenosis: Malacia   These infants demonstrate expiratory stridor, which results in episodes of oxygen desaturation, apnea, cyanosis, and bradycardia. Such episodes are often life threatening and associated with feeding and therefore called "dying episodes". The lumen of the trachea is compressed anterior–posterior in a scabbard-like deficiency. The real extent is assessed by *bronchoscopy under spontaneous respiration***. Since tracheomalacia can be self-limiting surgical intervention (e.g., aortopexy, tracheostomy, stenting) is only indicated in patients with repeated life-threatening symptoms.

24.3 Chest

Newborn Mastitis   Mastitis neonatorum is the result of an ongoing physiological swelling of the mammarian glands. It is triggered by the residual maternal estrogen hormone level. The swelling is usually painful and the whole gland is hardened. Trying to press out the colostrum can increase the frequency of infections, ending up quite often in localized abscess formation. First signs are high fever and inflamed and painful mammarian glands with discharge of pus and high fever. Mastitis neonatorum is treated by broad spectrum antibiotics *and incision and drainage of abscesses** (cave cosmetic and gland sparing incision techniques!).

Pleura Empyema   Accumulation of infected fluid within the pleural space is defined as empyema. The most common cause in children is infected parapneumonic fluid. Others include postoperative or posttraumatic (hematothorax) infections, or spreading from other infections like retropharyngeal or mediastinal abscesses. Usually, these children present with high fever, dull chest pain, cough, and dyspnea. Diagnosis is made by absent breathing sounds and dullness to percussion at the lung bases. In addition (massive) fluid collection in US scan or plain X-ray. All patients require antibiotics and *thoracocentesis**. In accordance to the clinical course pleural debridement by thoracotomy or more preferable thoracoscopy will be needed.

Hemato-/Pneumo-/Chylothorax   Pneumothorax is defined as an accumulation of free air, hemato- as accumulation of blood, and chylothorax as accumulation of chylus (lymphatic fluid) within the pleural space. A pneumothorax can happen spontaneously, by rupture of a subpleural bleb, secondary to an increased alveolar pressure (e.g., during mechanical ventilation). Or, even combined, hemato-/pneumothorax can be associated with a blunt or penetrating chest trauma and can be the result from a medical intervention like central venous catheter insertion or bronchoscopy. In tension pneumothorax the ipsilateral hemithorax is filled up with air/blood, the diaphragm is depressed, and the intercostal spaces on the ipsilateral side are expanded in comparison to the opposite side. Therefore, the mediastinal structures shift to the contralateral side causing respiratory compromise. Most common signs and symptoms are the sudden onset of dyspnea, lateralized chest pain, and diminished breath sounds on the ipsilateral side. *Patients with a (tension) pneumothorax require emergency evacuation of the air/blood****. A congenital or idiopathic chylothorax is noted in the first week of life. It is thought to be secondary to an injury to the thoracic duct or one of its branches during birth. Treatment starts with diet, octreotide acetate followed by evacuation of the chylus by either thoracocentesis or tube thoracostomy, and (finally) ligation of the thoracic duct.

Persistent Ductus Arteriosus Botalli (PDA)   During the fetal life, most of the blood circulates through the ductus arteriosus into the descending aorta. Postpartal, this circuit is functional and anatomically closed. The neonate with a persistent PDA, therefore, presents with dyspnea, rapid fatigue, intensive sweating as common signs of his/her heart failure. Therapeutic options are closure by *indomethacin medication**** or *surgical ligation**, via either thoracoscopic or open approach.

Esophagus Atresia (EA): Tracheo-Esophageal Fistula (TEF) Newborns with EA/TEF often have difficulties in clearing their saliva, demonstrate episodes of coughing, chocking, and even cyanosis quite shortly after birth. Attempts to feed the children result in immediate distress. In the clinical setting the diagnosis is confirmed by the failure to pass a firm NGT into the stomach. The classical antenatal sonogram shows the absence of air in the gastric area and the associated polyhydramnion. Postnatally, contrast studies (water-soluble contrast media, careful!), US, and (rigid) bronchoscopy are used to confirm the diagnosis. Common types of esophageal atresia and trachea-esophageal fistula are given: A: proximal esophageal atresia with distal trachea-esophageal fistula (TEF) (85–90 %); B: isolated esophageal atresia (5–7 %); C: TEF without esophageal atresia (2–6 %). Rare forms include atresia with proximal TEF (<1 %) and esophageal atresia with both proximal and distal TEF (<1 %). Associated anomalies (e.g., cardiac 27 %, urogenital 18 %, skeletal 12 %, vertebral 11 %, anorectal 12 %, gastrointestinal, and palate/laryngotracheal 8 %, VACTERL 19 %) are found in approximately half of these newborns. Some of them seem to be quite insignificant; however, a high proportion are even life-threatening and contribute directly to the high morbidity and mortality in this population. As soon as the diagnosis is confirmed, iv fluids and a *Replogle tube**** (sump suction catheter device) are administered, and the baby will be nursed in the supine or lateral position. In an otherwise healthy baby, *surgery is* performed ideally within the first 24 h**. Most preferable during an "elective" procedure since aspiration (pneumonia) and gastric acid reflux through the lower pouch, TEF are a constant risk. Using the classical approach the baby is positioned in a slightly right lateral elevated position with the right arm raised across the head. The right thoracotomy starts with a curved skin crease incision 1 cm below the angle of the scapula, extending from the anterior axillary line to the lateral margin of the erector spini muscles. After dividing the latissimus, the chest is opened through the fourth intercostal space. The pleura is carefully separated from the ribs to start an extrapleural approach (vs. transpleural approach) towards the TEF. The posterior mediastinal pleura is retracted forward until the azygos vein is visible, at the junction where it enters the superior vena cava. After mobilization the azygos vein is ligated and divided as it enters the cava. Now the fistulous communication between the trachea and distal esophagus is accessible. The distal esophagus and the TEF are identified, the fistula is ligated and cut off. To test TEF repair some N/S is installed into the thorax cavity and the anesthetist asked to exert positive air way pressure to see that no air bubbles leak from the suture line. Be aware, it is quite possible to mobilize the descending aorta in the erroneous impression that this is the distal esophagus!!. To identify the upper pouch the anesthetist is requested to push firmly on the reploge tube. The upper pouch is marked and dissected by bipolar diathermy. Important note: it is a general rule in pediatric surgery to mobilize only the proximal pouch and not the distal one!!. This is because the proximal esophagus can be mobilized better due to its superior intramural blood supply. Mobilizing the distal one instead can disrupt the tenuous bronchial arterial supply and lead to ischemia of the anastomosis. Finally, the two stumps are anastomized directly with fine interrupted polydioxane suture over a NGT placed into the lumen. If the procedure has been strictly extrapleural no chest tube is needed. If the repair has been transpleural or you are in any doubt, it is recommended to place a drain. Long gap EA with distal TEF should undergo cervical esophagostomy and feeding gastrostomy, accepting the need for an esophageal replacement surgery (e.g., extension/expander techniques (Foker), esophagus replacement, or limited (Thal) fundoplication at a later stage). A thoracoscopic approach is nowadays also feasible and safe. Serious complications are recurrent TEF (6–10 %), stenosis/stricture (15 %), dysphagia (10–20 %), GERD (up to 50 %), or anastomosis leak (10 %).

Congenital Diaphragmatic Hernia (CDH)   Failure of the pleuroperitoneal canal to close at 8–10 weeks of GA leads to a defect in the dorsolateral region of the diaphragm. Bowel loops returning from the yolk sac start to herniate through this defect into the chest and form the CDH. Eighty percent of CDHs happen on the left side, 19 % on the right, and 1 % is bilateral. Liver herniation, low lung-to-head-ratio, and made <25 weeks of GA are three important prenatal findings that identify those fetuses, who are likely to have a poor outcome with conventional treatment after birth. The posterolateral defect (Bochdalek hernia) is the most common type and it can range from a small defect to almost a complete agenesis of the diaphragmatic tissue. Others, less common, are the anteromedial defect (Morgagni hernia) or the central weakening of the diaphragm (diaphragmatic eventration). The management of the fetus with CDH should be carried out in a multidisciplinary team. It starts with prenatal counseling and discussion if prenatal or even fetal therapies (e.g., FETO, EXIT) are possible. The future management of the pregnancy and delivery is organized in a way that the birth can take place in a tertiary center. The transport into this institution should be most preferable "in utero". After birth, all efforts should be made to avoid gastric and bowel distension from mask ventilation. An endotracheal and a nasogastric tube are inserted. Pre- and postductal oxygen saturation can be measured to assess the degree of arterial oxygenation and ductal shunting. Surfactant might be administered, ventilator settings such as HFV, NO, and ECMO are chosen accordingly. The "honeymoon period" is a time when the neonate with a CDH demonstrates adequate oxygenation and low ventilator parameters in the absence of maximal medical therapy. It suggests that actually pulmonary tissue and function may be very compatible with life, but subsequent deterioration can always happen and be deleterious!! The pathophysiology of this phenomenon is complex but may relate to iatrogenic ventilator barotrauma and/or oxygen-induced injury via free radical release. The optimal time for surgery is after first medical stabilization. This delayed surgical repair is an attempt to improve the overall condition of the neonate, beforehand. *The key goal in management of CDHs is the surgical repair of the diaphragmatic defect, either in an open or -scopic (abdominal/thoracic) technique***. Briefly, the abdominal viscera/contents of the hernia are gently reduced. Visualization of the ipsilateral lung and the diaphragmatic defect and its margins. If the margins are mobilizable enough the defect is closed by interrupted nonabsorbable sutures. If the defect is too large, prosthetic material or an adjacent muscle flap might be used. Short- and long-term complications are given: chest deformities, pulmonary hypertension, recurrence, baro trauma, and infections.

24.4   Abdomen/Gastrointestinal Tract (GIT)

Hypertrophic Pyloric Stenosis   In hypertrophic pyloric stenosis the circular muscle of the pylorus is so hypertrophic that it narrows and elongates the pyloric channel. The usual onset of symptoms occur between 3 and 6 weeks of life. Vomiting, characteristically projectile and free of bile, next to dehydration and weight loss, due to inadequate fluid and caloric intake, soon become apparent. The visible gastric

peristalsis and the palpable pyloric tumor are other important clinical findings. Chloride depletion and metabolic
alkalosis are concomitant lab findings. The final diagnosis
nowadays is made by ultrasonography. If the pylorus presents as a hypoechoic ring with an echogenic center, the
pyloric diameter and length are enlarged and the muscle
thickness is 4 mm or more, the diagnosis of a hypertrophic
pyloric stenosis is confirmed. *Preoperative, electrolyte levels,
and dehydration need to be corrected**** before *Ramstedt's
pylorotomy** (splitting of the pylorus muscle until mucosa
bulges into the split incision) by an open, laparoscopic, or
Bianchi approach is performed. Complications are duodenal perforation, which is usually the result of excessive tissue separation at the distal end of the pylorus, or the
"recurrence" due to the incomplete splitting of the muscle
(in up to 8 % of cases).

Obstruction of the Intestine/Ileus   A simple bowel obstruction occurs when one end of the bowel lumen is obstructed.
This simple bowel obstruction may be complete or incomplete. In a closed loop bowel obstruction both the proximal
and the distal end of this (part of intestine) are obstructed.
Closed loop obstruction usually occurs when a loop of
bowel has herniated through a narrow orifice, such as an
indirect inguinal hernia or a mesenteric defect, or when
adhesive bands have formed (=incarceration). A volvulus
may produce a closed loop obstruction in the absence of a
compromised blood supply as well (=strangulation). Closed
loop obstruction can also occur in the large bowel when a
distal obstruction happens, and the colonic contents start to
distend this isolated loop/part more and more, because they
cannot decompress into the small bowel, because of the
intact ileocecal valve. In a closed loop obstruction, the
bowel grows progressively dilated from the accumulated
secretions. Over time, the increasing pressure within the

lumen is transmitted to the bowel wall and eventually exceeds the perfusion pressure of the circulation resulting in gangrene. Typical signs and symptoms are given: pain (dull, crampy), vomiting (greenish-brown, bilious, feculent odor), and abdominal distension. Auscultation of the abdomen reveals high pitched tinkles at irregular and random intervals, with occasional periods of hyperactive bowel sounds that lasts for seconds or minutes. Plain radiographs of the abdomen, supine and upright, are necessary; ultrasound scans can be helpful on the bedside. Common causes of bowel obstruction are given: intussusception, fecal impaction (e.g., NID), adhesions (e.g., due to previous surgeries, scars), inflammation/peritonitis (e.g., perforated appendicitis), enterocolitis, Hirschsprung's Disease, hernia, meconium ileus/plug, volvulus, malformations (e.g., atresia, duplication), and neoplasms. The principle surgical advice for all bowel obstructions is, "Never let the sun rise or set on a bowel obstruction". *The laparotomy/laparoscopy is always indicated as soon as possible***!*

Malrotation and Midgut Volvolus   During the fourth week of the embryonic life, the intestines move outside the abdominal wall and into the base of the umbilical cord. As soon as the bowel matures and enlarges (~tenth week of GA) the intestine returns back to the abdominal cavity. Rotation and fixation are completed 1 week later. The direction of the rotation during this process is 270° counterclockwise. Proper placement is evidenced and when the ligament of Treitz is fixed left to the spine and the cecum is located in the right lower quadrant. Since normal rotation is defined to be 270°, any rotation that is less has some elements of malrotation. Nonrotation or return of the gut to the abdomen without rotation is found in 0.5–2 % of cases and is rarely pathologic. Since malrotation can show various degrees of rotation, the exact placement of the GI tract can vary. However, the most common findings are that the duodenum does not cross the midline and that the cecum is high riding or superior to the transverse colon in the left upper quadrant. Not necessarily all patients become symptomatic, but most do so at a very young age. Bilious (green) vomiting is the leading symptom (>95 %) in patients with malrotation and midgut volvulus. The most common scenario is green vomiting for no reason in an infant who has (initially) a flat abdomen, is afebrile, and has not been previously ill. Soon the infant can become jittery, tachycardic, pale, and diaphoretic. Since unexplained bilious vomiting in an infant is a surgical emergency, an immediate upper GI study (most preferable) or a contrast enema is ordered to determine the position of the duodenojejunal junction (ligament of Treitz) and the position of the cecum in the RLQ. Ultrasound may suggest malrotation, if the superior mesenteric vein (SMV) lies not to the right of the superior mesenteric artery (SMA). If still in doubt, *quick and expeditious operative intervention must follow*, otherwise the baby might be dead within <6 h. Surgery is usually performed via an upper abdominal transverse incision. After entering the peritoneal cavity the ischemic bowel becomes visible, immediately. Midgut volvulus (MGV) is characterized by a 270° twist of the bowel around the axis of the superior mesenteric artery (SMA). The bowel is either normal, blue to black, or frankly necrotic. It is derotated counterclockwise (because MGV is always a clockwise twist of the bowel around the SMA axis), packed into warm saline gauze packs, and reperfusion is observed for several minutes. After the bowel has recovered a Ladd's procedure is performed (cutting off the Ladd's bands, returning back the bowel into the abdomen in nonrotated position by placing the entire small bowel on the right, the large bowel on the left, and the cecum in the left upper quadrant). The operation is concluded with an incidental appendectomy. If you encounter necrotic bowel during surgery, it has to be resected and a stoma created. If you have to resect a lot of bowel, you will have to face the short bowel syndrome and should decide accordingly. Midgut volvulus, in which the mesenteric blood supply to the bowel becomes twisted is the obvious example of strangulation obstruction. Another example is "closed loop obstruction". This strangulation obstruction occurs, when the circulation to a segment of intestine is impaired. The first step in sequence is venous compression, since arterial pressure is not yet compromised. The bowel wall and lumen become hemorrhagic with blood, the subsequent cessation of all blood flow produces the infarction and gangrene. This unique combination out of bacteria, toxins, blood, and necrotic tissue is particularly lethal, because the final result is septic shock and multiorgan failure with a high mortality rate. Since ischemia always progresses to gangrene, *prompt surgical intervention* *** and repair is key.

Meconium Plug Syndrome/Meconium Ileus (MI)   Is a bowel obstruction caused by inspissated meconium (higher protein, lower carbohydrate concentration, increased viscosity, decreased water content) in the newborn (with Cystic Fibrosis (CF)). In CF patients it is the earliest clinical manifestation. MI can either be simple (bowel dilatation, wall thickening, and congestion) or complicated (associated with volvulus, atresia, necrosis perforation, meconium peritonitis, or pseudocyst formation). Simple MI presents with abdominal distension at birth, failure to pass meconium, and bilious vomiting. Dilated loops of bowel become apparent and they have a doughy character that indents on palpation. Typically, the anus and rectum are narrow (nonused). On abdominal radiographs simple MI is characterized by unevenly dilated bowel loops with variable presence of air fluid levels. Sonographic characteristics include hyperechoic masses, dilated bowel, and nonvisualization of the gallbladder. Complicated MI presents more dramatically with abdominal wall erythema and edema and distension may be sufficiently enough to cause respiratory distress. There are signs of peritonitis and sepsis, a palpable mass can indicate a pseudocyst formation. Speckled calcifications on plain abdominal films are highly suggestive for an intrauterine perforation of the intestine and meconium peritonitis. A large dense mass with a rim of calcification is suggestive of a pseudocyst formation. Often the neonate is really sick and needs urgent resuscitation and management. If the infant shows no clinical or radiological signs of complications, and the infant is well prepared with *adequate fluid and electrolyte replacement as well as normothermia an enema is done under fluoroscopic control****. Thereby, under fluoroscopic control Gastrografin® solution is infused slowly and with low hydrostatic pressure through a catheter into the rectum. *Warm saline enemas containing acetylcysteine follow to complete the evacuation***. Usually semiliquid meconium passes out during the next 24–48 h. Radiographs are taken to confirm full evacuation and to exclude late perforation as clinically indicated. Serial enemas might be necessary, supported by oro-gastric administration of Gastrografin® and acetylcysteine. The major complication is rectal perforation. The main goal of surgical management in simple MI is the evacuation of the meconium from the lumen with preservation of as much bowel as possible. *Surgery is always indicated in all cases of complicated MI*** (progressive distension, signs of peritonitis, clinical deterioration). Surgical techniques include placement of indwelling ostomy tubes for postoperative bowel irrigation, decompression and/or feeding, resection of intestine followed by primary anastomosis or formation of a stoma, single or double barreled, in Bishop-Koop or Santulli technique.

Intussusception   It is the full-thickness invagination of the proximal bowel into the distal contiguous one. The proximal invaginating part is termed the intussusceptum, the distal receiving (=outer) part is the intussuscipiens. Most commonly affected are children between 3 months and 3 years of age. They usually present with crampy abdominal pain and distension, vomiting and dehydration, rectal bleeding, abdominal mass, and profound lethargy. Red currant jelly stools (=mixture out of intraluminal fluid, blood, and mucosal tissue fragments) are the most typical finding in these patients. Ileocolic – the ileum invaginates into the cecum or right colon – is the most common form of intussusception. Intussusception usually starts with a viral gastroenteritis or respiratory infection that results in a hyperplasia of the distal ileal lymphoid tissue. That hyperplasia is frequently blamed to initiate the process of intussusception (=leading point). The diagnosis is confirmed by contrast enema (fist or coiled spring sign) or ultrasound scan (target or bullet sign). After insertion of a *drip, rehydration, nasogastric and rectal tube decompression hydrostatic or pneumatic reduction**** is attempted. Maybe several attempts are needed (and allowed to do). However, *irreducibility, perforation, shock, and hemodynamic instability are clear indications for urgent operative treatment***. Gentle manipulation by pushing the intussceptum out of the intussusipiens (rather than by pulling it with traction) frequently results in successful reduction. If reduction is accomplished, no further intervention is required. If injuries to the bowel wall, necrosis or perforation, or a pathological leading point identified, resection and primary anastomosis are indicated.

Necrotizing Enterocolitis (NEC)/Focal Intestinal Perforation (FIP)   With regard to the neonate's intestine necrotizing enterocolitis (NEC) is the most common medical and surgical emergency. Focal intestinal perforation (FIP) appears to be a distinct clinical entity that occurs mainly in very low birth weight (VLBW) infants, where it finally accounts for the high percentage of gastrointestinal perforations. NEC is considered as a "disease of prematurity" with a high rate of morbidity and mortality. The onset of NEC is strongly associated with the initiating of feeding and its osmolarity. Compromised intestinal immune function, cytokines, and nitric oxide are other important factors. The most common sites of involvement are the terminal ileum, followed by the colon. The NEC can involve single or multiple segments, and nearly the entire intestine (pannecrosis). NEC cases usually have abdominal distension with an erythematous abdominal wall, signs of sepsis, (hemato)emesis, and (gross or occult) rectal bleeding. The abdomen may feel firm due to the abdominal wall edema. Characteristic findings in plain X-rays and ultrasonography are distended bowel, pneumatosis intestinalis, dilated bowel loops (fixed loop sign), portal venous air, pneumoperitoneum, and ascites. NEC usually is classified according to Bell: (I) infants with features suggestive of NEC. (II) infants with definitive NEC. (III) infants with evidence of bowel necrosis and clinical deterioration. *Nonoperative management of a NEC consists of nasogastric decompression, total parenteral nutrition, broad spectrum antibiotics, and bowel rest***. Major indications for surgery are deteriorating clinical course and abdominal wall erythema, free air in the abdomen, fixed loop sign, and/or an abdominal mass**.*

During surgery preserving as much viable intestine as possible is of key importance. Only perforated or clearly diseased/necrotic bowel should be resected. After resection, either a proximal stoma and anastomoses of the distal defunctionalized segments or multiple stomas are created. The stoma or mucous fistula can be brought out through your abdominal incision. Stoma closure will be performed after complete rehabilitation of the intestine. Common long-term complications include strictures and short bowel syndrome. In summary, despite the fact that most cases of early NEC can be managed successfully nonoperative, prompt surgical intervention is usually required for advanced or perforated NEC and virtually all FIPs.

Duodenal Atresia/Intestinal Atresia   In duodenal atresia prenatal ultrasound demonstrates a dilated fluid-filled stomach and a proximal duodenum in front of a polyhydramnion. Postnatally, the abdominal radiograph and or the ultrasonography show the classic double-bubble sign. An upper GI contrast study, next to the ultrasound scan can help with the differential diagnoses (duodenal stenosis, perforated web, annular pancreas, duodenal duplications, malrotation with Ladd's bands). Vomiting in patients with duodenal atresia is in the majority bilious, because 85 % of obstructions are distal to the entry of the bile duct into the duodenum. The most common genetic disorder associated with duodenal atresia is trisomy 21 (Down syndrome) in approximately one-third of patients. There are three major types: (I) represented by a mucosal diaphragmatic membrane, (II) represented by a short fibrous cord that connects the two ends of the atretic duodenum, (III) represented by a complete separation of the two duodenal ends. *Duodenoduodenostomy** with the Kimura diamond-shaped anastomosis is the treatment of choice. Therefore, a proximal transverse duodenal incision is anastomosed to a distal longitudinal duodenal incision. This operation can either be performed by open or laparoscopic approach. Mechanical intestinal "accidents" including vascular occlusions are most likely the cause for intestinal atresias. The most common side involved is the jejunum. Duodenal atresias are more common than ileal ones, whereas ileal atresias are more common than colonic ones. About 90 % of patients have single atresia, and the remaining may have multiple ones. A common classification for intestinal atresias is given: (I) mucosal web with an intact muscularis, (II) atretic segments separated by a fibrous band, (IIIa) atresia with a V-shaped mesenteric gap defect, (IIIb) "apple peel" deformity (in which the distal atretic segment receives a retrograde blood supply from the ileocolic or right colic artery), (IV) formed by multiple atresia with a "string sausage" effect. Neonatal small intestinal obstruction, bilious vomiting obstruction distal of the ampulla of Vater, maternal polyhydramnion (in the minority of cases !), a contrast enema showing a microcolon/unused colon, and, therefore, indicating the level of obstruction are typical findings to help with the final diagnosis. *An end-to-end or end-to-oblique anastomosis is performed whenever possible*. You might be in need to resect dilated abnormal atretic segments. By passage of injected air or saline or passage by a soft appropriately sized catheter the distal bowel should be evaluated for additional stenosis or atresia. Colonic atresias are usually part of a complex malformation. Many pediatric surgeons recommend to treat them with a (protecting) stoma.

Gastrointestinal Bleeding   Causes of upper GIT bleeding in infants and children are (newborn) hemorrhagic disease, swallowed maternal blood, esophagitis-gastritis, (stress associated peptic ulcer disease), and esophageal varices. In the lower GIT anal fissure, necrotizing enterocolitis, intussusception, Meckel's diverticulum, (juvenile) polyps, and inflammatory bowel disease. *Children with GIT bleeding might require blood replacement in the first instance***. However, replacement of one-half of their blood volume within 24 h and rebleeding during the same hospitalization are considered an absolute indication for your *surgical intervention***. For most diagnostic and therapeutic interventions, endoscopy is the gold standard approach. N.B.: Newborn hemorrhagic disease is a bleeding diathesis resulting from vitamin K deficiency. It presents as bruising gastrointestinal and umbilical bleeding and persistent oozing. Most newborns are vitamin K deficient and this deficiency might result in failure to produce clotting factors. And as a result, prothrombin time and activated partial thromboplastin time are prolonged, even when the platelet count and fibrogen level are normal. Breast milk does not have a sufficient quantity of vitamin K, *therefore intramuscular administration of vitamin K after birth** is preventive.

(Functional or Acute) Constipation/Intestinal Neuronal Dysplasia (IND)/Hirschsprung'S Disease (HD) "Difficulties" to open bowels and to defecate "normally" are quite common in children because their defecation intervals and pattern are very variable. In most cases they are associated with "chronic abdominal pain and discomfort". Correct diagnosis depends on a good history and physical examination (including rectal-digital palpation) as well as the selective use of contrast enemas, transit studies, anorectal manometry and rectal biopsies. Acute constipation suggests an organic cause (e.g., anal fissure, low fiber diet), whereas chronic constipation is usually functional. Functional constipation is represented by constipation, encopresis, and fecal incontinence. It is a disorder of delayed colonic motility in which no real organic or anatomic cause can be found. The best treatment approach is the combined, multidisciplinary implementation of defecation trials, dietary modifications, and laxatives. Psychosocial counseling and biofeedback training are often beneficial, use whatever works!! *In complex cases high irrigation enemas/clysma, manual rectal-digital removal of stool, and anal stretching might be necessary***. Intestinal neuronal dysplasia (NID) is a condition that resembles Hirschsprung's Disease. However, ganglia cells are present, but they are abnormal. Treatment consists *of laxatives and enemas, followed by*

*internal sphincter myotomy, if symptoms are persisting for a longer time**.* Congenital aganglionosis of the intestine is called Hirschsprung's Disease. In the majority of patients, the aganglionosis is found in the rectosigmoid, followed by the sigmoid the splenic flexure of the transverse colon, and the entire colon with a short segment of the terminal ileum is involved. The gross pathological features are dilatation and hypertrophy of the proximal colon with transition to normal sized or narrow (=transition zone) distal (aganglionic) bowel. The rectum in HD is empty and tight. Any rectal examination causes explosive passage of feces (or meconium in the newborn) and gas, providing acute relief for the patient. Diagnosis is confirmed by plain abdominal radiographs (distended bowel but no or only a small amount of air in the rectum), contrast enema (transition zone on the postevacuation film), anorectal manometry (absence of internal sphincter relaxation), and the rectal biopsy (absence of ganglia cells, increased acetylcholinesterase activity in the lamina propria and muscularis). HD enterocolitis and *toxic megacolon are the most emerging complications requiring prompt correction of the dehydration and electrolyte imbalance, rectal irrigation, and decompression of the intestine as well as broad spectrum antibiotics**.* Historically, the standard was to obtain a *diversion** proximal to the aganglionotic segment after making the diagnosis, followed by a *pull-through operation** when the bowel has a normal caliber, followed by the closure of the (protecting) stoma. However, most pediatric surgeons nowadays use a one-stage approach in the well-prepared patient. It can be done as an open, laparoscopic, transanal – or as a combination out of these methods – procedure (e.g., Soave, Swenson, Duhamel, Dela Torre).

Appendicitis The "typical" case presents with a gradual onset of periumbilical pain. The pain moves later into the right lower quadrant. Once the pain is located there, pain usually becomes worse and abdominal tenderness starts. "Mc Burney point" (1/3 of the distance from the anterior superior iliac crest in a direct line to the umbilicus), "rebound tenderness" (abdominal pain or tenderness elicited by the examiner with deep palpation followed by abrupt removal of the examining fingers), "Rovsing sign" (gentle palpation or percussion) of the left side of the abdomen (elicits pain at Mc Burney's point), or "psoas sign" (pain in the RLQ when activating the psoas muscle by pressing against the elevated right leg), etc., starts to get "positive". However, especially in children, the presentation can be very atypical, and atypical anatomic locations of the appendix can cause confusing physical findings. The final diagnosis is made by careful history taking, thorough repeated (!) physical examinations, and analysis of selected lab parameters like WBC and C-reactive protein. The finding of an enlarged, noncompressible appendix in an ultrasound scan is virtually diagnostic and especially helpful in adolescent girls to exclude tubo-ovarian pathologies. Differential diagnoses are various such as gastroenteritis, lymphadenitis mesenterialis, Meckel's diverticulitis, ovarian cysts, psoas abscess, pneumonia, etc. *Appendicitis can be operated on by either open or laparoscopic approach**. Nowadays, the laparoscopic approach with ligation of the stump with Roeder slings is the first choice in pediatric and adolescent surgery. In cases of perforated appendicitis with generalized or localized peritonitis, the peritoneal cavity is irrigated and drained with N/S during surgery, but no drain is left for the postoperative period. In these cases intravenous antibiotics (cephalosporine and metronidazole) are administered for several days. All other patients get only a single shot perioperative antibiotic prophylaxis.

Omphalitis/Vitelline Duct/Umbilical Hernia Omphalitis is an umbilical inflammation/infection in the newborn. Mild cases usually can be *managed by vigorous aseptic drying** and finally resolve spontaneously. Rarely, it progresses needing hospital admission, parenteral antibiotics, and surgical therapy. Extreme cases progress to necrotizing fasciitis requiring wide and fast (local) debridement. The most likely cause for a permanent or prolonged bilious or purulent discharge/drainage from the umbilicus is a vitelline duct anomaly. In such cases, the duct has not obliterated completely and a patent communication to the small intestine, vitelline cyst, or sinus persists. *All vitelline duct anomalies require surgical exploration and removal of all remnants including the intra-abdominal components**. If urine drains from the umbilicus a patent urachus or urachal cyst is the cause. After exclusion of a bladder outlet obstruction surgical exploration and removal of all remnants down to the bladder dome are indicated. Umbilical hernia is one of the most common pediatric surgical disorders. The majority of umbilical hernias close spontaneously by the age of 3–4 years. Incarceration or strangulation is very unlikely, thus umbilical hernia repair is an elective case.

Laparoschisis/Gastroschisis/Omphalozele A gastroschisis is located laterally, on the right side to the cord, which is inserting normally. There is no sac and the size of the defect is usually small. The content of the defect is usually intestine (containing fetal peritonitis due to the direct contact with the amniotic fluid), occasionally tubes and ovaries, but not liver. In an omphalocele, on the other hand, prolapsed liver is very likely, the defect size is much larger, there is a sac or at least its remnants and the cord inserts into this sac. In summary, omphalocele is a defect of the umbilical ring. Several genetic syndromes are associated with it, especially cardiac anomalies are quite common in infants with omphalocele. Gastroschisis is not associated with genetic syndromes, however, approximately 10 % of cases are associated with intestinal atresias. In both, the diagnoses can be made prenatally by ultrasound. Detection of a membranous sac and protrusion of the liver is associated with an omphalocele, whereas free floating bowel is associated to a fetus with gastroschisis. Detection of the abdominal wall defect in utero is important to search for additional anomalies, to plan timing, mode of delivery, and perinatal care. To allow early parental counseling and a discussion of potential termination of pregnancy in the case of multiple severe anomalies. Most studies show that cesarean section has no significant advantage over vaginal delivery, except in a fetus with a large omphalocele. Therefore, the mode and timing of delivery should be based on obstetrical factors and not on the presence and type of the abdominal wall defect. *Principles of immediate postnatal management in infants with abdominal wall defects are given: correcting hypovolemia, preventing hypothermia, and monitoring for signs of sepsis.* *** Since exposed bowel leads to an increased loss of insensible fluid and loss of heat, immediate management includes *placing the lower half of the infant, including all exposed viscera in a bowel bag, and placing the infant in a warmer place****. Initiate an intravenous access and fluid replacement, obtain an airway in case of respiratory distress, *place an orogastric tube to decompress the bowel*** and decrease the risk of aspiration, and last but not the least, administer intravenous antibiotics to decrease the risk of sepsis. Early bowel ischemia most likely results from strangulation caused by the too small abdominal wall defect. *Such small defects require immediate enlargement on the bedside by an incision relaxing both skin and fascia****. Generally, utmost care should be taken to avoid injury to the bowel, liver, and umbilical vein. The entire bowel (as far as possible) should be carefully inspected to rule out twisting as the cause of the vascular compromise. Placing the infant in left lateral decubitus position optimizes his/her venous return and cardiac output. After the emergency intervention with the "plastic bag" and "left side position- ing" as well as decompression of the GI tract by (minimum oral and anal) tubes (including instillation of mucolytics and laxatives), and evaluation for associated anomalies, *surgery for both, infants with gastroschisis or with omphalo- cele, is performed as soon as possible***. If the newborn is cardiorespiratory stable, in pediatric surgery centers sur- gery might be performed right in the delivery room. In summary, there are two options: primary or staged closure. In general, the whole-bowel content is reduced by gentle manual compression through the gastric and anal tubes. The viscera then are carefully reduced back into the abdominal cavity by closely observing the intra-abdominal pressure. If the intra-abdominal pressure can be main- tained on an acceptable level, primary closure can be started. The fascia (and the skin) is closed primarily by local flaps, prosthetic material, or fascia replacement by using remnants of the umbilical cord. *In a staged closure a rein- forced silatic silo**** (prefabricated or "homemade") is placed like a tent over the exposed viscera and attached to the fascia and skin around the defect. The tip of the silo is hooked up, vertically. Thus, the silo contents are reduced slowly and gradually back into the abdominal cavity. For the time, the silo protects the herniated bowel (from fluid and heat loss and mechanical irritation!) and redirects the pressure in the abdomen to promote the enlargement of the abdominal cavity. Whenever possible, the umbilicus is reconstructed at the initial stage. Since all children with abdominal wall defects have some type of malrotation, appendicitis will present atypically in the future and there- fore nearly all pediatric surgeons recommend its removal. N.B.: in cases where only nonoperative management is possible, the ancient method of using topical applications of agents promoting eschar formation might be used.

Groin Hernia/Inguinal Hernia (Strangulated/ Incarcerated) The failure of, or the incomplete obliteration of the processus vaginalis, leads to the development of hernias in children. Hernias in children have a high incidence (1–5 %, in premature infants up to 30 %) in common, almost all are indirect hernias, and boys outnumber girls. Sixty percent are located on the right, 30 % on the left side, and 10 % are bilateral. Most are asymptomatic, diagnosed occasionally as a bulge in the groin and these children are referred to for elective surgery. If the patient is irritable, in pain, presenting with signs of intestinal obstruction like abdominal distension, tenderness, vomiting and obstipation, physical examination shows an erythematous, tender, irreducible firm mass in the groin. Next to bowel, the ovary or the Fallopian tube becomes frequently incarcerated in females. If it cannot be *securely reduced immediately**, an incarcerated or strangulated hernia needs an emergency operation to reduce the content and release it from its strangulation****. The basic principle in repairing pediatric hernia is the high ligation of the sac. The approach can be open (still most common) or by laparoscope. Complications are bleeding, infection, injury to the cord structures, recurrence and iatrogenic cryptorchidism, atrophic testis.

Anal Fissure/Perianal Abscess/Fistula in Ano/Imperforate Anus Anal fissure (secondary to constipation) is the most common cause of bright blood in younger children. This fissure is usually found in the mucosa and skin lining of the anal canal in the posterior midline. Key symptoms are perianal pain and a small amount of hematochezia with every bowel movement. Since these children have learned to expect this pain every time when opening their bowels, they start to "avoid and postpone it" as long as possible, running into more and more constipation. *Generally, acute fissures are treated conservative with stool softeners and sitz baths, or surgically with a cut down of the fissure surface and anal stretching*.* Anal crypt and gland infection and occasionally a superinfected diaper rash are possible causes for a perianal abscess formation in children. *Perianal abscess is treated by incision and drainage and sitz baths*.* Is there a communication between an anal crypt and the perianal skin, *a fistula in ano** has formed. The main therapy is *fistulectomy*.* In infants the internal opening of the fistula is generally located opposite the external opening. Supralevatoric and other complex fistula are quite rare in children. Imperforate anus is a malformation of the anus with a wide spectrum of clinical presentations ranging from a fistula in the perineum to a completely blind ending rectum. These malformations are classified according to the gender of the patient, to low, intermediate or high, according to the level, the rectum terminates in relation to the puborectalis muscle complex. In addition, by the sort of fistula, running to either urogenital tract or the perineum. The most common defect in males is imperforate anus with a perineal fistula to the median raphe of the scrotum or the base of the penis. In females it is imperforate anus with a rectovestibular fistula. The incidence of associated malformations is high, most common are VACTERL, Down's Syndrome, Hirschsprung's Disease, and duodenal atresia. *Perineal anoplasty for low defects and colostomy followed by posterior sagittal* anorectoplasty (PSARP)** are the treatment of choice. One stage primary repair of high defects nowadays is also possible in selected neonates.

Biliary Atresia   Biliary atresia is a panductular obliterative process of the bile ducts resulting out of a sclerosing, inflammatory reaction starting most likely in utero, or just after birth. Most babies are of normal weight after their delivery and start thriving normally. Mild hepatomegaly is common. Stools may be pigmented for the first time, but then become acholic. Persistence of hyperbilirubinemia and jaundice (>2 weeks after birth) should prompt evaluation. If the hepatobiliary imaging scan and the ultrasonography of the liver and gall bladder support the diagnosis of biliary atresia, *exploratory laparotomy with introperative cholangiogram should be done. If indicated a Kasai procedure (hepatico-porto-enterostomy) should follow*.*

24.5 Urinary-Genitary Tract

Balanitis/Balanoposthitis The inflammation of the whole glans/penis tip alone is called balanitis. If the inner prepuce is involved, too, it is termed balanoposthitis. Most frequently it is caused by infection of retained smegma and urine, especially after repeated microtrauma after pulling back the foreskin rigorously. *The treatment consists out of ointment, penis bath, and gentle adhesiolysis and cleaning.* Circumcision *in the free interval*.*

Paraphimosis If the foreskin/prepuce is not pushed back correctly, e.g., after cleaning of smegma or after an erection, a paraphimosis can be the result. The glans will swell up, so that the preputial ring becomes too tight. This will lead to pain, vascular compromise, and finally necrosis. *Under general anesthesia the foreskin must be reduced into its normal position. This procedure usually requires the surgical cut off of the ring and/or a circumcision**.*

Zipper Injury   If young boys are in a hurry to "pee", they sometimes close their zipper too fast and inaccurately, finally squeezing in their foreskin. Since this injury is extremely painful, the *release*** should be done under sedation and strong analgesics minimum (better general anesthesia). With a (commercial) side cutting pliers the main body of the zipper should be torn off. *The tear in the foreskin will either be sutured or a circumcision will be done*** in due course.

Testicular Torsion/Torsion of the Testicular Appendix/Hydatide Torsion   In testicular torsion, the testicle twists around the spermatic cord causing immediately venous congestion, edema, and obstruction of the arterial blood flow, which, if left untreated, will lead to gonadal necrosis. Most frequently such cases occur in late childhood or early adolescence. In clinical practice almost all of these "young gentlemen" hide it behind as long as possible. But testicular torsion is an acute and painful unilateral swelling of the scrotum, with the affected testis elevated in its hemiscrotum. Diagnostics include Doppler ultrasound and nuclear scintigram. However, if in doubt, never delay *surgical exploration**** to make the final diagnosis. First, the torsion must be reversed. If the testis is still viable, it is fixed within the tunica vaginalis in a torsion-free, straight position. If it is nonviable, it should be removed. Second, to prevent torsion on the contralateral site, fixation on the contralateral site should be performed during the same surgery, or shortly thereafter in an elective operation. Eight to ten hours after the torsion, salvage of the testis is hardly possible. Most likely, prepubescent boys present with acute or gradual scrotal pain and tenderness localized in the upper pole of their testis. The twisted appendix/hydatide usually form a small tender nodule and presents as a bluish dot in the scrotal wall in front of a "normal" testis. *Conservative treatment consists of elevation, analgesics, and ice packs**. Because most cases resolve spontaneously, surgery is reserved only for selected cases. Epididymitis and orchitis are differential diagnoses and must be excluded.

Hydrocele If the processus vaginalis fails to obliterate completely, fluid starts to accumulate around the testis and its cord. This accumulation can be separated by septal walls and it is either constant or intermittent, or no communication into the peritoneal cavity will be found. Key clinical finding is the painless, transparent swelling of the entire or the hemi scrotum. Positive transillumination/diaphanoscopy by light and US are important for diagnosis. Our main surgical goal is to fenestrate the hydrocele wall and to resect it down to its borders. Subtile coagulation by diathermy is essential to avoid postoperative bleeding and hematoma. Small hydroceles in infants did not require any therapy at all. They will disappear over time in the majority of cases. However, constant, big, or recurrent hydroceles in older children and adolescents will be operated by *elective surgery**. Since the processus vaginalis is still open in young children in almost all cases, the inguinal approach is mandatory. In older children and adolescents, the scrotal approach can be considered, too. The so-called (ancient) "Winkelmann procedure" is contraindicated for children and adolescents at all age (increased risk of testicular compromise/necrosis!).

Obstructive Uropathies/Prenatal Hydronephrosis/Posterior Urethral Valves (PUV) The most common sites of congenital urinary tract obstruction are the ureteropelvic junction (stenosis of the renal pelvic outflow), the ureterovesical junction (all types of megaureter, vesicoureteral reflux), and the posterior urethral valves. The most common presentation of urinary tract obstruction is the prenatal hydronephrosis detected during the routine prenatal ultrasound screening. Prenatal hydronephrosis is defined by a pelvic anterior-posterior diameter greater than 8 mm at or beyond 24 weeks of GA, or an anterior-posterior pelvis-to-renal cortex ratio >0.5. A "dilatation" is identified much more often, then it will be finally a significant urologic abnormality. Clinical findings include flank pain accompanied by vomiting, urinary tract infection, hematuria, or an palpable abdominal mass due to the hydronephrosis. In addition, a postnatal ultrasound and a voiding cysturethrogram are of key importance in the postnatal management, as well as blood urea and serum creatinine. Later a nuclear renal scan might be needed as well. The most serious complication of an untreated urinary tract obstruction is the progressive loss of renal function, others are recurrent infection, stone disease, and failure to thrive. *Preservation of the renal function is the goal of any surgical intervention (e.g., antireflux surgery, reimplantation of the ureter, bladder drainage)***. Posterior urethral valves represent the most complex type of obstructive uropathies, leading rapidly to terminal renal failure. Prenatally, PUV presents with an oligohydramnion, postnatally with a bilateral hydronephrosis and dilated ureters, permanently filled, thickened bladder wall, and a dilated proximal urethra in the US scan. Pulmonary hypoplasia and potter facies are other characteristic clinical findings. Most important diagnostics are the lateral view in the voiding cysturethrogram (via the suprapubic catheter), the 99mTc-MAG3-scintigram, and the cysturethroscopy for direct visual inspection. Young's classification is given. Type I (most common): The valves are leaflets, like sails, separated by a slit-like opening, that extend distally and laterally from the verumontanum and fuses anteriorly at the 12 o'clock position. Type II (actually thought to be of little clinical significance): The valves extend proximally from the verumontanum and they are not obstructing. Type III: The valves are described as congenital urethral membrane that mimics a wind sock. Initially, respiratory support and fluid rescuscitation might be required, depending on the overall condition of the baby. Babies with significant hydronephrosis, acidosis, hyperkalemia, azotemia, or sepsis should have *prompt drainage of their bladder by urethral catheter, supravesical diversion, or vesicostomy****. Patients with good renal function and without infections may undergo *primary valve ablation via cystoscope****. All interventions should be done under antibiotic coverage. General complications are lifelong bladder dysfunction, voiding difficulties, vesico-ureteral reflux, and renal failure.

Imperforated   Hymen/Labial   Synechia/Hydrometrocolpos Occasionally, an imperforated hymen, adherent labia, or a transverse vaginal septum are diagnosed in the neonate. Most likely it will be diagnosed later in prepuberty. If significant mucous secretions occur, the bulging of the membrane between the labia, the distortion of the bladder and urethra may even lead to hydroureter and hydronephrosis. In the neonate, the hymen can rupture spontaneously following the massive impaction of mucous secretions. However, in the adolescent, the onset of the menstruation leads to a hematometrocolpos and lower abdominal pain and might require a *surgical opening**.

Ovarian Torsion/Ovarian Cysts   Typical findings are abdominal pain, most frequently focused in the left or right lower quadrant. Palpable mass in relation to the punctum maximum of pain. Opening bowels and formed stool are normal. Usually there is no fever. In ultrasound investigations usually a complex mass (=ovarian torsion; no blood supply in the US

Doppler) or a simple echo-free mass (=ovarian cyst) is found. Simple (fetal) ovarian cysts can have different, sometimes even giant sizes. They can rupture, spontaneously or delayed, or they can show bleeding inside the wall (hemorrhagic ovarian cysts, most frequently in puberty or adolescence). Ovarian cysts >4 cm, rapidly enlarging, or complex cysts do have a high probability of torsion. Torsion is the most common complication and can occur even in the fetus (=autoamputation of the ovary). *In the case of ovarian torsion, emergency (laparoscopic) exploration should be made immediately, the ovary derotated and every attempt to preserve this tissue****. Simple small cysts can be treated conservative, *bigger (>4–6 cm) and complex ones should be fenestrated via the laparoscopic approach**. Mesenteric cysts, urachal cysts, and intestinal duplications are part of the differential diagnoses.

24.6 Pediatric Surgical Emergency Interventions

Ventriculo-Peritoneal/External Shunt The classical way is to implant a system consisting of a silastic catheter with/ without a pressure valve, where the proximal tip is placed inside the ventricle and the distal one either in the peritoneal cavity (VP-shunt) or externally. The skull is usually accessed by a small burr hole (frontal or occipital), the lateral ventricle punctured by a cannula, and the catheter inserted in Seldinger technique. The distal tip is either connected to the external container or first tunneled under the skin and then placed into the abdominal cavity.

Foreign Body Extraction by Foley Catheter The lubricated Foley catheter is passed by at the level the foreign body stucks in the esophagus. Then the cuff is inflated and the foreign body is removed by gentle traction on the end of the Foley catheter.

Central Venous Line (CVL) A CVL is one option for venous access in critically ill children for measuring central venous pressure, administering medication, giving parenteral nutrition, or performing hemodialysis. Fast accessible puncture sites are Vv. jugularis ext/int, Vv. subclavia, Vv. cephalica/basilica, Vv. femoralis, and Vv. temporalis in smaller infants. The Seldinger puncture technique: (i) deep sedation, (ii) correct positioning of the patient, (iii) palpation of the access site and marking of the anatomical landmarks, (iv) disinfection and sterile covering, (v) preparation of the catheter set, (vi) puncture of the vessel and insertion of the guide wire, (vii) final placement of the catheter tip, (viii) fixation and dressing, (ix) control of the correct placement (e.g., ECG, X-ray, US). The tip must be located in the v. cava superior. Potential complications are hematoma, (hemato-) pneumothorax, fluido-thorax, pericardial effusion, or air embolism.

Tracheostoma Immature airway, obstructing congenital anomalies or acquired obstructions, tumors, and trauma are potential indications for tracheostomy in childhood. In principle, tracheotomy can be done by puncture/dilatation (Seldinger) or classic open surgical technique. Briefly, the open surgical technique: (i) under general anesthesia positioning of the patient: The shoulders are elevated on a roll, the head is hyperextended in the neck and supported by a doughnut-foam support to allow sufficient access to the surgical field. (ii) Surgical prep and drap of the entire neck from the lower lip down to the nipples. (iii) The transverse skin incision starts about a one finger width above the jugular notch, before it is extended through the subcutaneous fascia and platysma muscle. (iv) The anterior cervical fascia is opened vertically in the midline, in the same manner as the strap muscles. (v) After visualization of the trachea, the pretracheal fascia is lightly scored with the cautery to coagulate any tiny vessel. A nonabsorbable suture, each incorporating one or two tracheal rings is placed on either side of the midline and left 6–8 cm long. At the end of every case these sutures are taped securely to the chest wall as a guide to the tracheal incision in the event of a postoperative emergency like a cannula dislodgement. (vi) The endotracheal tube is prepared for removal, loosened, before a vertical incision is made through the trachea (rings 2, 3, 4) at the score mark level. To avoid misplacement a small catheter is inserted first into the tracheal lumen to serve as a guide over which the lubricated cannula is passed. (vii) The endotracheal cannula is removed, the ventilator connected to the tracheal cannula and when ventilation is satisfactory, the wings of the body of the cannula are secured to the patient. A fresh tracheostomy and the sutures should be left untouched for about 10 days. Potential complications are: early/late hemorrhage, cannula dislodgement/decannulation, cannula malplacement, or granulation tissue formation and obstruction. And, last but not least: tracheal stenosis formation.

Chest/Pleural Drain To evacuate a tension pneumothorax a large bore needle armed with a Heimlich valve is placed in the second intercostal space in the midclavicular line (Monaldi position). To drain pleural fluid the pleural space is punctured horizontally dorsal in the scapular line above the ninth rib. The fluid is either aspirated once or a catheter is inserted in Seldinger technique for continuous drainage.

The center of the fluid collection is best visualized by a transthoracic bedside ultrasound scan. For the classical continuous drainage the Bülau-position (fourth intercostal space in the midaxillary line) is preferred. Briefly, (i) the skin incision is made 1 cm below (ii) the intercostal muscles (fourth intercostal space) are separated and tunnel by blunt dissection until the pleura parietalis is reached. (iii) The pleura is perforated, the chest tube (mandarin and drain) inserted (there will be the sound like if you have a puncture in your tyre). (iv) The mandarin is removed and the tip of the tube pushed into place. (v) The water seal and the container are connected and the correct placement of the tube within the pleural space is checked by the oscillating air/blood tracers within the chest tube or by a X-ray film. (vi) The chest tube is fixed by sutures and dressed airtight. Complications: bleeding, injury of the lung, malplacement/occlusion of the tube, air leak, subcutaneous emphysema, fistula, and infection.

Transurethral/Suprapubic Catheterization The localization and volume of the bladder are localized by percussion or US, first. Transurethral approach: (i) preparation of your set. In newborns and infants a feeding tube is most preferable. (ii) Prep and drap of the genital area. (iii) Locate the meatus (more easy in boys then in girls) exactly. (iv) Lubricate the tip of the catheter and the urethra with local anesthetic jelly. (v) Insert the tube very carefully and gently into the up-lifted penile urethra (in boys). (Just pass it in girls, after separation of the labia and the clitoris.) (vi) When the tip reaches the proximal urethra, the penis is brought down to facilitate entry of the tip through the prostatic urethra into the bladder lumen. (vii) Fixation the tube to the penis shaft or the vulva by plaster stripes. Suprapubic approach: (i) Prep and drap the abdominopelvic area. (ii)

Under GA or deep sedation and local anesthesia a small skin incision is made over the pubic bone. (iii) The bladder is punctured by the cannula and the pigtail catheter introduced in Seldinger technique. (iv) The catheter end is connected to the urinary bag. (v) Fixation and dressing onto the lower abdominal wall.

Construction of a Silo if a prefabricated silo is not available, a sterile transparent plastic bag is used or created by suturing sheets together to form a "tent". The basis is sutured to the fascia/skin and the tip is twisted over the content with the walls being perpendicular to the abdominal cavity. The tip is hooked up. A gauze with antiseptics is placed around the basis of the silo. The silo is gradually reduced over the next days by twisting the tip or by placing a roller clamp at the appropriate level.

Bishop-Koop Enterostomy The distal chimney enterostomy, described by Bishop-Koop, involves resection with anastomosis between the end of the proximal and the side of the distal segment of the bowel (approximately 4 cm from the opening of the distal segment). The open end is brought out as the ileostomy. This technique allows normal gastrointestinal transit while providing a means for managing distal obstruction through the ileostomy.

Hydrostatic/Pneumatic Reduction of Intussusception Reduction is accomplished by inserting and securing a catheter into the rectum, taping the buttocks together in order to obtain an occlusive seal and installing either radiopaque fluid or air into the colon. Under fluoroscopic guidance pressure (not more than 150 mmHg) within the distal bowel pushes the intussuscipiens proximally. Complete reduction is confirmed only when air or contrast freely fills more proximal loops of bowel with reflux into the terminal ileum.

Incision and Drainage of Abscess Briefly, (i) incision site prepped and draped, (ii) (step) incision on the punctum maximum of the fluctuation (respection cosmetic areas), (iii) bacterial swab, if needed, (iv) press and rinse out all pus, (v) sharp and full debridement of the abscess wall, (vi) rinsing of the cavity with antiseptic solution and N/S, (vii) a (rubber) drain is placed into the cavity and fixed to the wound margin with a stay stitch, (viii) loose wound dressing with a gauze pack to allow outflow exsudate, (ix) over the next days, the drain is gradually removed and the former cavity of the abscess is flushed regularly, (x) the wound heals by secondary intention or is closed by secondary sutures.

Intraosseous Canulation In emergency situations the venous system may be collapsed and gaining intervenous access can be impossible. A quick and easy alternative in these cases is the placement of an intraosseous device. The two most common insertion sites are the proximal tibia just below the tibial tuberosity and, less commonly in infants the humerus at the level of the humeral head. Briefly, (i) insertion site prepped and draped, (ii) local anesthesia if appropriate, (iii) the ready needle and driver are positioned in a 90° angle to the bone, (iv) the needle is pressed into the skin (alternatively a small skin incision is made) until the tip is in safe contact with the bone, (v) the bone cortex is penetrated by squeezing the driver and applying gentle, steady downward pressure, (vi) a pop is encountered the medullary space has been reached, (vii) driver and stylet are removed and the catheter flushed to ensure its correct position, (viii) a standard gauze dressing is placed around the device. Complications are osteomyelitis, compartment syndrome, damage to the epiphyseal plate, iatrogenic fracture.

Catheterization of the Umbilical Vessels In neonates the umbilical vessels can be accessed directly in the first days of life. A few days later surgical cut down might be necessary. The umbilical artery can be used for blood pressure monitoring, blood sampling, and fluid or drug infusion, the umbilical vein for central venous pressure monitoring, blood sampling, fluid or drug infusion as well. Briefly, (i) the umbilical cord area is prepped and draped, (ii) the catheter set is opened and the catheter flushed with N/S and heparin, (iii) the umbilical stump is grasped and tape or a big suture is used to encircle the stump below skin level to prevent bleeding and to "stabilize" it, (iv) the stump is cut leaving enough length for easy manipulation during placement (and later fixation), (v) the arteries (small and thick walled) and the vein (larger and thin walled) are identified and gently dilated with a hemostat or forceps, (vi) the catheter is inserted into the lumen and temporarily fixed by the encircling suture, (vii) blood return is encountered and the catheter advanced to the corrected position (confirmed by X-ray), and (viii) if in correct place, the catheter is secured by a strong stay stitch suture.

Gastrostomy/Percutaneous Endoscopic Gastrostomy (PEG)/ Jejunostomy A gastrostomy is surgically or endoscopic percutaneously created gastro-cutaneous fistula that allows feeding or decompression. It is indicated in all patients with a functional gastrointestinal tract disorder enabling them to consume sufficient nutrition for growth and development. A feeding jejeunostomy is more advantageous in children with severe neurological impairment (e.g., coma) or high risk of aspiration (e.g., gastroparesis and reflux). Briefly, Stamm gastrostomy: (i) the incision site is prepped and draped, (ii) midline or left paramedian incision is made, (iii) the gastric wall is identified and opened, (iv) double purse string sutures are placed around the inserted tube creating a serosa lined tract, (v) the stomach is hooked up to the anterior abdominal wall to create a permanent adhesion. For the PEG technique: (i) the stomach is insufflated with air and transilluminated with a gastroscope pushed within the stomach, (ii) skin disinfection over the transillumination spot, (iii) a needle is placed percutaneously into the stomach, (iv) a guidewire is placed through the needle, endoscopically grasped, and brought out through the mouth, (v) the gastrostomy tube armed with a bolster is tied to the guidewire and pulled retrograde through the stomach and abdominal wall (vi) the correct position is visualized and confirmed, before the tube is fixed with a second bolster externally. A formal jejunostomy can be created via a second channel in the PEG system, as a Witzel fistula (comparable to the Stamm technique and via a needle jejunostomy). The most important point is that the tip ends at least 15 cm distal to the ligament of Treitz.

Chapter 25
Common Surgical Emergencies in Transplanted Patients

Nicola de'Angelis, Francesco Brunetti, and Daniel Azoulay

25.1 Introduction

The likelihood that an emergency surgeon will encounter a transplanted patient with a graft-unrelated surgical problem is ever increasing. This is due to two main reasons; first, organ transplantation has emerged as the preferred treatment modality for end-stage liver, kidney, heart, and lung diseases, with approximately 28,000 solid organs transplanted every year in the United States and in Europe, and a total estimate of 114,690 organs transplanted worldwide in 2012 [1]. Second, long-term graft survival has drastically improved over the last 10 years, entailing an ever-larger cohort of patients living and functioning under chronic immunosuppression.

N. de'Angelis (✉) • F. Brunetti • D. Azoulay
Department of Digestive Surgery and Liver Transplantation,
Henri Mondor Hospital, AP-HP, Université Paris Est – UPEC,
51, Avenue du Maréchal de Lattre de Tassigny,
94010 Créteil, France
e-mail: nic.deangelis@yahoo.it

© Springer International Publishing Switzerland 2017   457
S. Di Saverio et al. (eds.), *Acute Care Surgery Handbook*,
DOI 10.1007/978-3-319-15341-4_25

When considering the incidence of several common general surgical problems, it becomes apparent that, at some point, transplanted patients are likely to end up requiring surgical care outside of transplant centers, making it important for all surgeons to be familiar with the factors that may influence surgical outcomes along with issues that are likely to affect optimal timing of surgery and postoperative care in transplanted patients.

In general, surgical emergencies in the transplanted patient can be divided into two categories: problems directly related to the allograft, and those independent of the allograft. This latter category also includes traumatic injuries. Any problem directly related to the allograft should be referred to a transplant center immediately and simultaneously with the stabilization of the patient. Conversely, common surgical emergencies clearly independent of the allograft can be managed by the general surgeon, but they will require careful consideration of the patient's immunosuppressed state that might affect the clinical presentation as well as the response to treatment (Fig. 25.1). This chap-

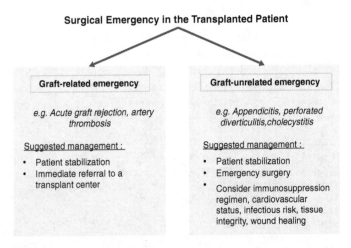

Fig. 25.1 Types of surgical emergencies in transplanted patients

ter will focus on the surgical management of common allograft-independent emergencies in transplanted patients.

25.2 Preoperative Considerations in the Transplanted Patient

Although the fundamental principles of surgery continue to apply, it is important to recognize the differences that exist between the transplanted patients chronically immunosuppressed and the general population. Transplanted patients have unquestionably more medical problems, particularly in regard to cardiovascular diseases. Moreover, the immunosuppression regimen can mask the presenting signs and symptoms of many disease processes, as well as interfere with the patient management for transplant-unrelated surgical procedures in terms of risk of drug interactions, adverse effects, wound healing, and postoperative complications [2].

In general, preoperative considerations are independent of the type of transplant and should start by assessing the underlying cardiac status of the patient [3]. Cardiovascular disease complications are a major cause of morbidity and mortality among transplanted patients, and particularly in renal-transplanted patients; thus, the major concern is the risk of a perioperative cardiovascular event [3–7]. It is noteworthy that immunosuppression can be considered a cardiac risk factor as least as important as hypertension or hyperlipidemia [4, 7, 8]. The administration of β-blockers to decrease perioperative cardiac morbidity should be considered in any transplanted patient about to undergo a major general surgical procedure [9].

Preoperative antibiotics have not been extensively studied in transplanted patients undergoing general surgery. However, transplanted patients should always be considered "at risk," since infection is an inevitable consequence of life-long immunosuppression. Current immunosuppressive regimens typically consist of two phases: induction phase and maintenance therapy. There are no uniform induction regimens, but most transplant centers use either high doses of conventional immunosuppressive agents, or polyclonal or monoclonal antibodies directed against T-cell antigens (more common in heart, lung, and kidney transplantation). Maintenance immunosuppression generally consists of a drug combination therapy, involving corticosteroids, calcineurin inhibitors, antiproliferatives, and mTOR inhibitors. With the standardization of immunosuppressive protocols, a pattern of susceptibility has been described, which appeared to be dependent on the dose, duration, nature, and temporal sequence of immunosuppressive therapy [10]. Thus, prophylactic antibiotics are virtually indicated in all cases, including clean cases, and during both induction and maintenance phases. As usual, broader spectrum coverage to include Gram-positive and Gram-negative bacteria is warranted for intra-abdominal procedures, given by infusion within 1–2 h before the surgical incision [3, 11].

Because most transplanted patients are maintained on chronic corticosteroids as part of their immunosuppressive regimen, the possibility of adrenal insufficiency is often raised when these patients develop emergent problems requiring surgical intervention. However, adrenal insufficiency has become less and less common, because the current doses of steroids used for the maintenance therapy have been markedly reduced compared with previous standards. As a consequence, the practice of administering a prophylactic supraphysiologic dose of corticosteroids peri-operatively (the so-called stress dose) appears to be unnecessary in most of the cases [12].

Finally, it must be considered that immunosuppressive therapy affects tissue integrity and wound healing. In particular, the use of glucocorticoids, even at low doses, is associated with consequent enhanced friability of skin, superficial blood vessels and intestinal wall, making a cautious and delicate handling of the tissues cardinal to avoid postoperative wound-healing complications. Moreover, the use of nonabsorbable sutures as well as keeping skin staples in place two to three times longer than usual are recommended in transplanted patients [3].

25.3 Traumatic Emergency in the Transplanted Patient

Transplanted patients represent only a small percentage of individuals seen in trauma centers, but they present with a peculiar condition in which the inflammatory responses following trauma injuries may be blunted by the long-standing immunosuppression [13]. Although there is a paucity of data in the literature, traumas in heart-transplanted patients have been generally associated with good graft outcomes (which is infrequently injured), whereas an increased potential for rejection has been reported in renal transplant patients [14]. Moreover, a higher rate of skeletal fracture has been suggested in transplanted patients compared to nontransplanted patients [15], while no increased risk of infection was observed in a recent retrospective study conducted in a large transplantation and Level I trauma center [16]. Only in few cases, mild damage to the grafts was radiographically observed, but patients did not manifest signs and symptoms of graft failure [16]. These data are encouraging and suggest that transplanted grafts are not at increased risk for injury following trauma.

25.4 Common Surgical Emergency in the Transplanted Patient

Gastrointestinal emergencies are highly frequent in transplanted patients and are associated with considerable morbidity and mortality [17–20]. The clinical presentation may be subtle or completely unexpected due to the masking nature of immuno-suppression, thus confirmatory imaging tests (e.g., computed tomography) should not be delayed in these patients. In general, treatment should be aggressive, since intestinal healing, as for any surgical sites, will be impaired and infection rates high. Surgery is most of the time the preferable treatment, since trans-planted patients are not good candidates for medical therapy in case of appendicitis, perforated ulcer, complicated diverticulitis, or any other condition that will require high degree of physio-logic wound-healing functions to repair without intervention.

Acute appendicitis after solid organ transplantation is a rare event, as documented by few case reports in the literature [21–23]. However, appendicitis in transplanted patients is commonly associated with delayed diagnosis, misdiagnosis, and compli-cated appendicitis, including rupture and gangrene. Moreover, if not aggressively treated, it can lead to substantial morbidity in the clinical setting of chronic immunosuppression. Laparoscopic appendectomy appeared to be safe and feasible in kidney-, pan-creatic-, and liver-transplanted patients, with intraoperative and postoperative outcomes similar to those procedures carried out in nontransplanted patients [21]. Conversely, some authors sug-gested conservative treatment, like radiological drainage, in transplanted patients with appendiceal abscesses to transform an emergency operation into an elective one in favor of a decreased morbidity [24]. However, the potential benefits of a medical management need to be balanced with the risks associated with delayed surgery in an immunosuppressed patient.

A higher incidence of diverticulitis, as well as more virulent disease, and more complicated recurrences are reported in immunocompromised and transplanted patients [25, 26]. The diagnosis and treatment of diverticulitis after solid organ trans-plantation are challenging, since maintenance immunosuppres-sive therapies may mask presenting symptoms and impair the ability to contain the infective process. This predisposes patients to an increased incidence of free peritoneal perforation or complicated disease in comparison to immunocompetent patients [25]. However, the incidence of colonic perforation after transplantation is rather low, involving 1–2 % of cases. Diverticulitis is the most common cause of perforations, followed by ischemic colitis and cytomegalovirus colitis, which can co-exist. Morbidity and mortality following emergency colectomy for complicated diverticulitis in immunocompromised patients are higher than those of immunocompetent individuals, ranging between 20 and 30 % [26, 27]. On the contrary, postoperative outcomes of elective procedures seem no different from those observed in nontransplanted patients [26]. The significant morbidity following sigmoid diverticulitis among transplant recipients has prompted consideration of pretransplant prophylactic surgery for patients with sigmoid diverticulosis proven by colonoscopy. In fact, this is a feasible approach only for kidney transplant candidates, since patients awaiting heart, lung, or liver transplantation are generally too sick to tolerate any major surgical procedures. Moreover, the incidence of sigmoid diverticulitis in transplant recipients (estimated at 1 %) may be too low to warrant prophylactic surgery as a routine protocol. Hartmann's procedure is the treatment of choice for diverticulitis complicated by perforation (Hinchey III and IV). The rate of stoma closure (i.e., Hartmann's reversal) observed in transplanted patients is comparable to that reported in the literature for immunocompetent patients [26, 28].

Peptic ulcer disease in transplanted patients represents another frequent gastrointestinal emergency associated with high mortality rate (up to 40 %). However, thanks to a deep screening of transplant candidates, and an active treatment of pre-existing disease with H_2-receptor antagonists or proton pump inhibitors, the incidence of peptic ulcer disease has drastically decreased. The relationship of corticosteroids with peptic ulcer disease is unclear; it appeared to be exacerbated by the immunosuppression regimen rather being a direct complication of steroid therapy. The prevalence of *Helicobacter pylori* infection in solid-organ transplant recipients is similar to that in nontransplant controls, and the incidence of *H. pylori*-related peptic ulcer disease and mucosa-associated lymphatic tissue lymphoma does not increase under the immunosuppressive treatment after transplantation [29]. Considering the excellent results of nonoperative ulcer therapy in transplanted patients, surgery should be limited to complicated or perforated cases. However, an early diagnosis and a prompt treatment are the key of success; thus, an exploratory surgery (either by laparoscopy or laparotomy) in patients with uncertain diagnosis might prove to be a better approach than wait for the symptoms to be aggravated.

Biliary tract diseases are among the most common problems in transplanted patients, with a prevalence of cholelithiasis as high as 30–40 % [17, 30, 31]. Despite actual controversies, this seems to be related to cyclosporine-induced perturbation of bile composition resulting in an increased prevalence of biliary stones formation [32, 33]. Clinically, the incidence of symptomatic cholelithiasis posttransplant is frequently observed in cardiac, lung, kidney, and kidney–pancreas-transplanted patients [31, 34–36]. Emergency surgery for acute biliary tree complications has been associated with high morbidity (up to 47 %) [30, 34] and mortality rates (up to 29 %) [30, 31], and thus, a prophylactic cholecystectomy in patients awaiting transplantation has been proposed as a strategy to avoid symptomatic gallstone diseases later on [37, 38]. However, this is still under debate and not routinely performed also because an emergency cholecystectomy can be highly problematic in patients with end-stage diseases.

Transplanted patients presenting with biliary symptoms should be treated promptly and aggressively. Laparoscopic cholecystectomy can be performed safely in lung- and kidney-transplanted patients, with outcomes that appeared comparable to nontransplanted populations [36, 39]. Conversely, heart-transplanted patients seem to be at higher risk when an emergency cholecystectomy is required, independently of the surgical approach (i.e., laparoscopic vs. open surgery) [30, 40], whereas pancreas-transplanted patients may require specific technical modifications in the laparoscopic cholecystectomy, which need to be carefully evaluated preoperatively. Finally, biliary problems in the liver-transplanted patient, such as strictures, cholangitis, abscesses, and liver bilomas, should be better referred to a center with experience in liver transplantation.

Ultimately, transplanted patients under immunosuppressive regimens are prone to wound healing impairment and secondary incisional hernia when exposed to surgery. Although no specific data are available about incisional hernias in transplanted patients subsequently undergoing emergency general surgical procedures, its incidence is expected to be higher than in the general population. In the literature, incisional hernias in liver-transplanted patients have been reported to be as high as 17 %, likely consequent to effects of immunosuppression, malnutrition, and end-stage liver disease [41]. The incidence of incisional hernia in renal-transplanted patients is lower, ranging from 3 to 4 % [42]. Several reports support that hernias repair by placement of prosthetic materials is safe also in transplanted patients despite the increased risk of infections [43, 44].

25.5 Conclusion

The general surgeon facing a transplanted patient with an allograft-independent surgical emergency needs to carefully consider the physiology of the transplanted organ, the pharmacology of the immunosuppressive drugs, and the underlying surgical conditions to be remedied [45]. Common surgical emergencies in transplanted patients are associated with considerable morbidity and mortality, but a multidisciplinary approach and an appropriate preoperative evaluation can anticipate excellent outcomes even in emergency settings. As a general rule, proceed with caution, apply evidence-based protocols, and expect the unexpected.

References

1. Mahillo B, Carmona M, Alvarez M, Noel L, Matesanz R. Global Database on Donation and Transplantation: goals, methods and critical issues (http://www.transplant-observatory.org). Transplant Rev. 2013;27(2):57–60.
2. Lin S, Cosgrove CJ. Perioperative management of immunosuppression. Surg Clin North Am. 2006;86(5):1167–83. vi.
3. Gohh RY, Warren G. The preoperative evaluation of the transplanted patient for nontransplant surgery. Surg Clin North Am. 2006;86(5):1147–66. vi.
4. Kasiske BL, Guijarro C, Massy ZA, Wiederkehr MR, Ma JZ. Cardiovascular disease after renal transplantation. J Am Soc Nephrol : JASN. 1996;7(1):158–65.
5. Desai S, Hong JC, Saab S. Cardiovascular risk factors following orthotopic liver transplantation: predisposing factors, incidence and management. Liver Int. 2010;30(7):948–57.
6. Luca L, Westbrook R, Tsochatzis EA. Metabolic and cardiovascular complications in the liver transplant recipient. Ann Gastroenterol. 2015;28(2):183–92.
7. Fellstrom B. Risk factors for and management of post-transplantation cardiovascular disease. BioDrugs. 2001;15(4):261–78.
8. Marcen R. Immunosuppressive drugs in kidney transplantation: impact on patient survival, and incidence of cardiovascular disease, malignancy and infection. Drugs. 2009;69(16):2227–43.
9. Auerbach AD, Goldman L. beta-Blockers and reduction of cardiac events in noncardiac surgery: scientific review. JAMA. 2002;287(11):1435–44.
10. Fishman JA, Issa NC. Infection in organ transplantation: risk factors and evolving patterns of infection. Infect Dis Clin North Am. 2010;24(2):273–83.
11. Bratzler DW, Houck PM, and Surgical Infection Prevention Guideline Writers, W. Antimicrobial prophylaxis for surgery: an advisory statement from the National Surgical Infection Prevention Project. Am J Surg. 2005;189(4):395–404.

12. Kelly KN, Domajnko B. Perioperative stress-dose steroids. Clin Colon Rectal Surg. 2013;26(3):163–7.
13. Giannoudis PV. Current concepts of the inflammatory response after major trauma: an update. Injury. 2003;34(6):397–404.
14. Mohammed EP, Venkat-Raman G, Marley N. Is trauma associated with acute rejection of a renal transplant? Nephrol Dial Transplant. 2002;17(2):283–4.
15. Barone GW, Sailors DM, Hudec WA, Ketel BL. Trauma management in solid organ transplant recipients. J Emerg Med. 1997;15(2):169–76.
16. Scalea JR, Menaker J, Meeks AK, Kramer ME, Kufera JA, Auman KM, Cooper M, Bartlett ST, Scalea TM. Trauma patients with a previous organ transplant: outcomes are better than expected-a retrospective analysis. J Trauma Acute Care Surg. 2013;74(6):1498–503.
17. Bhatia DS, Bowen JC, Money SR, Van Meter Jr CH, McFadden PM, Kot JB, Pridjian AK, Ventura HO, Mehra MR, Smart FW, Ochsner JL. The incidence, morbidity, and mortality of surgical procedures after orthotopic heart transplantation. Ann Surg. 1997;225(6):686–93; discussion 693–684.
18. Paul S, Escareno CE, Clancy K, Jaklitsch MT, Bueno R, Lautz DB. Gastrointestinal complications after lung transplantation. J Heart Lung Transplant. 2009;28(5):475–9.
19. Smith PC, Slaughter MS, Petty MG, Shumway SJ, Kshettry VR, 3rd Bolman RM. Abdominal complications after lung transplantation. J Heart Lung Transplant. 1995;14(1 Pt 1):44–51.
20. Steed DL, Brown B, Reilly JJ, Peitzman AB, Griffith BP, Hardesty RL, Webster MW. General surgical complications in heart and heart-lung transplantation. Surgery. 1985;98(4):739–45.
21. Wei CK, Chang CM, Lee CH, Chen JH, Yin WY. Acute appendicitis in organ transplantation patients: a report of two cases and a literature review. Ann Transplant. 2014;19:248–52.
22. Wu L, Zhang J, Guo Z, Tai Q, He X, Ju W, Wang D, Zhu X. Diagnosis and treatment of acute appendicitis after orthotopic liver transplant in adults. Exp Clin Transplant. 2011;9(2):113–7.
23. Quartey B, Dunne J, Cryer C. Acute appendicitis post liver transplant: a case report and literature review. Exp Clin Transplant. 2012;10(2):183–5.
24. Verzaro RM, Khan A, Falcone JL, Thai N, Shapiro R. Acute appendicitis in a kidney-pancreas transplant recipient: report of a case. Transplant Proc. 2006;38(9):3144–6.
25. Remzi FH. Colonic complications of organ transplantation. Transplant Proc. 2002;34(6):2119–21.
26. Reshef A, Stocchi L, Kiran RP, Flechner S, Budev M, Quintini C, Remzi FH. Case-matched comparison of perioperative outcomes after surgical treatment of sigmoid diverticulitis in solid organ transplant

recipients versus immunocompetent patients. Colorectal Dis. 2012;14(12):1546–52.

27. Catena F, Ansaloni L, Gazzotti F, Bertelli R, Severi S, Coccolini F, Fuga G, Nardo B, D'Alessandro L, Faenza A, Pinna AD. Gastrointestinal perforations following kidney transplantation. Transplant Proc. 2008;40(6):1895–6.

28. De'angelis N, Brunetti F, Memeo R, Batista da Costa J, Schneck AS, Carra MC, Azoulay D. Comparison between open and laparoscopic reversal of Hartmann's procedure for diverticulitis. World J Gastrointest Surg. 2013;5(8):245–51.

29. Ueda Y, Chiba T. Helicobacter pylori in solid-organ transplant recipient. Curr Opin Organ Transplant. 2008;13(6):586–91.

30. Richardson WS, Surowiec WJ, Carter KM, Howell TP, Mehra MR, Bowen JC. Gallstone disease in heart transplant recipients. Ann Surg. 2003;237(2):273–6.

31. Gupta D, Sakorafas GH, McGregor CG, Harmsen WS, Farnell MB. Management of biliary tract disease in heart and lung transplant patients. Surgery. 2000;128(4):641–9.

32. Hulzebos CV, Bijleveld CM, Stellaard F, Kuipers F, Fidler V, Slooff MJ, Peeters PM, Sauer PJ, Verkade HJ. Cyclosporine a-induced reduction of bile salt synthesis associated with increased plasma lipids in children after liver transplantation. Liver Transpl. 2004;10(7):872–80.

33. Moran D, De Buitrago JM, Fernandez E, Galan AI, Munoz ME, Jimenez R. Inhibition of biliary glutathione secretion by cyclosporine a in the rat: possible mechanisms and role in the cholestasis induced by the drug. J Hepatol. 1998;29(1):68–77.

34. Lord RV, Ho S, Coleman MJ, Spratt PM. Cholecystectomy in cardiothoracic organ transplant recipients. Arch Surg. 1998;133(1):73–9.

35. Takeyama H, Sinanan MN, Fishbein DP, Aldea GS, Verrier ED, Salerno CT. Expectant management is safe for cholelithiasis after heart transplant. J Heart Lung Transplant. 2006;25(5):539–43.

36. Taghavi S, Ambur V, Jayarajan SN, Gaughan J, Toyoda Y, Dauer E, Sjoholm LO, Pathak A, Santora T, Goldberg AJ, Rappold J. Postoperative outcomes with cholecystectomy in lung transplant recipients. Surgery. 2015;158(2):373–8.

37. Graham SM, Flowers JL, Schweitzer E, Bartlett ST, Imbembo AL. The utility of prophylactic laparoscopic cholecystectomy in transplant candidates. Am J Surg. 1995;169(1):44–8; discussion 48–49.

38. Kao LS, Kuhr CS, Flum DR. Should cholecystectomy be performed for asymptomatic cholelithiasis in transplant patients? J Am Coll Surg. 2003;197(2):302–12.

39. Jackson T, Treleaven D, Arlen D, D'Sa A, Lambert K, Birch DW. Management of asymptomatic cholelithiasis for patients awaiting renal transplantation. Surg Endosc. 2005;19(4):510–3.

40. Kras AL, Yo SW, Marasco SF, Wale R, Warrier SK. Elective versus emergency abdominal surgery following cardiac transplantation: a Victorian state transplant service experience. ANZ J Surg. 2013;83(11):833–7.
41. Janssen H, Lange R, Erhard J, Malago M, Eigler FW, Broelsch CE. Causative factors, surgical treatment and outcome of incisional hernia after liver transplantation. Br J Surg. 2002;89(8):1049–54.
42. Mazzucchi E, Nahas WC, Antonopoulos I, Ianhez LE, Arap S. Incisional hernia and its repair with polypropylene mesh in renal transplant recipients. J Urol. 2001;166(3):816–9.
43. Catena F, Ansaloni L, Leone A, De Cataldis A, Gagliardi S, Gazzotti F, Peruzzi S, Agrusti S, D'Alessandro L, Taffurelli M. Lichtenstein repair of inguinal hernia with surgisis inguinal hernia matrix soft-tissue graft in immunodepressed patients. Hernia. 2005;9(1):29–31.
44. Muller V, Lehner M, Klein P, Hohenberger W, Ott R. Incisional hernia repair after orthotopic liver transplantation: a technique employing an inlay/onlay polypropylene mesh. Langenbecks Arch Surg. 2003;388(3):167–73.
45. de'Angelis N, Esposito F, Memeo R, Lizzi V, Martìnez-Pérez A, Landi F, Genova P, Catena F, Brunetti F, Azoulay D. Emergency abdominal surgery after solid organ transplantation: a systematic review. World J Emerg Surg. 2016 Aug 30;11(1):43. doi:10.1186/s13017-016-0101-6.

Chapter 26
Emergency Management of Caustic Injuries

Mircea Chirica, Nicolas Munoz-Bongrand, Emile Sarfati, and Pierre Cattan

26.1 Introduction

Ingestion of corrosive agents, accidentally or with suicidal intent, is a rare but potentially devastating event [1]. Most patients present with mild injuries that resolve without sequels, but surgery is necessary in a small number of patients for the treatment of more severe injuries [1]. Emergency management of caustic injuries requires a multidisciplinary approach and involves emergency care physicians, surgeons, anesthesiologists, gastroenterologists, radiologists, otorhynolaryngologists, and psychiatrists [2].

M. Chirica MD, PhD (✉)
Department of Digestive and Emergency Surgery, University Hospital of Grenoble, Grenoble Alpes University, Paris, France
e-mail: mirceaxx@yahoo.com; mchirica@chu-grenoble.fr

N. Munoz-Bongrand • E. Sarfati • P. Cattan
Service de Chirurgie Générale, Digestive et Endocrinienne,
Hôpital Saint-Louis, 1, avenue Claude Vellefaux, Paris, France

© Springer International Publishing Switzerland 2017   471
S. Di Saverio et al. (eds.), *Acute Care Surgery Handbook*,
DOI 10.1007/978-3-319-15341-4_26

26.2   Epidemiology

In France, 15,000 new cases of caustic ingestion were reported in 1995 [1]. In the United States, more than 200,000 ingestions were reported in 2002, of which, 35,000 patients required hospital care [3]. In a recent report, 20 % of patients had severe involvement of the upper digestive tract and required emergency surgery for caustic injuries; mean age was 44 years, 55 % were men and 65 % of them had a psychiatric history of depression or schizophrenia [1]. Ingestion is usually intentional in adults (75 %), while accidents are more frequent in children [2–5].

26.3   Corrosive Agents

Most frequently ingested products are acids, alkalis, and oxidative agents (i.e., bleach). Strong acids have been reported to produce coagulation necrosis that lessens tissue penetration and decreases damage when compared to alkalis, which produce liquefaction necrosis resulting in immediate severe injuries at all levels of the gastrointestinal tract [2–5]. The pattern of ingestion varies geographically and is usually conditioned by local customs and the availability of a particular substance: acids are the frequently ingested substance in India, Turkey, and Taiwan, while bleach and alkalis are the leading cause in Europe and North America [3].

Ingested corrosives may cause severe hypocalcemia (phosphoric, hydrofluoric acids), hyponatremia (strong acids/alkalis), hypokalemia, and severe acidosis. Although the ingested quantity is directly related to the severity of the injuries, this information it is seldom available [2, 3].

26.4   Emergency Management

Four objectives must be achieved during the initial approach: (1) avoid aggravating caustic lesions; (2) control and treat organ failures; (3) address potential systemic effects; and (4) evaluate the extent of damage.

26.5   Initial Therapeutic Approach

26.5.1   Pre-hospital

During this phase, it is important to establish the diagnosis of caustic agent ingestion and identify the involved agent. The ingested product should be collected on the scene and brought to the emergency department. Evaluation of the ingestion scenario should include: (a) confirmation of caustic ingestion; (b) accidental or intentional ingestion; (c) detect co-ingestion of alcohol and/or drugs; (d) try to evaluate the ingested quantity (in adults assess normal sip (30–50 ml) versus large gulp (60–90 ml); (e) assess delay from ingestion [6]. It is important to identify additional risk factors such as extreme ages (young children, elderly), pregnancy, underlying disease, and the form of the ingested agent (solid, liquid, gel, vapors-concomitant aspiration) [6]. Strict supine position, provoked emesis, gastric lavage ingestion of diluents (milk, water) should be avoided because such maneuvers might induce repeat esophageal passage of the corrosive agent and aggravate caustic injuries. Attempts at pH neutralization with either a weak acid or alkali may increase damage by exothermic reaction and should be prohibited [6].

26.5.2 Emergency Department Management

After hospital admission, symptomatic treatment should be pursued while waiting to evaluate the severity of caustic injuries. Fiberoptic laryngoscopy is preferable to blind intubation for airway support; emergency tracheotomy may be necessary in difficult situations [6]. Poison Control Centers should be contacted at this point to assess potential systemic toxicity. Nasogastric tubes increase risks of gastric perforation and caustic pneumonia and should be avoided; their validity in preventing vomiting and stricture formation remains questionable [6]. The efficacy of proton-pump inhibitors, H2 blockers, corticosteroids, and broad-spectrum antibiotics has not been proven; systematic use should be avoided [3, 4].

26.5.3 Evaluation of the Severity of Caustic Injuries

26.5.3.1 Clinical Presentation

The clinical presentation depends on the type, amount, and physical form of the ingested substance. Solid agents adhere to the mouth and pharynx producing maximum damage at this level, while liquids transit rapidly and induce burns of the esophagus and the stomach. Clinical signs of peritonitis and hemodynamic instability requiring immediate surgery are infrequent. Hoarseness and stridor are suggestive of laryngeal or epiglottis involvement. Dysphagia, odynophagia, and drooling are symptoms of esophageal involvement; epigastric pain and hematemesis may be manifestations of stomach involvement. However, symptoms do not always correlate to the extent of gastrointestinal involvement and the absence of pain does not preclude significant damage [2–4]. Asymptomatic patients with unintentional ingestion of weak caustic agents usually do not have significant gastroesophageal injuries.

26.5.3.2 Laboratory Studies

Emergency blood tests should comprise serum levels of: Na^+, K^+, Cl^+, urea, creatinin, LDH, CPK, Ca^{2+}, Mg^+, WBC, hemoglobin, platelets, TP, lactates, and alcohol. β-HCG levels should be measured in young women. Correlation between laboratory values and the severity of caustic injuries is usually poor. High white blood cell counts (>20,000 cells/mm^3), elevated serum C-reactive protein levels, severe acidosis (pH < 7.22), renal failure, perturbation of liver function tests (ALT > 2 N), and low platelet counts were reported to predict transmural necrosis and poor outcomes [2–4]. Laboratory studies can be useful in patient monitoring and in guiding subsequent management [7].

26.5.3.3 Endoscopy

Endoscopy (3–6 h after ingestion) allows evaluating the extent and severity of caustic injuries [8–10]; several grading classifications have been proposed, most of which were derived from the Zargar classification [10]. Endoscopy used to be the cornerstone of management algorithms worldwide [2, 3, 5]. Patients with high-grade (3b) injuries are usually considered for surgery while nonoperative treatments are attempted for low-grade injuries (≤3a) [1]. The major drawback of endoscopy is its inability to predict accurately the depths of intramural necrosis; this may lead to futile surgery or inappropriate "wait and see" management [1, 11, 12]. Endoscopy reliably predicts risks of stricture formation during follow-up [9].

26.5.3.4 Computed Tomography

Computed tomography palliates shortcomings of endoscopy-based algorithms. CT use was helpful in guiding indications for esophagectomy in patients with grade 3b caustic esophagitis

[13]. In a recent study, CT outperformed endoscopy in selecting patients for surgery or nonoperative treatment [14]. Overall, recent data suggest that CT can replace endoscopy evaluation in the emergency management of caustic ingestion. The absence of post-contrast wall enhancement is the main criteria of full-thickness necrosis of the esophagus, the stomach, the duodenum and the bowel (Fig. 26.1). A management algorithm relying on both endoscopy and CT findings is presented in Fig. 26.2.

26.5.4 Nonoperative Management

A nonoperative approach can be offered to 70–80 % of patients after caustic ingestion. Patients eligible for nonoperative treatment may resume oral alimentation as soon they can swallow. After control of the psychiatric condition, patients with minor digestive tract involvement can be discharged as soon as they eat normally. Patients with severe injuries require close ICU monitoring immediately after ingestion; clinical and/or laboratory test aggravation (abdominal pain, rebound tenderness, shock, need for ventilatory support, renal failure, peripheral-blood leukocytosis, and/or acidosis) should prompt repeat evaluation (CT, endoscopy) to reassess the need for surgery.

26.5.5 Emergency Surgery

Emergency surgery is required in a small number of patients with full-thickness wall necrosis. In a recent report, emergency surgery was undertaken in 24 (20 %) of 120 consecutive patients managed with a combined CT-endoscopy algorithm [14]. Fiberoptic bronchoscopy should be performed on a systematic basis before surgery to rule out airway involvement. Laparotomy is the mainstay approach but laparoscopic exploration is feasible and safe [15]. The main emergency operations performed for the treatment of caustic injuries are detailed below.

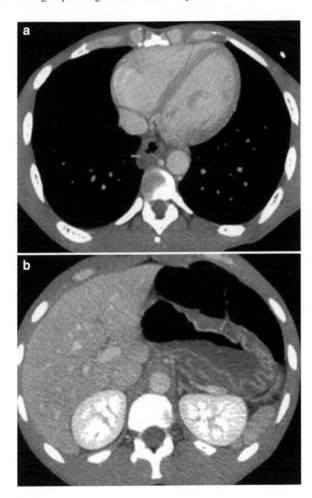

Fig. 26.1 Findings by computed tomography (CT). (**a, b**) Absence of transmural necrosis of the esophagus (**a**) and of the stomach (**b**). Post-contrast enhancement of the esophagus and the stomach is obvious (*arrows*) and the patient underwent successful nonoperative treatment. (**c, d**) Patient with transmural necrosis of the esophagus (**c**) (absence of esophageal enhancement, blurring of the esophageal wall and periesophageal fat) and the stomach (**d**) (absence of gastric wall enhancement); the pathology report confirmed transmural necrosis of the esophagus and the stomach

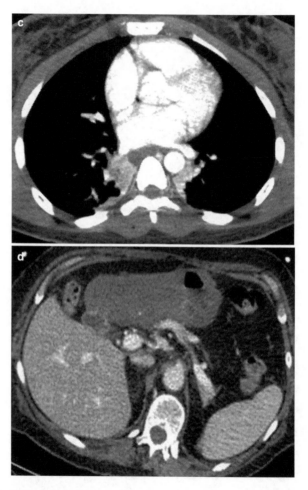

Fig. 26.1 (continued)

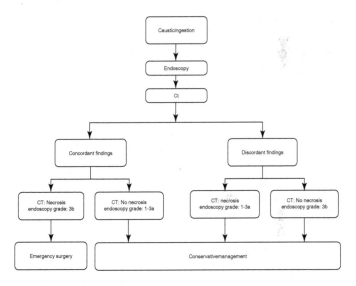

Fig. 26.2 Management algorithm for caustic injuries of the upper gastrointestinal tract

26.5.5.1 Oesophagogastrectomy (OGT)

OGT is the most frequently employed procedure; it is indicated when evaluation (CT/endoscopy) suggests transmural esophageal necrosis and laparotomy confirms transmural gastric necrosis. OGT is performed through a combined abdominal and cervical approach using an esophageal stripping technique. A cervicostoma and a jejunostomy are constructed at the end of the operation to avoid enteral nutrition while waiting for reconstruction [1]. Esophagectomy with gastric preservation is performed in the unusual situation of transmural necrosis confined to the esophagus; the operative technique and outcomes are similar to the OGT procedure. Positioning of a gastrostomy tube is recommended to avoid postoperative distension of the stomach.

26.5.5.2   Total Gastrectomy

Necrosis confined to the stomach should prompt total gastrectomy; partial gastric resections should be avoided because ongoing necrosis might compromise outcomes. Immediate reconstruction by esophagojejunostomy (EJ) should be attempted if patient condition allows; esophageal exclusion or external drainage can be performed as a damage control strategy [16]. EJ leakage in this setting (5–8 %) is in the range of EJ failure rates reported after gastrectomy for cancer. Feeding jejunostomy should be constructed systematically as esophageal strictures develop in most patients.

26.5.5.3   Extended Resections

Extended resections (beyond esophagogastrectomy) are required when caustic necrosis involves other abdominal organs [17]. Concomitant resection of the spleen, the colon, the bowel, and of the duodeno-pancreas was reported in up to 20 % of patients who underwent OGT [1]. Necrosis of the transverse colon is usually due to the direct extension of posterior gastric wall injuries to the mesocolon. Transmural duodenal necrosis is usually managed by pancreatoduodenectomy (PD), although the pancreatic parenchyma is seldom involved. If the patient condition allows, immediate pancreato-biliary reconstruction is recommended [18]. Bowel necrosis is usually related to intraluminal passage of caustic agent; massive bowel necrosis contraindicates resection because of poor patient survival and compromised nutritional and reconstructive issues. All obvious transmural necrosis injuries should be resected during the initial procedure; second-look procedures should be reserved to rare situations when ongoing necrosis is suspected [17].

26.5.5.4 Tracheobronchial Necrosis (TBN)

On rare occasions, esophageal necrosis may extend directly to the posterior aspect of the tracheobronchial tree. If TBN is certified, esophagectomy should be performed by a right thoracic approach to avoid further injuries and allow airway repair with a pulmonary patch technique [19].

26.5.5.5 Outcomes of Surgery for Caustic Ingestion

Immediate outcomes of surgery for caustic injuries are mainly conditioned by the extent of surgery. In a recent publication, mortality rates of gastrectomy, OGT, PD, and TBN for caustic injuries were 11 %, 14 %, 39 %, and 45 %, respectively; morbidity rates were 63 %, 65 %, 94 %, and 100 %, respectively [1]. The standardized mortality ratio (SMR) after emergency surgery for caustic injuries was 21.5 when compared with the general French population [1]. During follow-up, the ongoing decline in survival persists far beyond the emergency period. Roughly half of the patients die within 10 years of surgery because of operative complications, malnutrition, late morbidity, deterioration of the psychiatric condition, and suicide. After emergency surgery, only half of the patients eventually regain nutritional and respiratory autonomy. Factors with negative impact on long-term survival and functional outcomes include advanced age and the extent of the initial insult (as reflected by extended resection, emergency tracheotomy, and tracheal necrosis) [1].

26.6 Conclusion

Ingestion of caustic agents is a critical point in the lives of these patients because of the long-lasting effects on survival and functional outcomes. Efforts to improve outcome should be directed at avoiding unnecessary surgery in parallel with the development of public health prevention strategies aimed at limiting access to strong corrosive agents and at providing explicit information on their deleterious effects.

References

1. Chirica M, Resche-Rigon M, Bongrand NM, Zohar S, Halimi B, Gornet JM, et al. Surgery for caustic injuries of the upper gastrointestinal tract. Ann Surg. 2012;256(6):994–1001.
2. Contini S, Scarpignato C. Caustic injury of the upper gastrointestinal tract: a comprehensive review. World J Gastroenterol. 2013;19(25):3918–30.
3. Hugh TB, Kelly MD. Corrosive ingestion and the surgeon. J Am Coll Surg. 1999;189(5):508–22.
4. Keh SM, Onyekwelu N, McManus K, McGuigan J. Corrosive injury to upper gastrointestinal tract: still a major surgical dilemma. World J Gastroenterol. 2006;12(32):5223–8.
5. Ramasamy K, Gumaste VV. Corrosive ingestion in adults. J Clin Gastroenterol. 2003;37(2):119–24.
6. Bonavina L, Chirica M, Skrobic O, Kluger Y, Andreollo NA, Contini S, et al. Foregut caustic injuries: results of the world society of emergency surgery consensus conference. World J Emerg Surg. 2015;10:44.
7. Zerbib P, Voisin B, Truant S, Saulnier F, Vinet A, Chambon JP, et al. The conservative management of severe caustic gastric injuries. Ann Surg. 2011;253(4):684–8.
8. Zargar SA, Kochhar R, Mehta S, Mehta SK. The role of fiberoptic endoscopy in the management of corrosive ingestion and modified endoscopic classification of burns. Gastrointest Endosc. 1991;37(2):165–9.
9. Cheng HT, Cheng CL, Lin CH, Tang JH, Chu YY, Liu NJ, et al. Caustic ingestion in adults: the role of endoscopic classification in predicting outcome. BMC Gastroenterol. 2008;8:31.
10. Zargar SA, Kochhar R, Nagi B, Mehta S, Mehta SK. Ingestion of corrosive acids. Spectrum of injury to upper gastrointestinal tract and natural history. Gastroenterology. 1989;97(3):702–7.
11. Estrera A, Taylor W, Mills LJ, Platt MR. Corrosive burns of the esophagus and stomach: a recommendation for an aggressive surgical approach. Ann Thorac Surg. 1986;41(3):276–83.

12. Andreoni B, Farina ML, Biffi R, Crosta C. Esophageal perforation and caustic injury: emergency management of caustic ingestion. Dis Esophagus. 1997;10(2):95–100.
13. Chirica M, Resche-Rigon M, Pariente B, Fieux F, Sabatier F, Loiseaux F, et al. Computed tomography evaluation of high-grade esophageal necrosis after corrosive ingestion to avoid unnecessary esophagectomy. Surg Endosc. 2015;29(6):1452–61.
14. Do Dang G, L'Huillier M, Van Giai N, Van Orden JW. Coulomb sum rules in the relativistic Fermi gas model. Phys Rev C Nucl Phys. 1987;35(5):1637–45.
15. Di Saverio S, Biscardi A, Piccinini A, Mandrioli M, Tugnoli G. Different possible surgical managements of caustic ingestion: diagnostic laparoscopy for Zargar's grade 3a lesions and a new technique of "Duodenal Damage Control" with "4-tubes ostomy" and duodenal wash-out as an option for extensive 3b lesions in unstable patients. Updates Surg. 2015;67(3):313–20.
16. Chirica M, Kraemer A, Petrascu E, Vuarnesson H, Pariente B, Halimi B, et al. Esophagojejunostomy after total gastrectomy for caustic injuries. Dis Esophagus. 2013;27:122–7.
17. Cattan P, Munoz-Bongrand N, Berney T, Halimi B, Sarfati E, Celerier M. Extensive abdominal surgery after caustic ingestion. Ann Surg. 2000;231(4):519–23.
18. Lefrancois M, Gaujoux S, Resche-Rigon M, Chirica M, Munoz-Bongrand N, Sarfati E, et al. Oesophagogastrectomy and pancreato-duodenectomy for caustic injury. Br J Surg. 2011;98(7):983–90.
19. Benjamin B, Agueb R, Vuarnesson H, Tranchart H, Bongrand NM, Sarfati E, et al. Tracheobronchial necrosis after caustic ingestion. Ann Surg. 2015;263:808–13.

Chapter 27
Surgical Emergencies During Pregnancy

Goran Augustin

Acute abdomen can be defined as "any serious acute intra-abdominal condition attended by pain, tenderness, and muscular rigidity, and for which emergency surgery must be considered" [1]. Acute abdomen during pregnancy, without an obstetric cause, occurs in 1/500–635 pregnancies [2]. For some conditions, the predisposing factors are known in both the general and the pregnant population, such as acute cholecystitis. In other, such as acute appendicitis, the predisposing factors are not known.

G. Augustin
University Hospital Centre Zagreb and School of Medicine University of Zagreb, Kišpatićeva 12, 10000 Zagreb, Croatia
e-mail: augustin.goran@gmail.com

© Springer International Publishing Switzerland 2017   485
S. Di Saverio et al. (eds.), *Acute Care Surgery Handbook*,
DOI 10.1007/978-3-319-15341-4_27

27.1 Acute Appendicitis

27.1.1 Incidence

Acute appendicitis is present in 1/500–2000 pregnancies (which amount to 25 % of operative indications for the acute abdomen in pregnancy) [3].

27.1.2 History and Examination

The following features suggest acute appendicitis [3]: (1) severe abdominal pain, (2) pain in the right lower quadrant – the most reliable symptom, (3) nausea (nearly always present), (4) vomiting (2/3 of patients), and (5) after the third month of pregnancy, the pain could migrate progressively upward and laterally.

Abdominal tenderness is almost always present, rebound tenderness in 55–75 % [4], and abdominal muscle rigidity in 50–65 % of patients [3]. The psoas sign is observed less frequently during pregnancy when compared with the nonpregnant woman [5]. Fever and tachycardia may be present, but these are not sensitive signs.

27.1.3 Investigations

Leukocytosis is not diagnostic because it raises in the second and third trimesters and can reach $20 \times 10^9/l$ in early labor in normal pregnancy. A raised C-reactive protein (CRP) is not specific but the increase correlates with the disease severity. Neutrophil granulocytosis with left shift is diagnostic and indicates bacterial infection. Pyuria (pus in the urine) is observed in 10–20 % of patients [6]. This may also represent concurrent asymptomatic bacteriuria.

There are no Royal College of Obstetricians and Gynaecologists guidelines about the use of transvaginal ultrasound but it can define [7]: (1) the presence of adnexal or uterine pathology ruling out acute appendicitis, (2) free fluid in the pouch of Douglas, and (3) abnormal pathology in the ileocecal region – appendicitis, cecal tumors, or cecal diverticulitis.

Abdominal ultrasound is the modality of choice with variable sensitivity and specificity [8]. It has good accuracy in the first and second trimesters with less accuracy in the third.

Magnetic resonance imaging (MRI) is the modality of choice when the risk of radiation or the potential nephrotoxicity of iodinated contrast agents is a major concern [9, 10]. The patient's informed consent is mandatory; the safety of MRI for the fetus has not been proved according to the US Food and Drug Administration (FDA) guidelines and the American College of Radiology [9]. Thus, it is prudent to perform an MRI in pregnant patients only when ultrasound findings fail to establish a diagnosis.

The computed tomography (CT) scan is used when there is an uncertain clinical diagnosis or equivocal laboratory or ultrasound findings, or where access to MRI is limited. It is preferable to use the multidetector row CT scan with high-speed mode since it has half the radiation dose of the high-quality mode and its scanning parameters are otherwise identical.

27.1.4   Management

Management is surgical either by laparotomy or by laparoscopy. Even if the appendix appears normal, there are two reasons for removal: (1) early disease may be present despite its grossly normal appearance and (2) diagnostic confusion can be avoided if the condition recurs. Despite the surgical approach, the most experienced abdominal surgeon should perform the procedure to shorten the operation time and possible postoperative complications as much as possible.

Open appendectomy can be performed by: (1) muscle splitting incision (McBurney's incision), (2) midline vertical incision (this allows the surgeon to deal with unexpected surgical findings and for a Cesarean delivery if necessary), and (3) right pararectal incision. Despite the type of incision, the operation should be completed with minimal uterine manipulation.

Laparoscopic appendectomy is made in the first and second trimesters, and is recommended when the diagnosis is uncertain. The open (Hasson) technique is recommended and the cannula introduced 2–4 cm cranially from the palpable uterine fundus. It minimizes the complications of entering the abdomen and uterine or fetal injuries. If injury occurs, the ultrasound scan determines the presence of a fetal heart rate and residual amniotic fluid volume. With a live fetus and enough amniotic fluid, the gestation could be continued. Contamination of amniotic fluid with purulent or feculent material (possible chorioamnionitis) is addressed by the use of perioperative broad-spectrum antibiotics.

27.1.5   Prognosis

Pathological confirmation of inflamed appendix is found in about 67 % of patients [11]. Appendix in pregnant patient should always be removed since pregnancy is not affected by removal of a normal appendix [12].

Fetal mortality when the appendix is not perforated is 1.5–5 % [13, 14], while when perforated, fetal mortality rises to 20–35 % [13, 15]. Maternal mortality is less than 1 %. It is rare in the first trimester, and increases with advancing gestational age [12]. It is associated with: (1) a delay in surgery of more than 24 h [16, 17], and (2) appendiceal perforation – maternal mortality in up to 4 % [15, 18].

27.2   Acute Cholecystitis

27.2.1   Incidence

Acute cholecystitis is found in 1/1600–10,000 pregnancies. It is caused by gallstones in over 90 % of patients. The incidence of symptomatic and asymptomatic gallstones is 3.5–10 % in primiparous women, and up to 19 % in multiparous women [19].

27.2.2   History and Examination

Features suggesting acute cholecystitis are [20]: (1) a history of previous episodes of acute cholecystitis; (2) a history of nausea, dyspepsia, and an intolerance of fatty foods; (3) vomiting (in 50 % of patients); (4) abdominal pain in the right hypochondrium or epigastrium; and (5) pain also radiating to the back and around to the right scapula.

Abdominal tenderness on direct palpation and Murphy's sign are present. The rigid abdomen is found with gallbladder perforation and biliary peritonitis. Fever and tachycardia may not be present and so are not sensitive signs.

27.2.3   Differential Diagnosis

In decreasing incidence it includes: pyelonephritis, pancreatitis, peptic ulcer disease, acute appendicitis, pre-eclampsia, pneumonia, acute fatty liver of pregnancy, HELLP syndrome, myocardial infarction, and herpes zoster.

27.2.4   Investigations

Leukocytosis is not diagnostic because it is raised in the second and third trimesters and can reach $20 \times 10^9/l$ in early labor in normal pregnancy. A raised CRP correlates with the disease severity. Neutrophil granulocytosis with left shift indicates bacterial infection. Bilirubin and transaminases may be elevated, but are not specific. Raised alkaline phosphatase is also not helpful as estrogen causes elevation (levels may double during normal pregnancy). Serum amylase is transiently raised in up to 33 % in pregnant and nonpregnant women.

Gallstones are diagnosed by abdominal ultrasound in 95–98 % of patients [21]. If gallstones without wall thickening are found, then the diagnosis is biliary colic, not acute cholecystitis. In acute cholecystitis, findings include: (1) gallbladder calculi, (2) wall thickening (>3 mm), (3) pericholecystic fluid, (4) sonographic Murphy's sign (focal tenderness under the ultrasound transducer when it is positioned over the gallbladder), and (5) dilation of the intra- and extrahepatic ducts when the common bile duct is obstructed.

Magnetic resonance cholangiography is used if dilation of the intra- and extrahepatic ducts is found on abdominal ultrasound, especially when the cause of the dilatation is not certain.

27.2.5   Management

Medical treatment is commonly used initially, especially with biliary colic. It consists of a low-fat diet, analgesia, antibiotics, and anticholinergic antispasmodics such as dicyclomine. Patient should be admitted to hospital for a week, and then followed-up weekly. A second reason for conservative therapy is to delay surgery until the second trimester because the spontaneous abortion rate after open cholecystectomy is 12 % in the first, and only 5.6 % in the second trimester. Nonsteroidal anti-inflammatory drugs, such as ibuprofen, naproxen, or diclofenac can be used for pain relief. Paracetamol and weak opioids such as codeine are used if nonsteroidal anti-inflammatory drugs are not tolerated or are contraindicated. First-line treatments are ampicillin and sulbactam, cefoxitin, or cefuroxime (US FDA category B).

Recommendations for early and initial surgery are based on [22]: (1) reduced likelihood of recurrence – the recurrence rate during pregnancy is around 50 % [23]; (2) avoidance of medications during pregnancy; (3) elimination of potentially life-threatening complications – perforation, sepsis, and peritonitis; (4) lowering the incidence of gallstone pancreatitis, which causes fetal loss in 10–20 % of patients; and (5) lowering the incidence of spontaneous abortions, preterm labor, and preterm delivery.

Open cholecystectomy is performed by right subcostal incision or an upper midline incision. The Society of American Gastrointestinal and Endoscopic Surgeons (SAGES) published guidelines in 2007 that stated '*Laparoscopic cholecystectomy* is the treatment of choice in the pregnant patient with gallbladder disease, regardless of trimester' [24].

27.2.6   Prognosis

Prognosis is excellent because inflammatory disease is mostly away from the uterus. If outcomes are compared, laparoscopic access has significant advantages in all outcomes measured.

27.3 Intestinal Obstruction

27.3.1 Incidence

Intestinal obstruction is found in 1/1500–16,000 pregnancies
[25]. The most common cause are adhesions, present in
60–70%. They arise following previous abdominal or pelvic
surgery, or pelvic inflammatory conditions [26]. The second
most common cause is large bowel volvulus, which occurs in
25% of pregnant patients (it is the cause in only 3–5% of nonpregnant patients). Cecal volvuli are found in 25–45% of large
bowel volvuli. Other causes include small bowel volvulus (in
9%), intussusception (in 5%), and other rare conditions such as
hernia, cancer, and diverticulitis.

Rapid changes in uterine size can cause obstruction; at 16–20
weeks the uterus becomes an intra-abdominal organ, at 32–36
weeks the fetus enters the pelvic inlet, and at the puerperium the
uterus involutes and shrinks rapidly again. The redundant or
abnormally mobile colon is predisposed to torsion or twisting
because of uterine pressure [27].

27.3.2 History and Examination

Features suggesting intestinal obstruction are [26]: (1) previous
episodes of colicky abdominal pain; (2) abdominal pain is
observed in 90% of patients and may be constant or periodic,
mimicking labor; (3) nausea and vomiting; vomiting is not
always present, but if the obstruction is more proximal, vomiting occurs earlier; and (4) constipation, different from the usual
constipation in pregnancy; there is complete cessation of stool
and flatus.

The abdomen is distended and tender on palpation.
Hyperperistalsis is found early on, but later there is a complete

absence of peristalsis. Palpation of the uterus often causes pain secondary to transmitted pressure to the bowel, misleading that the problem is in the uterus. Rebound tenderness, fever, and tachycardia occur late and suggest peritonitis. Examine hernia orifices for protrusions and contents. If present and irreducible, incarcerated hernia is the cause of the obstruction. With digital rectal examination, the presence of intrarectal or perirectal masses, such as stenosis, rectal cancer, or rectal prolapse, should be confirmed or ruled out.

27.3.3 Investigations

Leukocytosis is not diagnostic because it is raised in the second and third trimesters and can reach $20 \times 10^9/l$ in early labor in normal pregnancy. The CRP correlates with the severity of obstruction, incarceration, and strangulation. Neutrophil granulocytosis with left shift is present. Electrolyte abnormalities are common due to dehydration, vomiting, and fluid shift into the bowel lumen. Elevated serum amylase is not specific.

The significant maternal and fetal mortalities associated with obstruction outweigh the potential risk of fetal radiation exposure. Plain abdominal X-rays are needed every 6 h if the obstruction is partial and in the absence of clinical improvement [26]. Contrast studies are needed if there is an absence of typical findings on plain abdominal films.

Colonoscopy can be therapeutic and result in the reduction of a sigmoid volvulus in 60–90 % of patients. The chance of reduction of cecal volvulus is low. There is more than a 50 % of recurrence of both sigmoid and cecal volvuli, which means that delayed surgery (fixation or resection) after delivery is mandatory [28]. Bloody intestinal contents or cyanotic mucosa suggests ischemia and are indications for emergent laparotomy.

27.3.4   Management

Medical management is started once the diagnosis is established, regardless of the completeness of the obstruction. Vomiting can cause large losses of fluid and electrolytes. Moreover, during obstruction a large volume of fluid is contained within the bowel lumen, and this contributes to dehydration and electrolyte disturbances. These should be corrected by intravenous infusion titrated against the laboratory findings. Nasogastric decompression eliminates the gastric contents, thus decreasing the incidence of vomiting and aspiration, and also decreasing abdominal pain caused by distension. During bowel obstruction, aerobic and anaerobic bacterial overgrowth occurs. The first-line treatment is a combination of clindamycin and cefazolin (US FDA category B), which should be started once the diagnosis is confirmed.

Surgery is indicated when: (1) medical therapy fails, (2) clinical, laboratory, or radiographic findings of disease progression; and (3) complete obstruction initially. A midline vertical incision is always used, except when an incarcerated hernia is the cause and the incision is made over the incarcerated hernia. The type of midline incision is made according to the estimated site; a medial midline incision for small bowel obstruction, and a lower midline incision for large bowel obstruction. Laparoscopic procedures are rarely performed. Laparoscopic cecopexy (anchoring the cecum to the lateral abdominal wall) can be made in a pregnant patient without a history of previous abdominal operations that could potentially cause adhesions.

27.3.5   Prognosis

The fetal mortality is 20–26%, and the maternal mortality is 6–20% [29].

27.4   Acute Pancreatitis

Acute pancreatitis occurs in 1/1000–3000 pregnancies [30], most commonly late in the third trimester and early postpartum. Pregnancy itself could be the cause due to increased intra-abdominal pressure on the biliary and pancreatic ducts. Other causes are: cholelithiasis (the most common cause – in at least 2/3 of patients) [30], alcohol abuse – the second most common cause [30], previous abdominal surgery, blunt abdominal trauma, infections (viral, bacterial, or parasitic), penetrating duodenal ulcer, connective tissue diseases, hyperparathyroidism, and hyperlipidemic pancreatitis [31].

27.4.1   History and Examination

Typical symptoms are the same as in nonpregnant patients. Patients may have a history of previous episodes of upper abdominal pain. There is severe epigastric pain radiating to the back, nausea and vomiting, and fever.

On examination, your patient may be lying in the fetal position with flexed knees, hips, and trunk. Bowel sounds are usually hypoactive, secondary to paralytic ileus. There is diffuse abdominal tenderness. There may also be Grey Turner's sign (bruising of the flanks) and Cullen's sign (bruising around the umbilicus).

27.4.2   Investigations

Leukocytosis is not diagnostic because it is raised in the second and third trimesters and can reach $20 \times 10^9/l$ in early labor in normal pregnancy. A CRP of 120 mg/l indicates necrotizing pancreatitis. Neutrophil granulocytosis with left shift is present. Serum levels of amylase and lipase may be raised; raised lipase levels are a better predictor of acute pancreatitis. Serial measurements on a daily basis reveal the progression/regression of the pancreatic inflammation. The amylase-creatinine clearance ratio is diagnostic [32]. It is low in normal pregnancy, but has a value of 5 % or more in pregnant women. Urea and electrolytes reveal acute prerenal insufficiency and electrolyte imbalance. Serum glucose confirms hyperglycemia or glucose intolerance. Hemoglobin and hematocrit levels confirm hemorrhage.

The American College of Obstetricians and Gynecologists have published the statement: "Women should be counselled that X-ray exposure from a single diagnostic procedure does not result in harmful fetal effects. Specifically, exposure to less than 5 rad (50 mGy) has not been associated with an increase in fetal anomalies or pregnancy loss" [33]. Plain X-ray will help to exclude other causes of acute abdomen (such as obstruction or pneumoperitoneum). Also, a sentinel loop may be present (an air-liquid level at the level of the jejunum) in the upper left abdomen, which suggests pancreatitis.

Transabdominal ultrasound confirms pancreatitis when there is (1) an edematous, enlarged pancreas, (2) pancreatic pseudocysts, (3) free intra-abdominal fluid and/or fluid in the omental bursa, and (4) thrombosis of the splenic vein due to compression.

CT with IV contrast may be used in complicated patients. There are no guidelines available that could help to minimize its use and the radiation exposure. Multidetector row CT with high-speed mode has half the radiation dose of the high-quality mode for otherwise identical scanning parameters.

27.4.3 Management

Initially, patients should be treated in intensive care. Vomiting and third space losses should be corrected by intravenous infusions. The replacement volume could be up to 10 l in total, depending on the severity of the pancreatitis and the laboratory findings. Current recommendations for nasogastric tube decompression are that it should be used only in patients with ileus or nausea and/or vomiting [34]. Pethidine (meperidine) or tramadol and not morphine should be used because these do not produce spasms of the sphincter of Oddi, which could exacerbate the pancreatitis [35]. Prophylactic antibiotics use is controversial, even in severe pancreatitis. Current recommendations for prophylactic use are [36, 37]: (1) severe acute pancreatitis (a CRP >120 mg/l), (2) pancreatic necrosis demonstrated by CT, and (3) persistent fever or signs of sepsis. Imipenem is the antibiotic of choice in patients who are not pregnant, but it is US FDA class C (animal studies have shown an adverse effect, but there are no adequate and well-controlled studies in pregnant women, or no animal studies have been conducted). So, as in acute cholecystitis, combination of antibiotics (e.g., clindamycin and cefazolin) is used.

Surgery is indicated in: (1) infected pancreatic necrosis, (2) a ruptured or infected pancreatic pseudocyst, and (3) severe hemorrhagic pancreatitis causing sepsis or hemodynamic instability. A right subcostal incision (it can be extended over the left hypochondrium) or extended upper midline laparotomy are used. The type of operation depends on the intra-abdominal findings. In necrotizing hemorrhagic pancreatitis, necrosectomy and drainage are performed. For an infected or ruptured pancreatic pseudocyst, open drainage is preferred. When biliary pancreatitis is proven, laparoscopic cholecystectomy with pre- or postoperative ERCP with endoscopic sphincterotomy is performed because of relapse rate up to 70 % [38].

Therapeutic delivery is the procedure performed primarily to cure refractory acute pancreatitis of any cause, especially hyperlipidemic before fetal complications (distress) ensue.

27.4.4 Prognosis

The maternal mortality rate ranges 0–37 %, while the perinatal mortality rate is 11 % [30].

27.5 Spontaneous Hepatic Rupture/Hepatic Subcapsular Hematoma

Spontaneous hepatic rupture and hepatic subcapsular hematoma occur mostly in the third trimester. They can either be a consequence of pregnancy or they can occur simultaneously with pregnancy. Pregnancy-related causes are: (1) intrahepatic cholestasis of pregnancy (progesterone-induced smooth muscle relaxation with biliary stasis), (2) acute fatty liver of pregnancy (moderate elevation of liver enzymes, significant coagulopathy, hypofibrinogenemia, hypoglycemia, and hyperbilirubinemia), and (3) HELLP (hemolysis, elevated liver enzymes, and low platelet levels) syndrome. Causes that occur simultaneously with pregnancy, but are not related are: (1) hepatic hemangiomas, and (2) hepatic tumors (benign or malignant).

27.5.1 History and Examination

There may be a history of pregnancy-induced hypertension with symptoms and signs: (1) related to pre-eclampsia: hypertension, swelling or edema, proteinuria, sudden weight gain, headache, changes in vision, racing pulse, mental confusion, difficulty breathing, and hyperreflexia; (2) nausea and vomiting; (3) abdominal pain in the right hypochondrium or epigastrium; (4) jaundice; and (5) collapse – late in the course of the disease, indicating hemorrhagic shock.

On examination there is: (1) a distended abdomen, (2) abdominal tenderness in the right hypochondrium, and (3) hemorrhagic shock (hypovolemic shock resulting from acute hemorrhage is characterized by hypotension, tachycardia, tachypnea, pale, cold, and clammy skin, and oliguria).

27.5.2 Investigations

Serial measurement of hemoglobin and hematocrit every 6–12 h if nonoperative management is indicated predicts rupture of the subcapsular hematoma. In the presence of adequate iron stores and iron intake, a pregnant patient's hematocrit level often falls below the normal range and is called "physiologic anemia of pregnancy." Hematocrit values of less than 30% are unusual. Leukocytosis is not diagnostic as it can be up to $20 \times 10^9/l$ at labor in normal pregnancy. Rising values indicate possible infection of the hematoma. Additional laboratory tests for known or unknown pregnancy-related diseases or the diseases that could complicate the course of this condition: serum liver transaminase and alkaline phosphatase levels; serum bilirubin and amylase; coagulation profile and platelet count; serum glucose. During normal pregnancy there is an increase in renal blood flow by about 60%, leading to an increase in the glomerular filtration rate. This has the effect of reducing serum blood urea nitrogen (BUN) and creatinine by half. Therefore, a relatively "normal" BUN and creatinine may reflect a seriously compromised renal function.

Plain abdominal X-ray eliminates other causes of acute abdomen (e.g., obstruction or pneumoperitoneum).

Abdominal ultrasound delineates a subcapsular hematoma or free intra-abdominal fluid and serial assessment every 6–12 h to define progression or rupture.

Abdominal CT is indicated in a stable patient with an uncertain diagnosis.

27.5.3 Management

Medical management is started as soon as the diagnosis of subcapsular liver hematoma or rupture without shock is established.

Treatment includes: (1) bed rest, (2) treatment of eclampsia, (3) fetal monitoring, (4) correction of coagulopathy, and (5) planned Cesarean section depending on the gestational age. If the fetus is around 20 weeks, then several weeks of observation (to enable fetal viability) is indicated if there are no indications for semi-elective or emergent operation. The right and left hepatic arteries, or both, can be occluded selectively by interventional radiological techniques.

Emergency surgery is indicated in hemorrhagic shock and includes: (1) resuscitation, (2) urgent total median laparotomy, (3) liver packing and transportation to specialized hepatobiliary centers, (4) hepatic resection, and (5) Cesarean section. Semi-elective surgery is indicated if ultrasound or CT progression of subcapsular hematoma is found. The bleeding with liver packing should be performed first. Local measures such as topical hemostatic agents and suture ligation of surface bleeders are of limited value especially when dealing with hemorrhage from large areas of denuded and friable liver in patients with associated clotting deficiencies. Then Cesarean section is made to save the baby and enable more space for definitive liver surgery if indicated.

27.5.4 Prognosis

Perioperative and postoperative mortality rates are 40–60 % for both mother and fetus [39].

27.6 Blunt or Penetrating Abdominal Trauma

27.6.1 Incidence

Trauma affects 6–7 % of pregnancies in the United States [40]. Most commonly it is blunt trauma such as motor vehicle accidents, physical violence (affecting 10 % of pregnant women), or accidental falls [41]. Less common penetrating trauma includes gunshot or stab wounds.

27.6.2 History and Examination

A history is usually easy, except when the injured patient is unconscious, in which case others should be consulted – friends, family, or passersby. The symptoms will depend on injured intra-abdominal organ: (1) placental abruption – vaginal bleeding (78 % of patients), uterine tenderness and back pain (66 % of patients), and uterine contractions (22 % of patients); (2) liver injury – right upper quadrant pain; (3) splenic injury – left upper quadrant pain; (4) perforation of hollow organs – diffuse abdominal pain; and (5) collapse occurs late in the course of the disease due to hemorrhagic shock.

Patient's blood pressure and heart rate are essential. The frequency of these measurements depends on the clinical condition of the patient. Find injury marks on the abdominal wall, such as seat belt marks, entrance and/or exit wounds, and contusions and/or hematomas. There will also be a distended abdomen, abdominal tenderness, or signs of hemorrhagic shock. Uterine contractions, uterine tenderness, or vaginal bleeding suggest severe direct fetal trauma.

27.6.3 Investigations

Hematocrit values less than 30 % are unusual. Serial measurement of hemoglobin and hematocrit every 6–12 h if abdominal pain persists without sonographic evidence of intra-abdominal hemorrhage is performed. Arterial blood pH and serum bicarbonate are important indicators of adequate tissue perfusion and oxygen supply, and a good predictor of fetal death. Additional laboratory tests for known or unknown pregnancy-related diseases or the diseases that could complicate the course of pregnant patients with trauma are measured: liver transaminases, alkaline phosphatase, bilirubin, and serum amylase; coagulation profile and platelet count; serum glucose. Positive Kleihauer-Betke test means direct blood contact between an Rh- mother and an Rh+ fetus. It determines the required dose of Rho (D) immune globulin to inhibit the formation of Rh antibodies in the mother and prevent Rh disease in future Rh+ children. Between 10 and 30 % of pregnant trauma victims have some evidence of fetal-maternal admixture of blood [42, 43].

X-ray examination is indicated for significant trauma, such as deformities, severe pain, or breathlessness in chest trauma. For nonsignificant trauma, X-ray examination could be delayed, unless there are persisting symptoms. For sprains and some nondisplaced fractures, immobilization is used initially and, in these more minor conditions, X-rays can be taken after 7 days if the pain or dysfunction persists.

Abdominal ultrasound may reveal a subcapsular hematoma of the liver or spleen, or free intra-abdominal fluid.

Fetal cardiotocography is significantly better for the diagnosis of placental abruption than ultrasound [44]. It is mandatory for the evaluation of a possible placental abruption, establishment of gestational age, assessment of amniotic fluid volume, and fetal well-being [42]. Significant fetal mortality may result even from minor trauma [45]. Monitoring of fetal heart rate should be initiated as soon as practicable in sufficiently advanced pregnancies (>20–24 weeks). The presence of contractions greater than one every 10 min indicates a 20 % risk of placental abruption [46]. For minor trauma, fetal monitoring is needed for 4–6 h. For major trauma with frequent uterine contractions, an abnormal fetal heart rate pattern, vaginal bleeding, or uterine tenderness, fetal monitoring is needed for a minimum of 24 h.

27.6.4 Management

Medical management includes [44]: (1) stabilization of the mother using supplementary oxygen, intravenous fluids (blood transfusion if indicated), (2) placing the mother in the left lateral position after 24 weeks gestation, and (3) the American College of Obstetricians and Gynecologists recommends giving D-immunoglobulin to all sensitized Rh- pregnant patients [47].

Surgery in hemorrhagic shock includes: (1) resuscitation, (2) urgent total median laparotomy, (3) liver packing and transportation to specialized hepatobiliary centers, (3) hepatic resection in a specialized center, (4) splenectomy in splenic rupture, (5) Cesarean section – if the gestation is over 24–28 weeks even during unsuccessful maternal resuscitation, when it should be performed within 5 min. *Damage control surgery* is rapid termination of an operation after control of life-threatening bleeding and intestinal spillage (systolic blood pressure <90 mmHg; T <34°C; activated partial prothrombin time >60 s; pH <7.2 or arterial base deficit ≥8; major intra-abdominal vascular injury; associated need for management of extra-abdominal life-threatening injury), followed by correction of physiological abnormalities, which precedes definitive management of initial injuries. In non-life-threatening conditions, standard procedures should be used as indicated: suturing of small and large bowel ruptures before peritonitis develops, bowel segment resections or stoma creation when peritonitis is present.

27.6.5 Prognosis

Trauma is the leading cause of nonobstetric maternal death [40].

Fetal injury in maternal penetrating trauma is high from both stab (42 %) and gunshot wounds (71 %) [48, 49]. The rate of fetal mortality after blunt maternal trauma is 3.4–38 % [40, 50], and is mostly a result of placental abruption, maternal shock, and maternal death. There are no strong clinical predictors of fetal death [51, 52]. A high injury severity score, low levels of hemoglobin, the need for a blood transfusion, and the presence of disseminated intravascular coagulation caused by an admixture of maternal and fetal blood are the most significant predictors of fetal mortality [53]. Even minor trauma can cause fetal death. Fetal outcome is highly dependent on gestational age and less so on the injury type, mechanism, or the severity of the injury. Women under 28 weeks' gestation have the highest risk of fetal, neonatal, or infant death [52]. Perimortem Cesarean section has a fetal survival rate of 50–70 % [54].

References

1. Stedman TL. Stedman's medical dictionary. 27th ed. Baltimore: Lippincott Williams & Wilkins; 2000.
2. Coleman NT, Trianfo VA, Rund DA. Nonobstetric emergencies in pregnancy: trauma and surgical conditions. Am J Obstet Gynecol. 1997;177:497–502.
3. Gomez A, Wood M. Acute appendicitis during pregnancy. Am J Surg. 1979;137:180–3.
4. Cunningham FG, McCubbin JH. Appendicitis complicating pregnancy. Obstet Gynecol. 1975;45:415–20.
5. Richards C, Daya S. Diagnosis of acute appendicitis in pregnancy. Can J Surg. 1989;32:358–60.
6. Bailey LE, Finley Jr RK, Miller SF, Jones LM. Acute appendicitis during pregnancy. Am Surg. 1986;52:218–21.
7. Caspi B, Zbar AP, Mavor E, Hagay Z, Appelman Z. The contribution of transvaginal ultrasound in the diagnosis of acute appendicitis: an observational study. Ultrasound Obstet Gynecol. 2003;21:273–6.
8. Puylaert JB, Rutgers PH, Lalisang RI, de Vries BC, van der Werf SD, Dörr JP, et al. A prospective study of ultrasonography in the diagnosis of appendicitis. N Engl J Med. 1987;317:666–9.

9. Kanal E, Borgstede JP, Barkovich AJ, Bell C, Bradley WG, Etheridge S, et al. American College of Radiology White Paper on MR Safety: 2004 update and revisions. AJR Am J Roentgenol. 2004;182:1111–4.

10. Singh A, Danrad R, Hahn PF, Blake MA, Mueller PR, Novelline RA. MR imaging of the acute abdomen and pelvis: acute appendicitis and beyond. Radiographics. 2007;27:1419–31.

11. Mourad J, Elliott JP, Erickkson L, Lisboa L. Appendicitis in pregnancy: new information that contradicts long-held clinical beliefs. Am J Obstet Gynecol. 2000;182:1027–9.

12. Halvorsen AC, Brandt B, Andreasen JJ. Acute appendicitis in pregnancy: complications and subsequent management. Eur J Surg. 1992;158:603–6.

13. Kammerer W. Nonobstetric surgery during pregnancy. Med Clin North Am. 1979;63:1157–64.

14. Babaknia A, Parsa H, Woodruff JD. Appendicitis during pregnancy. Obstet Gynecol. 1977;50:40–4.

15. Firstenberg MS, Malangoni MA. Gastrointestinal surgery during pregnancy. Gastroenterol Clin North Am. 1998;27:73–88.

16. Horowitz MD, Gomez GA, Santiesteban R, Burkett G. Acute appendicitis during pregnancy. Diagnosis and management. Arch Surg. 1985;120:1362–7.

17. Tamir IL, Bongard FS, Klein SR. Acute appendicitis in the pregnant patient. Am J Surg. 1990;160:571–6.

18. Mahmoodian S. Appendicitis complicating pregnancy. South Med J. 1992;85:19–24.

19. Basso L, McCollum PT, Darling MR, Tocchi A, Tanner WA. A study of cholelithiasis during pregnancy and its relationship with age, parity, menarche, breastfeeding, dysmenorrhea, oral contraception and a maternal history of cholelithiasis. Surg Gynecol Obstet. 1992;175:41–6.

20. Brunicardi FC, Andersen DK, Billiar TR, Dunn DL, Hunter JG, Pollock RE. Schwartz's principles of surgery. 8th ed. New York: McGraw-Hill Professional; 2004. p. 1199.

21. Chang T, Lepanto L. Ultrasonography in the emergency setting. Emerg Med Clin North Am. 1992;10:1–25.

22. Swisher SG, Schmit PJ, Hunt KK, Hiyama DT, Bennion RS, Swisher EM, et al. Biliary disease during pregnancy. Am J Surg. 1994;168:576–9.

23. Glasgow RE, Visser BC, Harris HW, Patti MG, Kilpatrick SJ, Mulvihill SJ. Changing management of gallstone disease during pregnancy. Surg Endosc. 1998;12:241–6.

24. Cosenza CA, Saffari B, Jabbour N, Stain SC, Garry D, Parekh D, et al. Surgical management of biliary gallstone disease during pregnancy. Am J Surg. 1999;178:545–8.

25. Ballantyne GH, Brandner MD, Beart Jr RW, Ilstrup DM. Volvulus of the colon: incidence and mortality. Ann Surg. 1985;202:83–92.

26. Perdue PW, Johnson HW, Stafford PW. Intestinal obstruction complicating pregnancy. Am J Surg. 1992;164:384–8.

27. Harer WB, Harer WE. Volvulus complicating pregnancy and puerperium. Obstet Gynecol. 1958;12:367–76.

28. Orchard JL, Mekha R, Khan H. The use of colonoscopy in the treatment of colonic volvulus: three cases and review of the literature. Am J Gastroenterol. 1984;79:864–7.

29. Connolly M, Unti J, Nora P. Bowel obstruction in pregnancy. Surg Clin North Am. 1995;75:101–13.

30. Ramin KD, Ramin SM, Richey SD, Cunningham FG. Acute pancreatitis in pregnancy. Am J Obstet Gynecol. 1995;173:187–91.

31. Herfort K, Fialova V, Srp B. Acute pancreatitis in pregnancy. Mater Med Pol. 1981;13:15–7.

32. Devore GR, Braken M, Berkowitz RL. The amylase/creatinine clearance ratio in normal pregnancies and pregnancies complicated by pancreatitis, hyperemesis, and toxemia. Am J Obstet Gynecol. 1980;136:747–54.

33. ACOG Committee on Obstetric Practice. Guidelines for diagnostic imaging during pregnancy. ACOG Committee opinion no. 299. Obstet Gynecol. 2004;104:647–51.

34. Loiudice TA, Lang J, Mehta H, Banta L. Treatment of acute alcoholic pancreatitis: the roles of cimetidine and nasogastric suction. Am J Gastroenterol. 1984;79:553–8.

35. Wu SD, Zhang ZH, Jin JZ, Kong J, Wang W, Zhang Q, et al. Effects of narcotic analgesic drugs on human Oddi's sphincter motility. World J Gastroenterol. 2004;10:2901–4.

36. Bang UC, Semb S, Nojgaard C, Bendtsen F. Pharmacological approach to acute pancreatitis. World J Gastroenterol. 2008;14:2968–76.

37. Xiong GS, Wu SM, Wang ZH. Role of prophylactic antibiotic administration in severe acute pancreatitis: a meta-analysis. Med Princ Pract. 2006;15:106–10.

38. Scott LD. Gallstone disease and pancreatitis in pregnancy. Gastroenterol Clin North Am. 1992;21:803–15.

39. Smith Jr LG, Moise Jr KJ, Dildy III GA, Carpenter Jr RJ. Spontaneous rupture of liver during pregnancy: current therapy. Obstet Gynecol. 1991;77:171–5.

40. Shah KH, Simons RK, Holbrook T, Fortlage D, Winchell RJ, Hoyt DB. Trauma in pregnancy: maternal and fetal outcomes. J Trauma. 1998;45:83–6.

41. Satin AJ, Hemsell DL, Stone Jr IC, Theriot S, Wendel Jr GD. Sexual assault in pregnancy. Obstet Gynecol. 1991;77:710–4.

42. Pearlman MD, Tintinalli JE. Evaluation and treatment of the gravida and fetus following trauma during pregnancy. Obstet Gynecol Clin North Am. 1991;18:371–81.

43. Goodwin TM, Breen MT. Pregnancy outcome and fetomaternal hemorrhage after noncatastrophic trauma. Am J Obstet Gynecol. 1990;162:665–71.

44. ACOG Committee on Obstetric Practice. Obstetric aspects of trauma management. Educational bulletin no. 251. Int J Gynaecol Obstet. 1999;64:87–94.

45. Esposito TJ, Gens DR, Smith LG, Scorpio R, Buchman T. Trauma during pregnancy: a review of 79 cases. Arch Surg. 1991;126:1073–8.

46. Dahmus MA, Sibai BM. Blunt abdominal trauma: are there any predictive factors for abruptio placentae or maternal-fetal distress? Am J Obstet Gynecol. 1993;169:1054–9.

47. American College of Obstetricians and Gynecologists (ACOG). Trauma during pregnancy. Technical bulletin no. 161. Int J Gynaecol Obstet. 1993;40:165–70.

48. Sandy EA, Koerner M. Self-inflicted gunshot wound to the pregnant abdomen: report of a case and review of the literature. Am J Perinatol. 1989;6:30–1.

49. Sakala EP, Kort DD. Management of stab wounds to the pregnant uterus: a case report and a review of the literature. Obstet Gynecol Surv. 1988;43:319–24.

50. Rogers FB, Rozycki GS, Osler TM, Shackford SR, Jalbert J, Kirton O, et al. A multi-institutional study of factors associated with fetal death in injured pregnant patients. Arch Surg. 1999;134:1274–7.

51. Theodorou DA, Velmahos GC, Souter I, Chan LS, Vassiliu P, Tatevossian R, et al. Fetal death after trauma in pregnancy. Am Surg. 2000;66:809–12.

52. El-Kady D, Gilbert WM, Anderson J, Danielsen B, Towner D, Smith LH. Trauma during pregnancy: an analysis of maternal and fetal outcomes in a large population. Am J Obstet Gynecol. 2004;190:1661–8.

53. Ali J, Yeo A, Gana TJ, McLellan BA. Predictors of fetal mortality in pregnant trauma patients. J Trauma. 1997;42:782–5.

54. Katz VL, Dotters DJ, Droegemueller W. Perimortem cesarean delivery. Obstet Gynecol. 1986;68:571–6.

Chapter 28
Geriatric Emergency Surgery

Torhild Veen, Jan Rune Aunan, and Kjetil Søreide

28.1 Introduction

Due to the progress in health and safety of living, elderly population is increasing worldwide. The rate of aged persons will accumulate in both developing and developed countries over the next decades. Currently, there are an estimated one billion people aged >60 years worldwide, and this is projected to increase to over two billion by year 2050, with a more than two- to three-fold increase in developing countries [1]. Associated with this change in demography comes also increased health care costs, added complexity in care and higher morbidity and mortality, in particular for patients presenting with emergency surgery conditions [2–4]. Thus, this chapter will give a brief overview of

T. Veen, MD • J.R. Aunan, MD • K. Søreide, MD, PhD (✉)
Department of Gastrointestinal Surgery,
Stavanger University Hospital, P.O. Box, 8100,
Stavanger, Norway
e-mail: ksoreide@mac.com

© Springer International Publishing Switzerland 2017   509
S. Di Saverio et al. (eds.), *Acute Care Surgery Handbook*,
DOI 10.1007/978-3-319-15341-4_28

issues in geriatric emergency surgery care that need to be taken into account by the surgeon.

28.2 Aging and Medical Conditions

With increasing age comes also an increased risk or susceptibility for certain diseases, including those that follow with added comorbidity, use of drugs and lifestyle risk factors. In most of the emergency general surgery conditions, the mortality also increases severalfold with each decade of age [5]. The biology of aging and its molecular hallmarks have been reviewed previously [6]. For surgeons it is of paramount importance to acknowledge that aging comes with specific concerns and added physiological challenges to specific organ systems and for the capacity to recover after an insult [7].

28.2.1   Role of Comorbidity

A number of preexisting comorbidities in the elderly presenting with an acute condition leads to increased postoperative complications and death [8]. A decreased cardiovascular and pulmonary reserve capacity results in tissue hypoxia that can be hard to detect. In the elderly, cardiogenic shock is often occult with a normal measured blood pressure due to stiff vessels and high vascular resistance [8] and shock (or hypoperfusion) starts at a higher blood pressure levels than in the young patient [9].

28.2.2   Renal Function and Reserve

Renal failure is also common and can be hard to detect due to the decreased muscle mass and creatinine levels in the elderly, making creatinine an unreliable predictor of renal function. Renal failure complicates hydration, medication dosage, and precludes the use of many commonly used drugs. Indeed, as such renal failure is associated with mortality [10].

28.2.3 Nutritional Status

Protein and caloric undernutrition is also prevalent, and the catabolic state associated with critical illness predisposes to rapid wasting, infections, and increased morbidity and mortality. This warrants early focus on nutritional support [8].

28.2.4 Cardiovascular Events and Drugs

Also surgery in the elderly is associated with postoperative complications like atrial fibrillation, myocardial ischemia, and respiratory failure. Coagulopathy is also common due to frequent use of warfarin and antiplatelet drugs in these patients [8].

28.2.5 Risk of Delirium

Postoperative delirium presents in about 10 % of patients after elective surgery and doubles to about 20 % after emergency surgery. Delirium is often underdiagnosed and it may delay rehabilitation.

Guidelines for prevention and improved treatment of delirium [11] advocate use of interdisciplinary teams, mobility and walking, avoiding restraints, sleep hygiene, and adequate nutrition, fluid, and oxygen. Postoperative pain control (preferably without opioids) is important for prevention.

28.3 Emergency Conditions for an Aging Population

Specific disease patterns emerge with increasing age. For example, the risk of fractures increases with age, and age- and gender-specific patterns demonstrate types, complexity, and need for operative treatment for long-bone fractures [12]. Further, risk of ruptured abdominal aortic aneurysms (rAAA) also demonstrates an age-specific increase [13], as does the risk of perforated peptic ulcer [14].

28.4 Assessment of Frailty in the Elderly and Risk Scores

With an aging population, it is necessary to find tools to evaluate risks for morbidity and mortality related to emergency surgery. The concept of *frailty* is described as "a state of reduced physiological reserve associated with increased susceptibility to disability" [15]. Frailty has been associated with worse outcome after surgery [16]. Frailty can be seen as a biological syndrome of decreased reserve or, as an accumulation of deficits in terms of medical, social, and functional deficits [16]. No available scores exist for the emergency setting. Existing scores have been investigated, but these either fail to predict accurately the outcome or they are cumbersome to use in a clinical setting. Scores developed for elective evaluation have been investigated for emergency abdominal surgery [17]. Among the six instruments, the Vulnerable Elders Survey (VES-13) predicted the 30-day mortality and morbidity best. In general, mortality increase with increasing age, higher ASA score, need for emergency procedures, and for palliative surgery associated with a malignancy [18]. Thus, the use of documented variables together with a clinical acumen are the best predictors at present.

28.5   Organization of Geriatric Emergency Services

Indeed, treatment elderly, frail patients is complicated, and organizing the treatment of geriatric patients has been a topic of debate. Specialized geriatric surgical units have been proposed as a solution [19]. Further, elderly surgical patients experience failure-to-rescue events at much higher rates than their younger counterparts, particularly for infectious and pulmonary complications [20]. Increased attention to the role of organizational dynamics in hospitals' ability to rescue these high-risk patients will establish high-yield interventions aimed at improving patient safety [21].

28.5.1   Geriatric Units and Multidisciplinary Care

The core of geriatric units should be a multidisciplinary approach including all subspecialties of surgery, and nonsurgical specialist such as anaesthesiologists, geriatricians, pharmacist, nutritionist, and physiotherapists [19]. Together they should conduct preoperative assessment for frailty, comorbidity, and polypharmacy, allowing for optimal presurgery fitness, and postoperative rehabilitation.

Trauma units designed to expedite the care of geriatric patients through a multidisciplinary approach have been successful [22]. Criteria for triaging, disposition, and admission were established between emergency department and surgeons. Orthopedic surgeons implemented strategies of operative management in 48 h. Internal medicine assisted in optimizing chronic disease and providing preoperative clearance with involvement of cardiology and anesthesiology [22]. Multidisciplinary teams included surgeons, physical therapists, occupational therapists, respiratory therapists, nutritionists, pharmacists, social workers, case managers, internists, a geriatrician, and physical medicine and rehabilitation for optimal and seamless care. A dedicated unit was established in the hospital, with a dedicated paging system. The geriatric trauma unit contributed to improved triage, improved quality of care, and safer discharge [22, 23].

28.6 Ethics, Limitations, and Boundaries for Geriatric Emergency Surgery

Some elderly patients with considerable comorbidity have a very poor prognosis with very limited chances for a functional recovery after an emergency surgery condition [24]. While the technical indication for surgery may be obvious, the overall approach to the specific patient may need a more differentiated approach [25]. Futility (defined as a very poor chance for survival or chance for recovery, or extremely high risk of ending up with permanent end-organ support in a high-dependent unit) may sometimes be clearly defined, but most often becomes a borderline decision between ethics, clinical predictions, and patient communication, for which no solid evidence currently exists. The number and severity of other underlying condition(s), as well as the treatment alternatives and their consequences, is a complex picture to interpret. Understanding the differences between Do Not Resuscitate (DNR), palliative care, hospice care, and symptom management in patients at the end of life is a critical skill set that is essential to all surgical care [26, 27], but specifically for geriatric surgical care and in the emergency setting.

References

1. Søreide K, Wijnhoven BP. Surgery for an ageing population. Br J Surg. 2016;103(2):e7–9. doi:10.1002/bjs.10071.
2. Desserud KF, Veen T, Søreide K. Emergency general surgery in the geriatric patient. Br J Surg. 2015. doi:10.1002/bjs.10044.

3. Rich PB, Adams SD. Health care: economic impact of caring for geriatric patients. Surg Clin North Am. 2015;95(1):11–21. doi:10.1016/j.suc.2014.09.011.

4. Bergenfelz A, Soreide K. Improving outcomes in emergency surgery. Br J Surg. 2014;101(1):e1–2. doi:10.1002/bjs.9347.

5. Havens JM, Peetz AB, Do WS, Cooper Z, Kelly E, Askari R, et al. The excess morbidity and mortality of emergency general surgery. J Trauma Acute Care Surg. 2015;78(2):306–11. doi:10.1097/ta.0000000000000517.

6. Aunan JR, Watson MM, Hagland HR, Søreide K. Molecular and biological hallmarks of ageing. Br J Surg. 2016;103(2):e29–46. doi:10.1002/bjs.10053.

7. Biffl WL, Biffl SE. Rehabilitation of the geriatric surgical patient: predicting needs and optimizing outcomes. Surg Clin North Am. 2015;95(1):173–90. doi:10.1016/j.suc.2014.09.004.

8. Menaker J, Scalea TM. Geriatric care in the surgical intensive care unit. Crit Care Med. 2010;38(9 Suppl):S452–9. doi:10.1097/CCM.0b013e3181ec5697.

9. Brown JB, Gestring ML, Forsythe RM, Stassen NA, Billiar TR, Peitzman AB, et al. Systolic blood pressure criteria in the National Trauma Triage Protocol for geriatric trauma: 110 is the new 90. J Trauma Acute Care Surg. 2015;78(2):352–9. doi:10.1097/ta.0000000000000523.

10. Yaghoubian A, Ge P, Tolan A, Saltmarsh G, Kaji AH, Neville AL, et al. Renal insufficiency predicts mortality in geriatric patients undergoing emergent general surgery. Am Surg. 2011;77(10):1322–5.

11. American Geriatrics Society Expert Panel on Postoperative Delirium in Older Adults. American Geriatrics Society abstracted clinical practice guideline for postoperative delirium in older adults. J Am Geriatr Soc. 2015;63(1):142–50. doi:10.1111/jgs.13281.

12. Meling T, Harboe K, Soreide K. Incidence of traumatic long-bone fractures requiring in-hospital management: a prospective age- and gender-specific analysis of 4890 fractures. Injury. 2009;40(11):1212–9. doi:10.1016/j.injury.2009.06.003.

13. Reite A, Søreide K, Ellingsen CL, Kvaløy JT, Vetrhus M. Epidemiology of ruptured abdominal aortic aneurysms in a well-defined Norwegian population with trends in incidence, intervention rate, and mortality. J Vasc Surg. 2015;61(5):1168–74. doi:10.1016/j.jvs.2014.12.054.

14. Thorsen K, Søreide JA, Kvaløy JT, Glomsaker T, Søreide K. Epidemiology of perforated peptic ulcer: age- and gender-adjusted analysis of incidence and mortality. World J Gastroenterol WJG. 2013;19(3):347–54. doi:10.3748/wjg.v19.i3.347.

15. Clegg A, Young J, Iliffe S, Rikkert MO, Rockwood K. Frailty in elderly people. Lancet. 2013;381(9868):752–62. doi:10.1016/s0140-6736(12)62167-9.

16. Robinson TN, Walston JD, Brummel NE, Deiner S, Brown CH, Kennedy M, et al. Frailty for surgeons: review of a national institute on aging conference on frailty for specialists. J Am Coll Surg. 2015;221(6):1083–92. doi:10.1016/j.jamcollsurg.2015.08.428.

17. Kenig J, Zychiewicz B, Olszewska U, Barczynski M, Nowak W. Six screening instruments for frailty in older patients qualified for emergency abdominal surgery. Arch Gerontol Geriatr. 2015. doi:10.1016/j.archger.2015.06.018.

18. Duron JJ, Duron E, Dugue T, Pujol J, Muscari F, Collet D, et al. Risk factors for mortality in major digestive surgery in the elderly: a multicenter prospective study. Ann Surg. 2011;254(2):375–82. doi:10.1097/SLA.0b013e318226a959.

19. Zenilman ME, Katlic MR, Rosenthal RA. Geriatric surgery—evolution of a clinical community. Am J Surg. 2015;209(6):943–9. doi:http://dx.doi.org/10.1016/j.amjsurg.2015.01.016.

20. Sheetz KH, Krell RW, Englesbe MJ, Birkmeyer JD, Campbell Jr DA, Ghaferi AA. The importance of the first complication: understanding failure to rescue after emergent surgery in the elderly. J Am Coll Surg. 2014;219(3):365–70. doi:10.1016/j.jamcollsurg.2014.02.035.

21. Ghaferi AA, Dimick JB. Importance of teamwork, communication and culture on failure-to-rescue in the elderly. Br J Surg. 2016;103(2):e47–51. doi:10.1002/bjs.10031.

22. Mangram AJ, Shifflette VK, Mitchell CD, Johnson VA, Lorenzo M, Truitt MS, et al. The creation of a geriatric trauma unit "G-60". Am Surg. 2011;77(9):1144–6.

23. Min L, Cryer H, Chan CL, Roth C, Tillou A. Quality of care delivered before vs after a quality-improvement intervention for acute geriatric trauma. J Am Coll Surg. 2015;220(5):820–30. doi:10.1016/j.jamcollsurg.2014.12.041.

24. Al-Temimi MH, Griffee M, Enniss TM, Preston R, Vargo D, Overton S, et al. When is death inevitable after emergency laparotomy? analysis of the American College of Surgeons National Surgical Quality Improvement Program database. J Am Coll Surg. 2012;215(4):503–11. doi:10.1016/j.jamcollsurg.2012.06.004.

25. Søreide K, Desserud KF. Emergency surgery in the elderly: the balance between function, frailty, fatality and futility. Scand J Trauma Resusc Emerg Med. 2015;23:10. doi:10.1186/s13049-015-0099-x.

26. Peschman J, Brasel KJ. End-of-life care of the geriatric surgical patient. Surg Clin North Am. 2015;95(1):191–202. doi:10.1016/j.suc.2014.09.006.

27. Dunn GP. Shared decision-making for the elderly patient with a surgical condition. Br J Surg. 2016;103(2):e19–20. doi:10.1002/bjs.10076.